Health in Japan

Health in Japan

*Social Epidemiology of Japan since the 1964
Tokyo Olympics*

Edited by

Eric Brunner

*Professor of Social and Biological Epidemiology,
Institute of Epidemiology and Health Care,
University College London,
London, UK*

Noriko Cable

*Senior Research Fellow,
Institute of Epidemiology and Health Care,
University College London,
London, UK*

Hiroyasu Iso

*Professor of Public Health,
Department of Social Medicine,
Graduate School of Medicine, Osaka University,
Osaka, Japan*

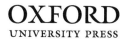
OXFORD
UNIVERSITY PRESS

OXFORD
UNIVERSITY PRESS

Great Clarendon Street, Oxford, OX2 6DP,
United Kingdom

Oxford University Press is a department of the University of Oxford.
It furthers the University's objective of excellence in research, scholarship,
and education by publishing worldwide. Oxford is a registered trade mark of
Oxford University Press in the UK and in certain other countries

First Edition published in 2021

Impression: 1

Published in the United States of America by Oxford University Press
198 Madison Avenue, New York, NY 10016, United States of America

British Library Cataloguing in Publication Data

Data available

Library of Congress Control Number: 2020944741

ISBN 978–0–19–884813–4

Printed and bound by
CPI Group (UK) Ltd, Croydon, CR0 4YY

Oxford University Press makes no representation, express or implied, that the
drug dosages in this book are correct. Readers must therefore always check
the product information and clinical procedures with the most up-to-date
published product information and data sheets provided by the manufacturers
and the most recent codes of conduct and safety regulations. The authors and
the publishers do not accept responsibility or legal liability for any errors in the
text or for the misuse or misapplication of material in this work. Except where
otherwise stated, drug dosages and recommendations are for the non-pregnant
adult who is not breast-feeding

Links to third party websites are provided by Oxford in good faith and
for information only. Oxford disclaims any responsibility for the materials
contained in any third party website referenced in this work.

Foreword

Japanese health success a challenge and an inspiration

Michael Marmot
Professor of Epidemiology and Public Health
Director, Institute of Health Equity
University College London

Why Japan? Why a volume about the health of one population, specifically, of the Japanese? Because there is so much to teach us about the causes of health and disease, particularly as non-communicable diseases and ageing populations have become of global importance. It is revealing to ask how Japan went from being a moderately healthy country, among the rich countries, to having the longest life expectancy in the world; exceeded now, only by Hong Kong.

My own interest in the health of the Japanese goes back to my PhD thesis in the 1970s, analysing data from the NiHonSan Study—a study of men of Japanese ancestry in Japan, Hawaii, and California. The background to the study was the high rates of stroke in Japan, decreasing across the Pacific to California; and ischaemic heart disease going the other way—higher in California. Acculturation to an American way of life was thought to be important; in particular making the transition to a Westernized diet. We found, though, that among men of Japanese ancestry in California, the more they were brought up and lived within Japanese culture and society the lower the rate of heart disease, regardless of level of plasma cholesterol, blood pressure, or smoking. Japanese culture and society seemed to hold secrets to better health.

When chairing the WHO Commission on Social Determinants of Health, published in 2008, I very much took the view that the health of a society told us something important about the nature of that society. It follows that the good health of the people of Japan is telling us something important about Japanese society and culture.

That said, we should be wary of jumping to simple conclusions. To take three examples on which this book sheds light. First, Japanese life expectancy improved rapidly from the 1960s on, and overtook that of other advanced countries. Initially the improvement in health seemed to fit with inclusive growth: improvement of GDP and relatively narrow income inequalities. After the Japanese economic bubble burst at the end of the 1980s, GDP growth slowed and income inequalities grew somewhat bigger, yet health continued to increase. Much to look at.

Second, there was concern that as Japan westernized so its pattern of health and disease would take on a Western hue. Too simple. Not only did stroke mortality decline markedly, so too did age-standardized mortality from ischaemic heart disease. Japan experienced improvement in 'its' distinctive disease, stroke, but also in the 'western' disease, ischaemic heart disease. Here, proximate causes, as well as social determinants might be important. Availability of refrigerators meant that salting of foods for preservation was less imperative. The resultant reduction of salt intake will have played a role in reduction of high blood pressure and hence of cerebro- and possibly of cardio-vascular disease. Westernization of diet will have contributed to rising levels of plasma cholesterol. But the Japanese diet is not Western and ischaemic heart disease declined, from a low level.

Third, the status of women: slow progress in gender equity might be a challenge to simple notions of why women in Japan have extraordinarily long life expectancy compared to women elsewhere. Certainly, from my studies of Japanese-Americans on, I have looked to the cohesive nature of Japanese society as providing explanations for improvements in health in Japan; and giving lessons that may be widely applicable to other societies.

Foreword

Keizō Takemi
Member of the House of Councillors
World Health Organization Goodwill Ambassador for Universal Health Coverage

We are witnessing a turning point in the world. This book was primarily written before COVID-19 overwhelmed the world. It is published amidst the first wave of the pandemic and its aftermath in many countries, and will be read in a world changed by the COVID-19 storm. Globalization in the twenty-first century connected societies, economies, and communities, and collectively brought wealth and longevity around the world. Japan positions itself as the front-runner of such trend and embarks on a social experiment showing the world that creating an active and healthy ageing society is the way forward for a sustainable human society with a growing number of silver citizens. In this context, what will be the significance of this publication based on Japanese experience? I think Japan has presented many miracles in global public health. The first miracle is the remarkable health development during the 20 post-war years leading up to the 1964 Tokyo Olympics. Japan successfully controlled many infectious diseases and realized universal health insurance coverage. Such successes served as the basis of further economic prosperity and political stability. The second miracle is the continued improvement of health indicators despite 30 years of economic slump after 1990 when Japan's over-inflated stock market and real estate bubble burst. The third miracle is the Japanese society's resilience displayed after the Great East Japan earthquake on 11 March 2011, and we see this resilience again in the COVID-19 response during the first half of 2020. What are the background factors of such miracles? Are they changing, if so, in what direction? These are all legitimate questions. I am thankful to the contributors of this book, who have been engaged in research and practice related to the social determinants of health in Japan, for highlighting how the health behaviours of individuals can impact society. At the same time, the COVID-19 pandemic has uncovered some of the vulnerabilities of our society, such as the immaturity of Japan's digital health information systems and incomplete integration of public health and curative services.

Internationally, Japan has advocated the concept of human security. This concept is meant to challenge the limitation of international political order based on individual sovereign states, by delineating an alternative thinking to directly connect individuals at microscopic level and society at macroscopic level. More specifically, we have led and advocated universal health coverage based on our solid experience. Also, we have stressed that integration of all health-related socio-economic policies is indispensable to achieve the Sustainable Development Goals. From now on, various changes triggered by the COVID-19 pandemic will inevitably impact individuals, local communities, and nations as a whole. In such a changing world, Japan strives to be a nation that humbly addresses human vulnerability and offers solutions to global issues.

Preface

Japan was the first Asian country to reach European and North American levels of economic development. Around the time of the first Tokyo Olympics, Japan's economy reached a similar size to the UK's, and the country had made the epidemiological transition from infectious to non-communicable disease as the major cause of adult mortality. The next 60 years witnessed astonishing changes in demographics, health, and social norms. Massive gains in life expectancy and unprecedented super-ageing of the population have produced a taste of the global future. In 1964, the 65+ age group was 6% of the population, in 2020 it is 28%. Japan's fertility rate dropped way below replacement level in 1975, a decade or two ahead of China and South Korea, and the population has been shrinking since 2009.

Headline health trends are remarkable. The world-beating gains in life expectancy are well known. Japan continues to have the lowest heart attack rate in the world. The stroke death rate has been cut to European levels and continues to decline. Japan's cancer mortality rates are lower than the UK, the US, and France, and the trend is downward. The health record is, as we would expect, not perfect: the suicide rate is high and the quality of care for people with serious mental illness remains problematic.

Twenty years ago, it became clear that Japan had entered a new era. Having achieved, by 1990, its post-war aim of becoming an economic and technological powerhouse, social change was now on the national agenda. The homogeneous male breadwinner system of secure, pensioned employment began to lose ground to more precarious working arrangements and rapidly-rising participation of women in the labour market. The ageing demographic poses another social challenge, as the three-generation family has all but disappeared following urbanization and the fading of traditions about family and gender roles.

The two periods, 1964–1990 and 1991–2020, are distinctive. There was high economic growth and low inequality in the earlier period, but in the later low-growth period social and economic inequalities have tended to increase. The two roughly 30-year periods offer a natural epidemiological experiment, with the health and wellbeing of the Japanese people at risk. The results of this before-and-after natural experiment are described in this book. Overall, there is good evidence that population health continues to improve and inequalities in health and wellbeing have remained small. Japanese society remains cohesive and resilient through the period of social change. That resilience is reflected in the low COVID-19 death rate to date, described in the prologue.

The authors contributing to this book are leading epidemiological researchers based in universities across Japan. The editors thank them all. Almost all authors are contributors to the annual Osaka seminar on the social determinants of health organized by Osaka University and University College London. The three-day seminar has attracted 100 or more participants every year since 2010 to lectures and discussions on the state of the evidence and how it might be translated into policy. The seminar's success has motivated this book as a summary and a synthesis of a growing body of research in social epidemiology in Japan. We hope it may influence as well as inform our readers.

EB, NC, and HI
London and Osaka
June 2020

Contents

Prologue

Hiroyasu Iso, Noriko Cable, and Eric Brunner

The 2020 Global COVID-19 Pandemic

As we write this prologue (15 June 2020), SARS-CoV-2 is challenging profoundly human health, healthcare systems, social and economic activity all over the world. The longer-term direct and indirect health effects of this virus will be complex because of its particular biological features. Health inequalities are likely to widen because probability of infection and, once infected, vulnerability to severe coronavirus disease (COVID-19), mortality, and prolonged health effects is tightly linked to existing social disadvantage. Hard hit may be young workers, lone mothers, those in precarious employment, individuals on low incomes, older people, and those with existing ill-health. The post-pandemic exit strategy in Japan and elsewhere will determine the shape of re-construction, not only citizen's health, social behaviour, healthcare, economy, and environment but also systems and technologies to combat and prevent further pandemics.

The Japanese Epidemic: January–February 2020

The first Japanese case of COVID-19 was a bus driver who served tourists from Wuhan on 18 January. COVID-19 was declared a designated infectious disease on 28 January under the Infectious Disease Control Act 2014, which gives power for compulsory hospitalization and quarantine. The case cluster on the *Diamond Princess* cruise ship docked at Yokohama prompted the policy of containment and contact tracing of passengers and crew between 1 and 27 February. Quarantine was applied to incoming tourists and repatriated Japanese residents from China in late January and early February, and the border was closed to travellers from Hubei in China and Daegu in South Korea. The Expert Group on Novel Coronavirus Disease Control was set up and met for the first time in mid-February to advise on managing the COVID epidemic.

Testing for COVID-19 infection was scaled up more slowly than in other rich countries. In Japan, around 160/100,000 people had been tested by early

May, while other major economies (although not the UK) had built capacity to test at five times that rate. Under-testing early in the epidemic may explain why the doubling time for cases was estimated at eight days in Japan, when it was two days in China and South Korea, and three days in Europe.

With relatively little testing, it is unclear how Japan's epidemic evolved in the first four months of 2020. The World Health Organization situation report for 7 May classified Japan (15,463 confirmed cases, 2019 population 126,161,000) as having 'clusters of cases', suggesting some successful containment and far less intense spread than countries with a classification of 'community transmission'. The number of confirmed cases in the US (1.2 M), UK, Spain, and Italy (each >200,000) was much larger.

Japan's COVID-19 deaths to this date are similarly much fewer, 551 compared with >25,000 in the UK, Spain, and Italy, and 65,000 in the US. Almost all pneumonia deaths in Japan were viral RNA polymerase chain reaction (PCR) tested before or after death, reducing the likelihood of under-reporting.

Japan's 469 public health centres are the community bases for prevention and response to infectious disease. Nurses and doctors working at these centres conduct telephone counselling, deliver behavioural control messages, and collect detailed contact-tracing information. During the first phase of the epidemic, PCR tests in national and prefecture laboratories were limited to those who had a fever ($\geq 37.5^\circ$C) lasting 4+ days, plus fatigue or breathing difficulty, or those who had recently returned to Japan or were close contacts of known cases. The first epidemic wave was controlled substantially by this strategy.

The second epidemic wave emerged in early March. Before this time, clusters of COVID-19 cases had been contained, but infected individuals were now escaping surveillance and not quarantined. Asymptomatic or not-yet symptomatic cases were probably missed at airports. Insufficient testing was a contributory factor. Isolated cases became the majority, together with increasing numbers of in-hospital or in-facility clusters involving physicians, nurses, and care providers as well as patients. This situation strongly suggested person-to-person spread. Some public health centres faced overload in their infection control activities. Prime Minister Abe requested closure of all primary, secondary, and high schools from 2 March.

Postponement of 2020 Tokyo Olympics and State of Emergency: March–May 2020

On 24 March, the Tokyo Games, due to open on 24 July, were postponed until July 2021. The Olympic Committee statement explained the need to 'safeguard the health of the athletes, everybody involved in the Olympic Games, and the international community'. Abe declared a state of emergency in seven prefectures on 7 April, extended to the whole country on 16 April. With the authority of their position, and without legal enforcement, prefectural governors advised schools, public facilities, and some businesses to close.

The national government pledged JPY100,000 (£770, US$920) to every citizen for support during lockdown. Cash payments were made to small- and medium-sized businesses: JPY 2M (£15,420, US$18,390) for companies, JPY 1M (£7710, US$9190) for independent traders. Interest-free unsecured loans were made available. The collapse of small businesses, which employ 70% of Japanese workers, may raise the rate of psychiatric disease and suicide, as followed the 2008 global financial crisis.

COVID-19 was a legally designated infectious disease. However Japanese lockdown strategy was largely voluntary and prefectures could relax the advised shutdown of local businesses. The constitution guarantees individual freedoms and rights, and although non-food shops, bars, and restaurants were asked to close, some remained open. Citizens were requested, without legal enforcement, to stay at home in order to reduce human contact by 80%, i.e., to avoid crowded, confined (poorly ventilated) places, and close contact, the so-called 'three modes of density' outside the household. Remote working and online education were highly recommended.

Japan's government wanted to balance health and economic protection with safeguards for privacy and preventing stigmatization of patients, health and care workers, and their families. The 'soft' strategy was much different from the lockdown strategies in China, Europe, and the US. South Korea also adopted a softer strategy, but with extensive PCR testing, closed borders, contact tracing over the mobile phone network, and compulsory home quarantine for carriers and anyone coming within 2 metres of a carrier.

Epidemic Preparedness

The state of emergency was declared in Japan on 7 April, six weeks later than in South Korea (23 February), where the first case was identified on 20 January. Several factors may be considered to explain the delay. First, unlike in South Korea, there were no cases or deaths due to severe acute respiratory syndrome (SARS) in the 2003 epidemic or Middle East Respiratory Syndrome (MERS) in 2015 in Japan. Second, PCR testing capacity was limited and the potential impact of COVID-19 may have been underestimated. Third, the Expert Group giving scientific advice to the government about the COVID-19 epidemic met for the first time on 16 February. Fourth, although legislation for special measures was passed on 13 March, the emergency did not come into force for three weeks.

The COVID-19 Emergency

In early April, the Japanese Medical Association, alarmed that healthcare might be overwhelmed by the increasing number of in-hospital clusters, suspended outpatient activity, non-urgent operations, and screening examinations. In mid-April, PCR testing was extended beyond public health centres to walk-in and drive-through sites in order to reduce transmission. Prefectures prepared facilities including hotels, special clinics, and hospitals for triage of infected patients. In retrospect, there were some localized difficulties with hospital admission but capacity was sufficient to respond to need for beds for COVID-19 patients. Less than half of available beds were used in Tokyo, Osaka, and other large cities at the height of admissions.

The emergency was lifted on 25 May. The daily number of confirmed new cases had fallen from hundreds in mid-April to around 30. According to the 29 May report from the Expert Group, the cumulative number of infected patients was 16,550, of whom about one-third were admitted to hospital (n=5627). Certainly, Japan avoided a major epidemic (Figure P.1). The small number of Japanese COVID-19 deaths to date is likely due to several factors.

- Provisional data show a low 30-day mortality rate after severe disease (24% among mechanically ventilated patients).
- The Japanese value social cooperation, and most have a high level of health literacy and respect for official guidance.
- Collective resilience and individual endurance in the face of disasters is high, as demonstrated in the months after the 2011 Great East Japan Earthquake and Tsunami.
- The universal healthcare system provides good access to clinics and hospitals.

The COVID-19 crisis is expected to continue until at least one effective and safe vaccine is developed. Availability of drug treatment would make coexistence with SARS-CoV-2 easier. Meanwhile, avoidance of the three modes of density, use of facemasks, and careful and frequent washing of hands will remain important defences.

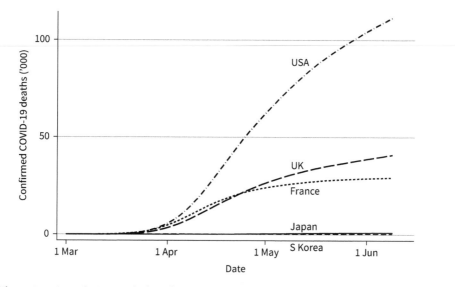

Figure P.1 Cumulative total of confirmed deaths from COVID-19, Japan and selected countries, 1 March–9 June 2020.

The accumulated total of test-confirmed COVID-19 deaths on 9 June was 916 in Japan, 40,597 in the UK and 111,007 in the US. Trend lines are smoothed using locally weighted regression.

Source: Roser M, Ritchie H, Ortiz-Ospina E, Hasell J (2020). Mortality data published by European Centre for Disease Prevention and Control. Available at: https://ourworldindata.org/coronavirus [last accessed 21 July 2020]. ©CC-BY.

The Future

The pandemic in Japan and across the world darkens the future with increased uncertainty. Sustained economic recession would increase unemployment and reduce income. Socially, Japanese men and women have been thrown together at home by the lockdown. The negative consequences of possible increased divorce, domestic violence, and child abuse remain to be determined. These negative effects may be highly unequal, according to age, region, and socioeconomic status. The biggest economic impact could be among the poorest and most vulnerable groups, increasing health disparities in Japan. Persisting economic stagnation or decline is likely to lead to increased mental health problems and suicide, substance abuse, and reduced life expectancy. These hazards point to the need for public health professionals to make their voices heard in the policy-making process.

On the bright side, positive change in the social environment may be accelerated. Business, administration, education, and the national government have all promoted home working, tele-meetings, and online systems for banking and administrative tasks. With the COVID-19 crisis, changes are being made more enthusiastically and widely than ever before. One revolutionary change in the Japanese system, discussed early in the epidemic, is reduction in the traditional time-wasting company stamp-seal (*hanko*) custom for document certification. Other improvements to work-life balance might include cutting long and inefficient working hours, long face-to-face meetings, enhancing the status of women in the workforce, and gender balance in housework. At the same time positive social relationships cultivated by traditional modes of relaxation and communication can be preserved. Importantly, reform of legislation, public health, and healthcare systems will be needed to increase pandemic preparedness.

It is too early to evaluate Japan's soft strategy for combating COVID-19, which involves little legal enforcement, and much reliance on cultural self-restraint, cooperation, and disaster resilience. There is, however, good reason to believe that Japan can keep its top position in the life expectancy ranking in the world when the pandemic is over.

Contributors

Jun Aida, Associate Professor, Department of International and Community Oral Health, Graduate School of Dentistry, Tohoku University, Sendai

Shiho Amagasa, JSPS Research Fellow, Department of Preventive Medicine and Public Health, Tokyo Medical University, Tokyo

Sachiko Baba, Assistant Professor of Bioethics and Public Policy, Department of Social Medicine, Graduate School of Medicine, Osaka University, Osaka

Eric Brunner, Professor, Institute of Epidemiology and Health Care, University College London, London. Visiting Professor, Osaka University

Noriko Cable, Senior Research Fellow, Institute of Epidemiology and Health Care, University College London, London. Visiting Associate Professor, Osaka University

Takeo Fujiwara, Professor, Department of Global Health Promotion, Tokyo Medical and Dental University, Tokyo

Yoshiharu Fukuda, Professor, School of Public Health, Teikyo University, Tokyo

Tomoya Hanibuchi, Associate Professor, Department of Frontier Science for Advanced Environment, Graduate School of Environmental Studies, Tohoku University, Sendai

Hideki Hashimoto, Professor, School of Public Health, the University of Tokyo, Tokyo

Ayako Hiyoshi, Associate Professor, Clinical Epidemiology and Biostatistics, School of Medicine Sciences, Örebro University, Örebro. Department of Public Health Sciences, Stockholm University, Stockholm

Kaori Honjo, Professor, Department of Social and Behavioral Sciences, Osaka Medical College, Osaka

Mariko Inoue, Associate Professor, School of Public Health, Teikyo University, Tokyo

Shigeru Inoue, Professor, Department of Preventive Medicine and Public Health, Tokyo Medical University, Tokyo

Hiroyasu Iso, Professor of Public Health, Department of Social Medicine, Graduate School of Medicine, Osaka University, Osaka

Yuri Ito, Associate Professor, Department of Medical Statistics, Research and Development Centre, Osaka Medical College, Osaka

Norito Kawakami, Professor, Department of Mental Health, Graduate School of Medicine, the University of Tokyo, Tokyo

Hiroyuki Kikuchi, Assistant Professor, Department of Preventive Medicine and Public Health, Tokyo Medical University, Tokyo

Shinsuke Koike, Associate Professor, Institute for Diversity & Adaptation of Human Mind, the University of Tokyo, Tokyo

Katsunori Kondo, Professor, Department of Social Preventive Medical Sciences, Centre for Preventive Medical Sciences, Chiba University, Chiba. Head, Department of Gerontological Evaluation, Center for Gerontology and Social Science, National Center for Geriatrics and Gerontology, Obu

Naoki Kondo, Associate Professor, School of Public Health, the University of Tokyo, Tokyo

Kotatsu Maruyama, Associate Professor, Graduate School of Agriculture, Ehime University, Ehime

Yusuke Matsuyama, Assistant Professor, Department of Global Health Promotion, Tokyo Medical and Dental University, Tokyo

Hiroki Nakatani, Project Professor, Keio University Global Research Institute, Keio University, Tokyo

Tomoki Nakaya, Professor, Department of Frontier Science for Advanced Environment, Graduate School of Environmental Studies, Tohoku University, Sendai

Nobutoshi Nawa, Assistant Professor, Department of Medical Education Research and Development, Tokyo Medical and Dental University, Tokyo

Bernard Rachet, Professor, Inequalities in Cancer Outcomes Network (ICON), Department of Non-Communicable Disease Epidemiology, Faculty of Epidemiology and Population Health, London School of Hygiene and Tropical Medicine, London

Michikazu Sekine, Professor, Department of Epidemiology and Health Policy, University of Toyama, Toyama

Akihito Shimazu, Professor, Faculty of Policy Management, Keio University, Kanagawa

Kokoro Shirai, Specially Appointed Associate Professor of Public Health, Department of Social Medicine, Graduate School of Medicine, Osaka University, Osaka

Takahiro Tabuchi, Deputy Head, Department of Cancer Epidemiology, Cancer Control Centre, Osaka International Cancer Institute, Osaka

Akizumi Tsutsumi, Professor, Department of Public Health, Kitasato University School of Medicine, Sagamihara

Kazumasa Yamagishi, Professor, Department of Public Health Medicine, Faculty of Medicine, University of Tsukuba, Tsukuba

1

Excellent Population Health, Low Economic Growth

Eric Brunner, Noriko Cable, and Hiroyasu Iso

1.1 Introduction

The 1964 Summer Olympics were the first held in Asia and the first to be watched around the world by live satellite broadcast. The International Olympic Committee chose Tokyo at their 1959 meeting because Japan was so well on the road to recovery after the immense destruction caused by World War II. Growth was almost 10% per year between 1955 and 1975. Japan's achievements over the past 60 years have been remarkable and fascinating in many dimensions.

The outstanding health of the people of Japan is a phenomenon that deserves investigation. Life expectancy jumped to the top of the country rankings by the mid-1970s and stayed there, even during the three recent decades of economic stagnation. In contrast, life expectancy growth in the UK and US stalled after the financial crisis of 2008. There is no intrinsic biological reason why Japanese people should be healthier than others (see Section 1.2.7). Instead, it appears that Japanese culture and social institutions are resilient in respect of the health of its population in good times and bad. Japan is affluent. Japan also has a history of disruption—natural and man-made shocks such as the 2011 earthquake and tsunami, the burst economic bubble in 1990, and the financial crises that followed.

Trends in headline health statistics allow us to examine the proposition that the health of Japanese people is better protected than in other countries, including the UK. More specific questions relate to changes in health trends following the economic turning point when Japan's boom years came to a close. Has progress in the health status—wellbeing and mortality rates—of the Japanese slowed, in comparison to the three decades before 1990? More

Eric Brunner, Noriko Cable, and Hiroyasu Iso, *Excellent Population Health, Low Economic Growth* In: *Health in Japan*. Edited by: Eric Brunner, Noriko Cable, and Hiroyasu Iso, Oxford University Press (2021). © Oxford University Press. DOI: 10.1093/oso/9780198848134.003.0001.

subtly, we can ask in what way trends in inequalities in health have changed since 1990. The chapter also summarizes some of the factors in Japanese culture and social arrangements which shape its population's health from the perspective of social epidemiology.

1.2 Health: Big in Japan

1.2.1 The Ageing Demographic

At the time of the first Tokyo Olympics, Japan was a young nation (Table 1.1). For each person 65 and over there were six children and teenagers. Today, 56 years later, there are not one, but ten, older people for every six children and teenagers. The super-ageing population shift in Japan is large and extremely rapid compared to other countries. The proportion of Japanese aged 65 and over is already more than one quarter, while in the UK, the older population is expected to exceed 25% only in 2050.

Contraction of the younger population contributes to the large demographic shift. The fertility rate decreased after the baby booms of 1948 and 1973 to a low of 1.26 births per woman in 2005, far below 2.1, the approximate level needed for population replacement (Chapter 2). The fertility rate is an important policy target as Japan searches for answers to its labour shortage. Although the fertility rate increased to 1.43 in 2017, it remains below the average of 1.66 for high income countries.[1]

Table 1.1 Population and age structure in 1964 and 2020, Japan and UK

	Population (million)	0–19 years (%)	65+ years (%)	Ratio of older:younger
Japan				
1964	97.4	37.6%	6.0%	0.16
2020	126.5	17.0%	28.4%	1.67
UK				
1964	53.9	30.9%	12.1%	0.39
2020	67.9	23.1%	18.7%	0.81

Data from United Nations, Department of Economic and Social Affairs, Population Division (2019). World Population Prospects 2019.

1.2.2 Wellbeing and Happiness

Vital statistics such as birth and death rates can be compared across countries and cultures. In contrast, comparison of subjective measures of health needs understanding of cultural specifics. Much of the research on wellbeing and happiness has been conducted in the US. Americans, with a primarily individualistic self-identity, tend to describe momentary happiness emotions in an independent way, in terms of personal achievement, self-esteem, and excitement. In contrast, Japanese express an interdependent self, focusing on social harmony, interpersonal relationships, and sense of calm.[2]

East Asian and Western concepts of happiness and wellbeing are not identical.[3] Wellbeing refers to the overall cognitive evaluation of life, and compared to Americans, Japanese tend to pay more attention to their social environment, and give value to adjusting behaviour to circumstances and expectations of others. Wellbeing therefore depends partly on self-awareness and social responsiveness. In this respect, wellbeing has a collective dimension in Japanese culture. The social expectations and obligations that underlie this aspect of wellbeing point to complexities such as a need for caution, and recognition that positive emotions such as happiness are not permanent.

In Japan, accordingly, wellbeing questionnaire scores tend to be lower than in Western countries. The difference probably reflects the importance of modesty and social harmony to the collectively oriented Japanese self. Standard Western psychometric scales measure the European-US concept of wellbeing, which appears partly incomplete by East Asian cultural norms. The American 'satisfaction with life scale', for example, is based only on evaluating individualistic statements: 'In most ways my life is close to my ideal; The conditions of my life are excellent; I am satisfied with my life; So far I have gotten the important things I want in life; If I could live my life over, I would change almost nothing'.[4]

Globalization has brought cultural change to Japan, for example in the form of increased attention to personal achievements rather than relationships in the workplace and other social settings. In an experimental study, the group assigned to imagine and describe an 'achievement scenario' reported lower wellbeing after the exercise than the group assigned to the 'relationship scenario'.[2]

These researchers further identify a tendency among the Japanese to negative appraisal of individualistic behaviours in others. Individualism implies egotistic independence, bringing with it a risk of social disconnection. The *hikikomori* disorder, disturbed social withdrawal which may continue for ten years or more, is considered by some researchers to be an extreme response to modernization, as Japan moves towards individualistic values.[3]

As Japanese culture adapts to global influences, individual assessments of wellbeing may change because increasing value is given to achievements, over relationships. Social inequality in wellbeing will not necessarily increase, as long as value continues to be attached to equality in opportunity for self-realization and personal achievement.

A large representative survey series assessed wellbeing i.e. subjective health, at three-year intervals from 1986 to 2013. The proportion self-rating their current health 'good' or 'fairly good' at each survey wave estimates the trend in wellbeing in the population over the period spanning the economic boom and the low-growth decades starting in the 1990s (Figure 1.1). A sense of good health was reported by half of the population at that time, declining to about 40% after 2004 (the low proportion in 1986 may be the product of a low response rate). These figures are similar to those in the UK Household Longitudinal Study, although respondents were asked a different question, to rate their 'satisfaction with their general health'. The proportion answering 'mostly' or 'completely' satisfied in 2010–2013 in the UK was 48%. It is unclear whether the sense of national wellbeing is higher or lower among the Japanese compared to the British.

The difference in wellbeing across the income distribution at each survey wave provides a measure of the health inequality trend. Relative and absolute inequalities in wellbeing were largely stable between 1986 and 2013.

1.2.3 Life Expectancy and Mortality Trends

Japan's worldwide lead in demographic transformation is well known. Life expectancy at birth increased in the past 50 years by more than 2.5 years per decade. In 2017 it was 81.1 in men and 87.3 in women, compared to 67.7 and 72.9 years in 1965.

By 1964, deaths due to tuberculosis, diarrhoea, and other infectious diseases in children and young adults had declined to a low level.[5] Non-communicable disease mortality then became the main determinant of the life expectancy trend (Figure 1.2). Declining death rates from stroke and stomach cancer were particularly important after 1964. These favourable trends have continued for 50 years (see Figures 11.1 and 12.2). Heart attack and coronary death rates were already low five decades ago and have declined further.

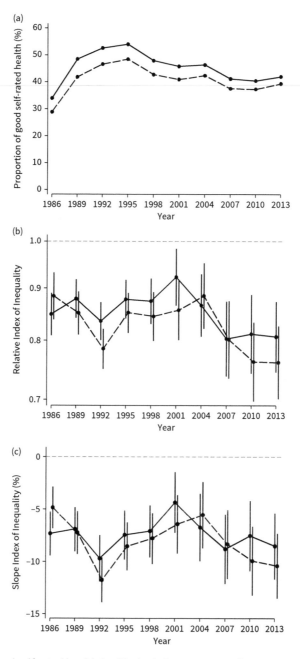

Figure 1.1 Good self-rated health (wellbeing), Japan, men and women, 1986–2013, age-standardized. A: prevalence B: relative inequality C: absolute inequality

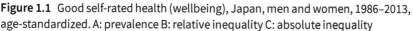

Men: solid line; women: dashed line. A: Overall prevalence of good health defined as answering 'good' or 'fairly good' to the question 'What is your current health (condition)?' on a five-point scale. Inequality based on equivalized household income before tax. Estimates and 95% confidence interval adjusted for age, household clustering, survey year, prefecture, marital status. Sample size: 371,710 men, 393,858 women. B: relative index of inequality (log binomial function). C: slope index of inequality.

Source: Honjo and Hiyoshi, unpublished analysis of Comprehensive Survey of Living Conditions. Methods in Hiyoshi et al, J Epidemiol Community Health. 2013;67:960-965

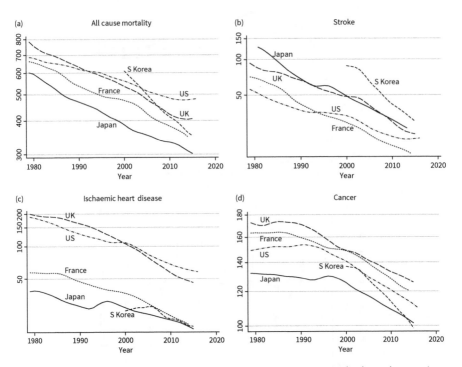

Figure 1.2 Age-standardized mortality rates per 100,000, Japan and selected countries, 1979–2016

Rates are standardized to the WHO World Standard Population (2001) and displayed on a log scale. Trend lines are smoothed using locally weighted regression. Downloaded Korean data for the years before 2000 is of uncertain quality (Hyeon Chang Kim, personal communication).

Source: Data from World Health Organisation Mortality Database. https://www.who.int/healthinfo/statistics/mortality_rawdata/en/

Life expectancy gains slowed down in the years after 1990. Between 1970 and 1989 life expectancy at birth increased by an average of 3.3 years per decade among men and 3.7 years among women. Between 1990 and 2010 the increases were 1.9 and 2.4 years per decade respectively.[6] The gains slowed by 40% in men and 35% in women. The reduction in the rate of improvement is smaller in Japan than in the UK and US after the 2008 financial crisis. In the UK, the average increase life expectancy dropped from about 2.5 years to about 1 year per decade (comparing 2000–2009 with 2010–2016). The decline was more dramatic in the US, from about 2 years in the first decade of the Millennium to zero in men and 0.3 years per decade in women. There is a clear contrast in the size of the change in rates of life expectancy improvement in Japan after 1990 (about 40% reduction) and the US/UK after 2009 (60–100% reduction).

1.2.4 Ischaemic Heart Disease and Stroke

The epidemiology of ischaemic heart disease and stroke in Japan is unusual. Rates of fatal stroke were extremely high in the 1950s, 60s, and 70s. The declining stroke mortality rate, now down to European levels (Figures 1.2 and 11.1), made an important contribution to the rise in Japanese longevity (Chapter 11).[7] As noted in Section 1.2.3, fatal heart attacks were rare and decreased further.

The pattern of high stroke and low heart disease rates and their trends has been traced to a small number of diet-related risk factors, particularly salt intake, and cigarette smoking (Figure 11.2). High blood pressure is the major modifiable risk factor for stroke, and was common in Japan before refrigeration replaced salt preservation of food. Post-war public health campaigns suggested cutting the high salt level in miso soup and other staple Japanese foods. Conversely, blood cholesterol levels were low compared to Western countries and then increased in the 1980s. Risk factor screening for people over 40 was introduced in 1983 (see Section 1.3.2).

The widespread belief that the traditional high fish, low meat diet is instrumental in the low risk of heart attack in Japan fits well with the epidemiological evidence.[8] The beneficial effects on heart disease risk of long chain omega-3 fatty acids in oily fish may not be as large as once thought. A systematic review of trials of 12+ months duration (total N>100,000 participants) finds little effect of fish oils on cardiovascular health.[9] Nevertheless, oily and white fish is valuable as a source of protein and meat substitute.[10]

1.2.5 Cancer

Cancers of the stomach, bowel, breast, and lung are important causes of death globally, and in Japan. Age-standardized total cancer mortality has declined in Japan, especially since the late 1990s (Figure 1.2). The rate has declined among women since 1960—few Japanese women smoke—and since 2000 in men also, as smoking prevalence has declined (Chapter 12). Cancer research in Japan is well developed, with cancer registries across the whole country since 2016 collecting data on incidence, survival and mortality, and social inequalities in cancer outcomes.[11] Screening for stomach, cervical, lung, breast, and colorectal cancer is available in every municipality. National guidelines are available, but recent evidence suggests local cancer screening services vary in quality.[12]

Stomach cancer mortality peaked about 1960 when the age-standardized rate was double that in the UK, US, and Australia. Japanese rates are now a quarter of the 1960 peak, but they remain above rates in the West (Figure 12.2). Japan introduced nationwide mass screening in 1983, and survival rates are reportedly high (Chapter 12). Hygiene appears to have played a part in the decrease from the high early rates. Bacterial stomach infection with *Helicobacter pylori,* a risk factor for stomach cancer, is believed to have been common during and after World War II. Treatment and eradication of this infection is considered to be cost-effective in high-risk populations.[13]

1.2.6 Dementia

Super-ageing Japan is at least 20 years ahead of the UK in population structure. It has universal social care policy for older people based on insurance.[14] Japan has a three-fold greater population aged 65+ (36 M versus 13 M, Table 1.1). The prevalence proportion of dementia rises exponentially from 65 to 90, overall about 15% of the 65+ population.[15] This estimate suggests there are over 5 M people living with dementia in Japan, compared with about 1 M in the UK.[16] It is unclear why dementia should be more common in Japan, compared to the UK and the US. The pattern of causes is similar: Alzheimer's disease 67%, vascular dementia 19%, Lewy body dementia 5%, mixed dementia 4%. If the excess of disease is real, international comparative studies could identify the reasons for this.

Long-term-care insurance was introduced in 2000, as a national system providing substantial consumer choice over personal care arrangements (Chapter 8). Individuals are able to choose home care provided by family, care worker or nurse, day care or institutional care. Support is provided according to level of need with modest copayment, capped to prevent hardship.

1.2.7 Why Should the Health of the Japanese Be Any Better than Others?

Essentially, health is the result of interactions between genes and environment. It could be that the Japanese population is healthy because it is well-adapted to its living environment. Recurrent famines during the past 300 years may have favoured the survival of those with genes for efficient fat storage[17] but it is not clear how such traits would promote health in a rich country such as Japan. The tendency of South Asians to accumulate abdominal fat and to have high risk of type 2 diabetes is consistent with this idea. Obesity prevalence is relatively low in Japan, at least partly because the food culture discourages over-eating. (Chapter 11). Another genetic adaptation that might support a long lifespan could be evolved resistance to infectious disease.[18]

There is no evidence for specific 'Japanese genetic' adaptive mechanisms explaining its good population health today. Societal development in the past century has produced a living environment that is radically different from the Japanese evolutionary past in many ways. Prevalence of obesity and infectious diseases is low, and it is unclear what biological advantage might explain the good health of the population when non-communicable disease is predominant. Intolerance to alcohol is common among East Asians, due to a variant alcohol dehydrogenase gene. Low alcohol consumption may explain why the Japanese breast cancer mortality rate is low.[19,20] Migration studies support the view that living environment and health behaviours are the key influences. Groups of Japanese ancestry living in Honolulu and San Francisco have cardiovascular risk levels that are closer to those of the host rather than source population.[7]

1.3 Social Determinants of Health in Japan

Few will disagree with the statement that most Japanese people are healthy and live a long life. To understand what this means, how, and in what way, the Japanese have been so successful in this respect, social epidemiologists look to the impacts of the social system, and living and working conditions on health (Figure 1.3). A growing body of research on the 'causes of the causes'[21] in Japan coincides with the economic slowdown since 1990. Considering its age demographic, low fertility rate, and low economic growth, Japan offers us some important evidence and ideas about societal arrangements compatible with a sustainable and healthy future.[22]

1.3.1 Health Inequalities

Health inequality, the degree of systematic difference in health across social groups (higher status linked almost always to better health outcomes),

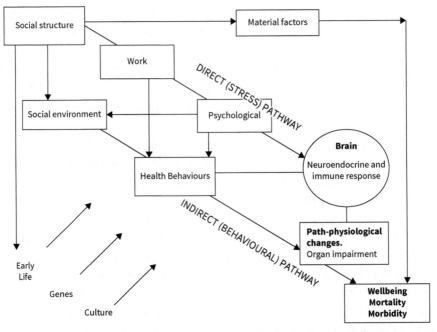

Brunner and Marmot, in SDOH, 2nd edition, OUP 2006

Figure 1.3 Social determinants of health, research model

Associations (links) between the boxes are hypotheses to be tested with cross-sectional, prospective (follow-up), and longitudinal analyses on study participants.

Source: Reproduced with permission from Brunner EJ, Marmot MG. Social organisation, stress and health. In Marmot, MG, Wilkinson RG (Eds.). Social Determinants of Health (2nd ed). Oxford: Oxford University Press 2006.

is most important. Together with headline statistics on life expectancy and death rates from the major causes, measures of health inequality provide a digestible summary of national health status. Disadvantaged groups cannot be identified with average figures. Absolute poverty has become a rare condition in rich countries including Japan. Relative poverty, defined in relation to the median wage, remains associated with poor physical and mental health and shorter life expectancy, even in the wealthiest countries that have comprehensive welfare systems. Generally, health inequalities are seen in all countries, whether on the basis of income, wealth, occupation, or other measures of access to resources. Social epidemiologists share the view that health inequalities are undesirable, unfair, and at least partly preventable (Box 1.1). Reduction of health inequality has been a public health objective in Japan since 2012 (Chapter 10).

Box 1.1 Whitehall II cohort study

The social determinants of health research model (Figure 1.2) was developed to summarize thinking about research strategy in the Whitehall II study.[23] The study recruited 10,308 male and female civil servants. They have been followed since 1985 with repeat clinic examinations and questionnaires. The figure shows a representation of the social determinants of health concept. Two main pathways are hypothesized to link social structure with common causes of morbidity (illness) and mortality, and wellbeing: direct, stress mechanisms, independent of smoking and other health behaviours, and indirect, behavioural mechanisms. 'Material' pathways, absolute poverty, and hazards such as heavy manual labour are not of great importance to office workers with secure employment and pension rights. The research model is a guide for building hypotheses to test using multiple waves of risk factors and health data collected from participants, linked together with medical records and death certificates. Evidence from the study contributes scientific support for public health policy.

1.3.2 Public Health and Prevention

Prefectural-based public health centres were established in Japan after World War II, and in 1980 there were 855, funded nationally and by prefectures. Centres controlled tuberculosis, and they continue to have responsibility for communicable, intractable, and mental diseases, and environmental health problems. Screening for cardiovascular disease (CVD) and cancer was introduced by municipalities at local public health or medical centres in 1983. The work of municipalities expanded to include maternal and child health, rehabilitation and care of the elderly, as well as prevention of CVD and cancer in cooperation with prefectural public health centres. The number of municipal health centres increased to 2,456 in 2017 and that of prefecture-based public health centres has been reduced to 469. In 2008, health insurers replaced the municipalities for health checkups, individual counselling, and referral to local physicians for the prevention and control of lifestyle-related disease including diabetes, hypertension, dyslipidaemia, and CVD, with an emphasis on metabolic syndrome. Public health centres are central to further reduction in non-communicable disease.

1.3.3 Medical Care

Japan has universal health care funded by a mixture of taxation, insurance, and copayments. Outpatient, inpatient, prescription, and dental services are covered (70–90%). The level of copayment depends on age and income.[24] The patient journey differs from the UK's National Health Service (NHS) system because there is direct access to hospital care. Japan has a network of public health centres (Section 1.3.2), but few specialist family physicians to guide and regulate access to hospitals. Continuity of care based on primary care medical records is not provided nationally.

Acute care performance assessed by mortality rate is good. In 2008, hospital mortality after major surgery (1.28%) was similar to that in the US (1.23%).[25] This comparison may be slightly optimistic because the potential complication of clinical obesity is common in the US and rare in Japan. Evaluation of the performance of the Japanese public health clinic system is less favourable. Control of hypertension and diabetes and its complications was found to be less than optimal despite universal health cover.[25,26] Lack of continuity of care based on medical records may be an important explanation.

1.4 History and Culture

1.4.1 Japanese Origins

The Japanese people has its origin in three source populations, Ainu, Mainland Japanese, and Ryukyuan (Okinawan). Its pre-historic origins are partly understood. Paleolithic hunter-gatherer people from Southeast Asia, the first human inhabitants, arrived about 40,000 years ago before Japan was separated from the mainland by rising sea-levels. They established one of the oldest pottery cultures in the world, the Jōmon, some 12,000 years ago. A second more recent wave of migration around 2,000 to 3,000 years ago brought rice farming, metalwork, and weaving from the Asian continent to Japan, and transition to the Yayoi culture.[27,28]

Genetic analysis has been used to study the Jōmon–Yayoi transition. One technique is to analyse DNA sequences on the male Y chromosome, which are stable (no recombination) at conception. These sequences provide markers of origin and similarity.[29] Admixing (inter-breeding) of indigenous Jōmon and incoming Yayoi is evident. Uncertainty remains about

Yayoi origins. Ancestral groups probably made the crossing from Korea to Kyushu. Genetic and anatomical markers are equally compatible with origins in northeast Asia, with evidence of gene flow from peoples migrating from areas now part of eastern China and Russia to Hokkaido, probably via Sakhalin Island and Kamchatka Peninsula.[27] The net result of the ancient and more recent migrations is the large Mainland Japanese or Yamato population group descended from Jōmon and Yayoi, the Ainu in the north descended from Jōmon and Northeast Asian peoples, and the Ryukyuan people in the south. There is some genetic similarity between the Ainu and Ryukyu populations, despite the 2,000 km distance between their locations, which remains unexplained.

1.4.2 A Brief Cultural History

Japan adopted the Chinese writing system in the fifth and sixth centuries, at the same time that Taoism, Buddhism, and Confucianism crossed the Korea Strait. Chinese civilization influenced Japanese culture for fourteen centuries, up to the Meiji restoration, seen particularly in the influences of Confucianism. This system had several dimensions, including those of moral, social, political, and quasi-religious thought. Japanese Confucianism differed from the Chinese form in two major respects.[30] First, unlike the absolute power of the many Chinese dynasties, the Japanese imperial family is from a single continuous historical line, that shared power with others. Second, Japanese Confucianism placed emphasis on loyalty, duty, and martial skills, as embodied in the samurai, whereas China developed a civil society with wider access to education.

The Tokugawa era (1603–1867) was a period when Japan developed even under a condition of self-imposed isolation during 1639 and 1854. A small Dutch trading base in Nagasaki (Dejima) was one of few external connections. The feudal military government was headed by the Shōgun, always from the Tokugawa clan. The Emperor in Kyoto, a pope-like figure, remained symbolic ruler, but political power was in the hands of the Shōgun and his lords (daimyō) supported by their elite samurai warriors, who alone could carry a sword. Beneath them in the hierarchical and hereditary class system were first farmers and peasants, second craftsmen, third merchants, and fourth outcasts (burakumin) who worked in occupations connected with death such as butcher and undertaker. Japan had a distinct and detailed social structure in this period, unlike China. The daimyō took much of the rice crop, partly to pay to his landless samurai to protect his domain.[31] There was minimal social mobility. Merchants, ranked beneath craftsmen and farmers, who became wealthy could enter the upper classes by buying land and marrying their child into a samurai family.[32]

During these 250 years, Japan's culture became unified. Edo, now Tokyo, grew to a city of a million, similar in population to London. The dual rule of Emperor and Shōgun had upheld an armed peace.[31]

1.4.3 Modernize or Die

The start of Japan's transition to a modern state is popularly represented by the arrival of Commodore Perry's black ships in Tokyo Bay in 1853.[30] A trade treaty imposed by the Americans followed five years later, ending the long period of national isolation. Equally important was the secret sea journey of five young samurai from Yokohama to London in 1863, in the rebellious period at the end of the Shogunate. The Choshu Five studied Western science and technology at University College London and it appears also sought to buy weapons to pursue the overthrow of the Tokugawa clan. After their return, the Five were important in the modernization process. Hirobumi Ito and Kaoru Inoue later became the first prime minister and foreign secretary in the new Meiji restoration government (1885).[33]

Japan's turn towards Western ideas produced a rapid transformation after the Meiji Emperor was installed in 1868. The feudal system was abolished, occupational choice and marriage was freed of class restrictions, universal education was introduced, and industrialization and conscription began. With the end of samurai privilege to carry weapons, their role as a class changed to business and administration and to building zaibatsu, large industrial conglomerates such as Sumitomo and Mitsubishi.[30] All this was a nationalist project, motivated by observation of Western economies and European empires. It was considered necessary for Japan's survival.[32]

After 1894, imperial Japan engaged in several wars in the Asia-Pacific region. The end of the empire came in 1945 with the incendiary bombing of Tokyo on 10 March and atomic bombing of Hiroshima and Nagasaki on 6 and 9 August. Some 300,000 people died as a result of these attacks.[32]

The second major transformation of modern Japan began to crystallize during the seven years of US occupation. The 1947 constitution guaranteed individual rights, governance by the people, demilitarization and pacifism. The 1952 Treaty of San Francisco was the formal end of empire. A network of public health centres was set up. Benedict's respected anthropological study summarizes the national response to defeat as a recognition that militarism had been a failure and an error, requiring a new way of life that will earn the respect of other nations.[31]

1.4.4 Continuity and Change

During the economic growth period before 1990, Japanese achievements in population health were linked by observers to the positive influences of its social structure.[7] The hierarchical but interconnected society was based on class, gender, and age, with roots in the feudal system of the Tokugawa era. Confucian culture remained important in the Meiji, Taishō, and Shōwa eras (1868–1912, 1912–1926, 1926–1989) and its influence continued after 1945 because the men in power had been educated before the war.

The system of harmony, cooperation, and respect was first learnt within the family, in preparation for the transition to school, followed by paid work for men, and homemaking for women. Networks of clearly defined and orderly relationships provided a strong basis for the huge task of post-war rebuilding and modernization. Construction of housing, sanitation, roads, high-speed railways, schools and universities, factories and offices, health centres and hospitals, was a remarkable feat of planning and resource allocation for a large and expanding population, increasing from 94 M in 1960 to 118 M in 1980.[34]

Aspects of social behaviour are likely to have contributed to the extraordinary rate of improvement in the health status of the population. A characteristic that stands out is industriousness. Attitude surveys show the commitment to work, company, and national productivity goals well exceeded Western levels.[30] Extensive overtime, with a considerable proportion unpaid, short holidays, and a deep-rooted culture of presenteeism remain standard. Surprisingly, these work arrangements coincided with a period of rapidly improving population health (Chapter 6).[35] Long working hours are a risk factor for death from heart attack,[36] however this is not a common event in Japan, despite *Karōshi* (Figure 1.1c and Chapter 11).

Karōshi, death from overwork, and *karōjisatsu*, work-related suicide, are well-known and disturbing aspects of Japanese culture (Chapter 6). The economic downturn after 1997 appears to have triggered a sharp rise in suicide rates (Figure 1.4) in middle-aged men in particular.[37] Legal restriction

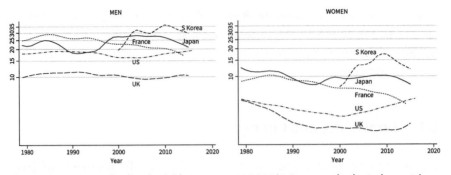

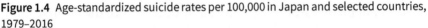

Figure 1.4 Age-standardized suicide rates per 100,000 in Japan and selected countries, 1979–2016

Rates are standardized to the WHO World Standard Population (2001) and displayed on a log scale. Trend lines are smoothed using locally weighted regression. Downloaded Korean data for the years before 2000 is of uncertain quality (Hyeon Chang Kim, personal communication).

Source: Data from World Health Organisation Mortality Database. https://www.who.int/healthinfo/statistics/mortality_rawdata/en/

of overtime was only introduced in 2019, limiting overtime hours to 45 per month and 360 per year. It may be understood that Japanese long-hours culture produces victims who sacrifice their lives for the benefit of other citizens.

Work-related deaths are most common in managers, executives, and men made redundant.[37,38] *Karōshi* and honour/status-related suicide among male white collar workers contributes to the low social inequality in male mortality in Japan.[39] This pattern differs from that in Western countries, where workers in routine occupations are at higher mortality risk than executives, partly as a result of poorer working conditions including long working hours.[40]

1.4.5 Gender

The post-war generation is now in positions of influence. Education has changed to reflect more liberal and individualistic values. One indicator of change, at the time of writing, is that there are several women in the Japanese cabinet.

The male breadwinner, female homemaker role was an enduring feature of Japanese life in the second half of the twentieth century. Anecdotally, a financial journalist observed that she did not recall meeting any Japanese women working in a senior government or business position in Tokyo in the 1990s, unless they were working for a foreign company.[41] In 2018, women's participation in the labour force in Japan was 51%, similar to France (50%), but below the UK (57%) and US (56%).[42]

This statistic, however, does not tell us how many Japanese women work in full-time, skilled, professional, and well-paid jobs. The gender pay gap (25%) remains much larger than the OECD average.[43]

The paradox of the gender difference in health in Japan is considerable. As noted in Section 1.2.3, women's life expectancy was 87.3 years in 2017 compared to 81.1 in men. The gender difference increased between 1975 and 2000. Women's life expectancy advantage has dropped since then from 6.9 to 6.2 years, but is still higher than in the UK. If social status is important, the position of Japanese women may have been misjudged by Western observers, for example, in relation to financial status, social support, and sense of personal agency (Chapter 3). Smoking rates do contribute to gender inequality in health: in 2018, few women smoked (7%), compared to men (29%). Smoking rates in 1965 were respectively 16% and 82%. Compounding this, there is evidence that smoking-related hospital stays and mortality tend to be higher in male compared with female smokers.[44]

1.5 Economic Growth and Income Inequality

Wealth and income are important factors influencing health and wellbeing.[45] In parallel with Japan's health success, its economic performance, until 1990, is often referred to as a miracle.[30,41] This loose term does not do justice to the national determination to recover and to live again after defeat.[31] Japan's economy overtook the UK's in 1967 and was double the size six years later (Figure 1.5). It remained the world's second largest economy after the US, until overtaken by China in 2010.

In the mid-1980s, admiration and interest in Japanese economic growth became mixed with some worry about possible Japanese dominance over older Western economies.[46] However, the Japanese asset bubble burst in 1990 and since then economic growth has been slow. Figure 1.5 shows the major change in the Japanese trend-line after 1990, in units of current US$, for international comparison. This measure of average 'standard of living' is a problem because it does not take account of national differences in the cost of living, and it is sensitive to the US$ exchange rate.

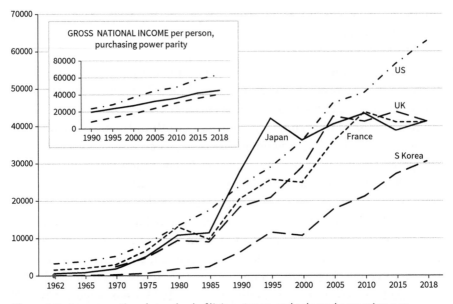

Figure 1.5 Average national standard of living, Japan and selected countries: per person, 1960–2018

Main graph, Gross National Income (GNI) per person, 1960–2018, Atlas method (current US$) converts local currency to US$ at average annual conversion rate. Inset graph, GNI per person, 1990–2018, purchasing power parity (current international $) accounts for national differences in prices. Data shown for all available years.

Source: World Bank http://datatopics.worldbank.org/world-development-indicators/themes/ economy.html (accessed 4 September 2019)

Another measure of living standards is available from 1990, which takes account of differences in the cost of housing, goods, and services. Figure 1.5 inset graph shows, after purchasing power adjustment, that the average standard of living in Japan continued to rise during the 'lost decades', but at a slower rate than in the US and Korea. It seems that the usual representation of Japan's recent economic trajectory may be too negative.

Income inequality is an important index of social conditions.[47] In the period of high economic growth, Japanese incomes were more equal than in the west, suggesting that inequality is not a necessary condition for economic success.[7] The most recent measures of income distribution after tax (Table 1.2), indicate that Japan is more equal than the UK and the US, but more unequal than Nordic countries. At the same time, there are vulnerable groups with a high poverty rate such as single parent families (Section 18.3.2) that fall outside the social protection system.

Table 1.2 Income inequality in Japan, South Korea, Nordic countries, UK, and US, 2015

	GINI coefficient, net income	Share of income received. top:bottom fifth	Income share received by top fifth
Denmark	0.26	3.7	35.2%
Finland	0.26	3.7	37.2%
Sweden	0.28	4.2	36.9%
France	0.30	4.4	41.2%
Japan	0.34	6.2	39.7%
Korea	0.35	6.9	39.7%
UK	0.36	6.1	41.6%
US	0.39	8.3	46.5%

Disposable income data for 2015 from representative surveys. Countries ranked in ascending order of GINI coefficient (range 0–1: low is more equal).

Income share received by top fifth of households for 2006–2008 (latest data for Japan 2008).

1.6 Conclusion

Our proposition at the start of this chapter was that the health of Japanese people is better protected than in other countries. Trends in headline health statistics for Japan over the past 60 years are undeniably good. Japanese life expectancy at birth and the all-cause mortality rate have continued to improve.

The positive role of Japanese cultural and societal factors is evident in the natural experiment of the economic boom years (1960–1990) and later decades of low growth after 1990. According to mortality statistics, Japan's health continues to be resilient. Softer statistics for Japanese self-rated health suggest inequalities in wellbeing have not widened during recent decades of low economic growth and slightly increasing net (after tax) income inequalities. In contrast, trends in the UK and US health statistics in the years following the financial crisis of 2008 worsened considerably.

References

1. World Bank Databank. Available at: https://databank.worldbank.org/home.aspx [last accessed 18 February 2020].

2. Uchida Y. Personal or interpersonal construal of happiness: a cultural psychological perspective. *Int J Wellbeing* 2012;2:354–69.

3. Ryff CD, Love GD, Miyamoto Y, Markus HR, Curhan KB, Kitayama S, et al. Culture and the promotion of well-being in east and west: understanding varieties of attunement to the surrounding context. In: Fava GA, Ruini C, (eds), *Increasing Psychological Well-being in Clinical and Educational Settings*. Dordrecht: Springer 2014:1.

4. Diener E, Emmons RA, Larsen RJ, et al. Satisfaction with life scale. *J Pers Assess* 1985;49:71–5.

5. Adair T, Kippen R, Naghavi M, et al. The setting of the rising sun? A recent comparative history of life expectancy trends in Japan and Australia. *PLoS One* 2019;14(3):e0214578. doi: 10.1371/journal.pone.0214578.

6. Human Mortality Database. Available at: https://www.mortality.org [last accessed 18 February 2020].

7. Marmot MG, Davey Smith G. Why are the Japanese living longer? *Br Med J* 1989;299:1547–51.

8. Iso H, Kobayashi M, Ishihara J, et al. Intake of fish and n3 fatty acids and risk of coronary heart disease among Japanese: the Japan Public Health Center-Based (JPHC) Study Cohort I. *Circulation* 2006;113(2):195–202.

9. Abdelhamid AS, Brown TJ, Brainard JS, et al. Omega-3 fatty acids for the primary and secondary prevention of cardiovascular disease. *Cochrane Database Syst Rev* 2018;11:Cd003177. doi: 10.1002/14651858.CD003177.pub4.

10. Brunner EJ, Jones PJ, Friel S, et al. Fish, human health and marine ecosystem health: policies in collision. *Int J Epidemiol* 2009;38(1):93–100.

11. Ito Y, Nakaya T, Nakayama T, et al. Socioeconomic inequalities in cancer survival: a population-based study of adult patients diagnosed in Osaka, Japan, during the period 1993–2004. *Acta Oncol* 2014;53(10):1423–33. doi: 10.3109/0284186x.2014.912350.

12. OECD. *OECD Reviews of Public Health: Japan*. Paris: OECD Publishing 2019.

13. Pasechnikov V, Chukov S, Fedorov E, et al. Gastric cancer: prevention, screening and early diagnosis. *World J Gastroenterol* 2014;20(38):13842–62. doi: 10.3748/wjg.v20.i38.13842

14. Tamiya N, Noguchi H, Nishi A, et al. Population ageing and wellbeing: lessons from Japan's long-term care insurance policy. *Lancet* 2011;378(9797):1183–92. doi: 10.1016/s0140-6736(11)61176-8

15. Ikejima C, Hisanaga A, Meguro K, et al. Multicentre population-based dementia prevalence survey in Japan: a preliminary report. *Psychogeriatrics* 2012;12(2):120–3. doi: 10.1111/j.1479-8301.2012.00415.x

16. Ahmadi-Abhari S, Guzman M, Brunner EJ, et al. Temporal trend in dementia incidence since 2002 and projections for prevalence in England and Wales to 2040: modelling study. *BMJ* 2017;358:j2856. doi: 10.1136/bmj.j2856

17. Neel JV. Diabetes mellitus: a 'thrifty' genotype rendered detrimental by 'progress'? *Am J Hum Genet* 1962;14:353–62.

18. Wells JC. Ethnic variability in adiposity and cardiovascular risk: the variable disease selection hypothesis. *Int J Epidemiol* 2009;38(1):63–71. doi: 10.1093/ije/dyn183

19. Ugai T, Kelemen LE, Mizuno M, et al. Ovarian cancer risk, ALDH2 polymorphism and alcohol drinking: Asian data from the Ovarian Cancer Association Consortium. *Cancer Sci* 2018;109(2):435–45. doi: 10.1111/cas.13470

20. Ugai T, Milne RL, Ito H, et al. The functional ALDH2 polymorphism is associated with breast cancer risk: a pooled analysis from the Breast Cancer Association Consortium. *Mol Genet Genomic Med* 2019;7(6):e707. doi: 10.1002/mgg3.707

21. Marmot M. Achieving health equity: from root causes to fair outcomes. *Lancet* 2007;370(9593):1153–63.

22. Brunner E, Hiyoshi A, Cable N, et al. Social epidemiology and Eastern wisdom. *J Epidemiol* 2012;22(4):291–4. doi: 10.2188/jea.je20120079

23. Marmot M, Brunner E. Cohort Profile: the Whitehall II study. *Int J Epidemiol* 2005;34(2):251–6.

24. Ikegami N, Yoo BK, Hashimoto H, et al. Japanese universal health coverage: evolution, achievements, and challenges. *Lancet* 2011;378(9796):1106–15. doi: 10.1016/s0140-6736(11)60828-3

25. Hashimoto H, Ikegami N, Shibuya K, et al. Cost containment and quality of care in Japan: is there a trade-off? *Lancet* 2011;378(9797):1174–82. doi: 10.1016/s0140-6736(11)60987-2

26. Tanaka H, Tomio J, Sugiyama T, et al. Process quality of diabetes care under favorable access to healthcare: a 2-year longitudinal study using claims data in Japan. *BMJ Open Diabetes Res Care* 2016;4(1):e000291. doi: 10.1136/bmjdrc-2016-000291

27. Jinam T, Nishida N, Hirai M, et al. The history of human populations in the Japanese Archipelago inferred from genome-wide SNP data with a special reference to the Ainu and the Ryukyuan populations. *J Hum Genet* 2012;57(12):787–95. doi: 10.1038/jhg.2012.114

28. Metropolitan Museum of Art, Department of Asian Art, New York City. Available at: http://www.metmuseum.org/toah/hd/jomo/hd_jomo.htm; https://www.metmuseum.org/toah/hd/yayo/hd_yayo.htm [last accessed 23 March 2020].

29. Rasteiro R, Chikhi L. Revisiting the peopling of Japan: an admixture perspective. *J Hum Genet* 2009;54(6):349–54. doi: 10.1038/jhg.2009.39

30. Jaques M. Japan: modern but hardly western. In: *When China Rules the World*. 2nd ed. London: Penguin 2012.

31. Benedict R. *The Chrysanthemum and the Sword*. Cleveland: Meridian 2005.

32. Buruma I. *Inventing Japan*. London: Phoenix 2003.

33. Embassy of Japan. Available at: https://www.uk.emb-japan.go.jp/en/event/2013/choshu/info.html [last accessed 18 February 2020].

34. UN Department of Economic and Social Affairs 2019. Available at: https://www.un.org/development/desa/en/ [last accessed 23 March 2020].

35. Kawakami N, Araki S, Takatsuka N, et al. Overtime, psychosocial working conditions, and occurrence of non-insulin dependent diabetes mellitus in Japanese men. *J Epidemiol Community Health* 1999;53:359–63.

36. Kivimaki M, Nyberg ST, Batty GD, et al. Job strain as a risk factor for coronary heart disease: a collaborative meta-analysis of individual participant data. *Lancet* 2012;380(9852):1491–7. doi: S0140-6736(12)60994-5 [pii];10.1016/S0140-6736(12)60994-5 [doi]

37. Chang SS, Gunnell D, Sterne JA, et al. Was the economic crisis 1997–1998 responsible for rising suicide rates in East/Southeast Asia? A time-trend analysis for Japan, Hong Kong, South Korea, Taiwan, Singapore and Thailand. *Soc Sci Med* 2009;68(7):1322–31. doi: 10.1016/j.socscimed.2009.01.010

38. Wada K, Kondo N, Gilmour S, et al. Trends in cause specific mortality across occupations in Japanese men of working age during period of economic stagnation, 1980–2005: retrospective cohort study. *BMJ* 2012;344:e1191. doi: 10.1136/bmj.e1191

39. Tanaka H, Nusselder WJ, Bopp M, et al. Mortality inequalities by occupational class among men in Japan, South Korea and eight European countries: a national register-based study, 1990–2015. *J Epidemiol Community Health* 2019;73(8):750–8. doi: 10.1136/jech-2018-211715

40. O'Reilly D, Rosato M. Worked to death? A census-based longitudinal study of the relationship between the numbers of hours spent working and mortality risk. *Int J Epidemiol* 2013;42(6):1820–30. doi: 10.1093/ije/dyt211

41. Tett G. Womenomics: cracks are beginning to show in Japan's glass ceiling. *FT Weekend Magazine*, 20 July 2019.

42. TheGlobalEconomy.com. Available at: https://www.theglobaleconomy.com/rankings/Female_labor_force_participation/ [last accessed 18 February 2020].

43. OECD. https://data.oecd.org/earnwage/gender-wage-gap.htm [last accessed 18 February 2020].

44. Case A, Paxson C. Sex differences in morbidity and mortality. *Demography* 2005;42(2):189–214. doi: 10.1353/dem.2005.0011

45. Lutz W, Kebede E. Education and health: redrawing the Preston Curve. *Popul Dev Rev* 2018;44(2):343–61. doi: 10.1111/padr.12141

46. Katzner DW. Explaining the Japanese Economic Miracle. *Japan and the World Economy*. 2001;13:303–19.

47. Wilkinson R, Pickett K. *The Inner Level*. London: Allen Lane 2018.

2

Women, Men, and the 'Missing' Babies

Sachiko Baba and Hiroyasu Iso

2.1 A Decline in Fertility Rates and the Missing Third Baby Boom

Fertility is influenced by social, economic, and health transitions[1] and affects the composition of the population. Fertility decline is a serious demographic challenge for high- and middle-income countries; continuing low fertility contributes to accelerate the increases in the population of older people. The total fertility rate, described as the fertility rate, for short, in this chapter, signifies the average number of children that would be born to a woman over her lifetime. Conversely, the birth rate signifies the total number of live births per year per 1,000 population. In this chapter, we focus on the fertility rate by overviewing its trend and surrounding factors.

2.1.1 Two Baby Booms, and the Missing Third Baby Boom

Japan has experienced two short baby booms, which were indicated by the number, not the rate, of live births (Figure 2.1). The first baby boom was from 1947 to 1949, with the annual number of live births exceeding 2.5 M. The second, which was mainly generated by those born in the first, occurred from 1971 to 1974, with the annual number of live births reaching more than 2 M.

Since the second baby boomers were generated from the first baby boomers when they reached reproductive age, the third baby boomers were expected. However, more than 40 years have passed without a third baby boom, even if pregnancies that ended in abortion or stillbirth are considered[2] and those born in the second baby boom have already reached or surpassed reproductive age. Trends in the fertility rate since the mid-2000s appears to be stable or slightly increased, yet this is a reflection of further declines in women of the reproductive age (denominator) than the live births (numerators). The

Sachiko Baba and Hiroyasu Iso, *Women, Men, and the 'Missing' Babies* In: *Health in Japan*. Edited by: Eric Brunner, Noriko Cable, and Hiroyasu Iso, Oxford University Press (2021). © Oxford University Press. DOI: 10.1093/oso/9780198848134.003.0002.

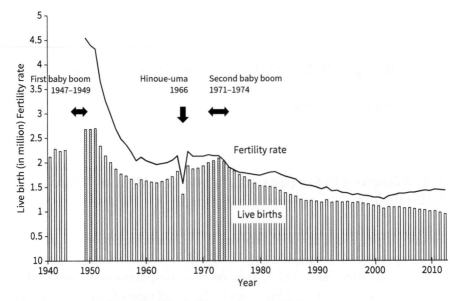

Figure 2.1 Live births and fertility rate in Japan, 1940–2017

Number of live births: shown in millions. Fertility rate: annual average number of live births per woman over her lifetime. It is calculated as the sum of age-specific fertility rates between 15 and 49 years old. Data not available for 1944–1946.

Source: Data from Statistics of Japan. Summary of results of National Census 2015. http://www.stat. go.jp/data/kokusei/2015/kekka/pdf/gaiyou1.pdf

number of live births was 946,065 in 2017,[3] representing only 0.75% of the total population.

2.1.2 Fertility Trends in Japan and Neighbouring Countries: Republic of Korea and China

The first baby boom in Japan was the result of a high fertility rate after soldiers returned home from World War II. Legalization of induced abortion introduced in 1949[2] may have contributed to the short-lived nature of the baby boom. The fertility rate fell below the replacement level of 2.1 in 1957, but it increased again with economic growth in the 1960s, leading to the second baby boom that started in 1971 and which, like the first, was quite short, ending in 1974.[4] Two events potentially contributed to the end of this second baby boom. The first was an economic recession in Japan, starting with the oil crisis in 1973.[4] The second was the introduction of the national policy to suppress potential population explosion declared at the First Japan Population Conference in 1974 by promoting no more than two children per family.[5]

Between the two baby booms, in 1966, there was a sharp one-year drop in the fertility rate and live births. The fertility rate fell to 1.58,[3] which was 74% of the rate in the previous year. This was due to the superstition-induced trend, called *hinoe-uma*, coming from a sexagenary (60-year) cycle according to the year of birth. The same calendar system is also used in Korea, Vietnam, and China;[6] however, the supersition that women born in the year of *hinoe-uma* would have bad tempers and make their husbands unhappy[7] is unique in Japan.

The Republic of Korea (South Korea, thereafter) experienced a high fertility rate during 1955–1963.[8] After that, South Korea's birth control policy contributed to a considerable decrease in the fertility rate, from 6.10 in 1960 to 1.63 in 1995 (Figure 2.2).[9] Their birth control policy aimed to promote smaller households by offering lower tax rates and prioritizing public housing for those who accepted sterilization after having two or fewer children.[10,11] An upward trend in fertility rates was observed around the 1980s, possibly generated by the birth cohort born around 1955. Despite small ups and downs, the fertility rate in South Korea has been generally decreasing; the country has had a lower birth rate than Japan since 2001.

During the 2000s, South Korea experienced small one-year peaks in the fertility rate according to zodiac animals in 'the year of the *golden pig*' in 2007 and 'the year of the *black dragon*' in 2012.[12] However, South Korea's fertility

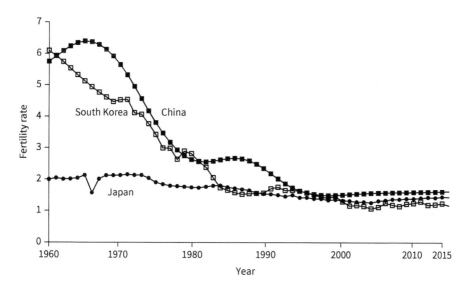

Figure 2.2 Fertility rates in Japan, South Korea, and China, 1960–2015

Source: World Bank. [https://data.worldbank.org/indicator/SP.DYN.TFRT.IN?locations=JP-CN-KR]
Licensed under a Creative Commons Attribution 4.0 International License

rate hit 0.98 in 2018 and is the only country in the world to have a fertility rate less than one.[13]

In the case of the Republic of China, a national famine occurred from 1959 to 1961, triggering a population boom after the event.[14] The highest fertility rate (6.40) was observed in 1965. After implemntation of the one-child policy in 1979, the rate steadily decreased until 1982. A smaller second upward trend in the fertility rate in 1988 was observed, possibly generated from the cohort born around 1965. After that, the fertility rate decreased again in China, even after the ending of the one-child policy in 2015.

The fertility rate of China in 2015 was 1.6,[14] slightly higher than that of Japan in the same year. Nevertheless, the adult population aged between 16 to 59 years had already started to decrease from 2012,[15] with no apparent upward trend in China's fertility rate observed since 1990. Similarly to its neighbouring countries, China has its own beliefs related to zodiac animals, such as preferences for dragons and pigs and avoidance of sheep as birth years.[16,17]

2.2 Why Are the Number of Babies Declining in Japan?

We can offer three explantions for Japanese low fertility, including: increased numbers of induced abortions and decreased numbers of pregnancies. These can be considered separately or in combination. Marriage rates are also decreasing in number and if not, are delayed.

2.2.1 Is Induced Abortion Increasing?

In 1948, three years after the end of World War II, Japan legalized induced abortion and sterilization(Box 2.1) with the Eugenic Protection Law, which coexists with criminal law. This law was initially introduced 'to prevent the live births of abnormal infants from the eugenic point of view' and to protect the health of women.[18] It was primarily used to force pregnant women to obtain an abortion, or to force a man or a woman to undergo sterilization if they or even their relatives had psychiatric diseases, mental disorders, hereditary diseases or anomalies, mental retardation, or leprosy, regardless of the person's consent.[18] These eugenic items were removed from the law in 1996, but over time, 58,000 abortions and 165,000 sterlizations were forcefully and involuntarily conducted.[18,19] Induced abortion was also permitted for pregnant women in the case of rape.

> ### Box 2.1 Involuntary sterilization
>
> The Japanese Diet enacted legislation in 2019 to pay 3.2 million JPY (approximately £21,600, if £1=150 JPY) to each person who underwent forced, involuntary sterilization under this law, for compensation. Most cases, approximately 165,000 people, were women with disabilities. Available at: https://www.japantimes.co.jp/news/ 2019/04/24/national/japan-passes-bill-pay-survivors-forced-sterilization-eugenics-law-%C2%A53-2-million/#.Xnlubaj7SF4 [last accessed 23 March 2020].

In 1949, the law was revised to permit inducing abortion for economic reasons. The number of induced abortions then increased dramatically, from 101,061 in 1949 to 320,150 in 1950. Conversely, live births over the same period decreased from 2,696,638 to 2,337,507, with the end of the post-war baby boom in 1950.[2,20]

Figure 2.3 shows trends in the abortion rate per 1,000 women of reproductive age and the induced abortion ratio per 1,000 live births since 1949. The prevalence of abortion among reproductive-aged women reached a peak in 1955 and then the numbers steadily decreased. The induced abortion ratio per 1,000 live births increased from 1949 to 1957, and then decreased until the mid-1970s, except for the year of *hinoe-uma*, in 1966.

Since the late 1950s, as opposed to a consistent decrease in the prevalence of abortion, the induced abortion ratio per 1,000 live births was stable until the mid-1980s, which can be explained by the rapidly declining number of live births (denominator) compared with the reducing numbers of abortions (numerator). This means that more Japanese opted out of having babies by refraining from sexual intercourse or using contraception.[8,19] All of these figures (number, rate, ratio) decreased again in the 2010s; the recent abortion rate in Japan (6.4 per 1,000 women) is lower than that of other countries.[20,21] Large numbers of abortions in Japan, until the mid-1950s, were due to unemployment,[22] as well as many unwanted pregnancies as a result of rape and prostitution during the unstable post-war period.[22] Induced abortion was also regarded as a main form of birth control.[23]

Teenage girls are a high-risk population for abortion worldwide, and Japan is no exception.[18] However, women of advanced age are also at high risk, which is unique in Japan as the indued abortion ratio per 1,000 live births among women aged 45 to 49 years was five times as high as that in all ages.

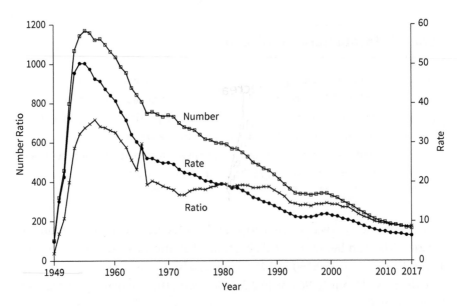

Figure 2.3 Abortion in Japan 1949–2017

Number of abortions (thousands), rate: abortion rate (per 1,000 women aged 15–49 years). Ratio: abortion ratio (per 1,000 live births). Year: calendar year until 2001; fiscal year (April–March) from 2002.

Source: data from Report on Public Health Administration and Service. https://www.mhlw.go.jp/toukei/saikin/hw/eisei_houkoku/17/; Statistics of Japan. Summary of results of National Census 2015. http://www.stat.go.jp/data/kokusei/2015/kekka/pdf/gaiyou1.pdf

This is probably because longer-acting and more highly effective contraceptive methods have not been used among married couples (see Section 2.2.3).[18]

Induced abortions are performed by a certified obstetrician, as surgical abortion using a hard metal currette,[24] while the World Health Organization recommends less invasive techniques, which include i.e. the use of pharmacological drugs or vacuum aspiration. National health insurance or private insurance in Japan does not cover the cost of abortion, nor do any charity organizations. Typical abortion procedures in Japan cost around 200,000 JPY (£1,300), implying that socially disadvantaged women would have limited access to abortion.

In South Korea, induced abortion is illegal except for medical reasons. An estimated induced abortion rate was as high as 29.8 per 1,000 reproductive-aged women in 2005, but significantly decreased to 19.7 in 2011 and 4.8 in 2017.[25] In the case of China, induced abortion was legalized in 1953[26] and abortions were widely carried out for unauthorized pregnancies after the one-child policy was introduced in 1979.[14,26] The abortion rate reached its highest level in the early 1980s (560 per 1,000 women) and went down sharply to

180 per 1,000 women after the relaxing of the family planning policy in the 2000s.[14]

2.2.2 Is Sexual Activity Decreasing in Japan?

Japanese people do not appear to have frequent sexual intercourse. According to a worldwide survey by a condom company in 2005, the frequency of sex among Japanese was 45 times per year, regardless of marital status, which is by far the least frequent, compared with 103 times as the worldwide average, 118 among UK residents, and 96 among Chinese.[27] Moreover, a study using national fertility surveys revealed that the prevalence of heterosexual inexperience among those of reproductive age, regardless of marital status, increased from 21.7% in 1992 to 24.6% in 2015 for women, and from 20.0% to 25.8% for men.[28]

Possible causes for infrequent sexual activity, especially among Japanese men, is social disadvantagement due to being unemployed, on temporary/part-time work, or having low income.[28] Possible explanations among couples also include advanced age, the extremely long working hours of men, having one or more children under the age of three, stress among spouses, or marital conflicts.[29] Another plausible reason might be the increased use of the Internet and social network services, leading the unmarried to live in a virtual world and making them less motivated to engage in direct human contact or sexual intercourse.

2.2.3 Country Profiles of Contraceptive use

The prevalence for modern contraceptive use was much lower in Japan (44.4%) than in developed (61.0%) or even developing countries (56.4%) (Table 2.1). However, this low prevalence has continued for a long time, and seems to scarcely affect the recent fertility trend. Contraception in Japan is relatively expensive. The most popular method in Japan was the male condom (40.7%).[30] Condoms are the cheapest form of contraception and are easily accessible as they can be purchased in drug stores and 24-hour convenience stores without a prescription. On the other hand, the use of oral contraceptives or an intrauterine device (IUD) in Japan was very low. Oral contraceptives have been approved since 1999, but they require prescription by an obstetrician and are not covered by Japanese national health insurance

Table 2.1 Prevalence (in %) of contraception use by type among women who are married or in a union, across selected countries

	Any modern methods	Sterilization: female	Sterilization: male	Birth control pills	IUD	Male condom	Calendar methods
Developing countries	56.4	20.6	1.9	7.5	14.7	6.3	2.3
Developed countries	61	8.4	5.3	17.7	8.9	18.4	5.3
Japan (in 2005)	44.4	1.5	0.4	1.0	0.9	40.7	11.8
South Korea (in 2009)	70.1	5.9	16.8	2.0	12.8	24.3	–
China (in 2006)	84.0	28.7	4.5	1.2	40.6	8.5	9.3
UK (in 2008/9)	84.0	8.0	21.0	28.0	10	27.0	6.0
France (in 2008)	74.1	3.8	0.8	40.6	18.9	7.9	0.4
US (in 2006/10)	70.4	22.1	11	16.3	5.2	11.8	–

Source: data from United Nations Department of Economic and Social Affairs. World Contraceptive Patterns 2013. http://www.un.org/en/development/desa/population/publications/family/contraceptive-wallchart-2013.shtml

if the use is not for medical purposes. Injectable or implanted contraceptives have not been approved in Japan. Emergency contraceptive pills also require prescription and are expensive, costing around 12,000 JPY (£80). Sterilization has not been widely taken up, probably because of the history of involuntary sterilization.

However, Table 2.1shows that in South Korea, male condoms and male sterilization were popular as contraceptive methods. In conrast, the use of the birth control pill or an IUD was lower than that for male contraception, but higher than the Japanese figure. This possibley reflects a male-dominant culture where men take the initiative to control reproduction.

In China, IUDs for women with one child, abortions for unauthorized pregnancies, and sterilization for both men and women with two or more children were said to be the core strategies,[35] reflected in a high prevalence of modern contraceptive use (84.0%). The most common contraceptive method was the IUD (40.6%), followed by female sterilization (28.7%).

2.2.4 Does Assisted Reproductive Technology (ART) Help Low Fertility in Japan?

Assisted reproductive technologies (ARTs) (e.g. in vitro fertilization (IVF), intracytoplasmic sperm injection, frozen embryo transfer) enable pregnancy without sexual intercourse. In Japan, there were 54,110 live births from ARTs in 2016, which amounted to 5.5% of all births that year.[30] Among all ARTs, 83% were frozen embryo transfers.[31] Japan's high prevalence of ART might be related to delayed marriage, financial support from the government, and a substantial number of ART clinics. However, ARTs haven't compensated for the decrease in sexual activity to generate more births. In contrast, the prevalence of ART in South Korea was 0.7%[12] and only 358 organizations are authorized for IVF in China.[32]

2.3 The Role Played by Marriage in Japan

Given that birth outside of marriage is very rare in Japan (i.e. 2.3% in 2015), timing of marriage can play a significant role in fertility rates. The number of people remaining single has been increasing in both sexes.[33] Among those who were aged 35 to 39 years, 35.0% of men and 23.9% of women were unmarried in 2015, in contrast to 14.2% and 6.6% in 1985. In addition, the proportions of households with children have been decreasing from 46.2% in 1996 to 24.1% in 2013,[33] as opposed to an increase in proportions of households with one child only, which were 35.2% in 1996 and 45.2% in 2013.

A possible reason why women are choosing to remain single was suggested by a Japanese sociologist to be due to high expectations for their potential spouse.[34,35] As more Japanese women have acquired higher education and have been participating in the labour market, they have been enabled to support themselves financially. However, traditionally, Japanese married women have been financially dependent on their spouse (see also Chapter 3); unmarried working women prefer their potential spouse to be in a higher financial status than theirs. A Dutch sociologist counterargued against this by indicating five factors to cause both men and women to remain single or have fewer children:[36] 1) the very high direct cost of children (due in part to a competitive education system), combined with very low government financial support for families; 2) a very high opportunity cost of having children, owing to considerable normative obstacles that prevent women from staying in the labour market; 3) the persistence of unequal gender norms regarding the division of paid and unpaid work, including care for children and elderly parents, which makes marriage an unattractive option for single women; 4) increasing uncertainty with respect to financial security; and 5) other norms, including consumerism, individualism, and the acceptability of remaining childless. Although some factors can be observed in other societies, all of these factors coexist in Japan as well as in South Korea and reinforce their negative impact on fertility.[36]

2.4 How Could Japan Stop the Trend of 'Missing' Babies? Our Suggestions

In earlier sections, we have discussed the fertility decline and the missing third baby boom, followed by some possible explanations for the low fertility rates. In 2015, Japanese Prime Minister Shinzō Abe proposed the introduction of *yume o tsumugu* (dream-weaving) childcare support policy to help raising the fertility rate to the government-defined 'desired birth rate' of 1.8.[37] This idea was included in the second of Mr Abe's 'three arrows', now referred to as 'Abenomics'. The government's proposed childcare support policy focuses on stabilizing employment in the young generation, promoting a better work–life balance, and providing childcare. In 2019, the government proposed free nursery and kindergarten provision.[38] These proposals are expected to mitigate some of the factors regarding delayed marriage and childless or one-child families described in the previous section. However, it may be difficult to change other factors such as conventional norms. Here, we make three suggestions to increase fertility rates in Japan.

First, relevant strategies to increase fertility rates and population size in Japan should be formed using scientific evidence and implemented. As stated previously, the government set the goal to raise the fertility rate to 1.8. Even if this 'desired rate' is achieved, the population in Japan would inevitably continue to decrease, given the replacement level being 2.1. Moreover, the number of older people in Japan surpass the number of working-age adults, which is likely to lead to further shrinkage in its population size. Currently, the Japanese government is only allowing immigration for the purpose of working alongside tight restrictions.[39] The goal to achieve an increase in the number of live births could be reset by allowing more immigrants of reproductive age and children, while supressing the speed of population shrinkage by maintaining the fertility rate among Japanese.

Second, fertility should be discussed not only in terms of population or economic policies, but also in the context of health and welfare policies. Reproduction is primarily for individuals. A pregnancy ending in abortion is often unplanned in the background of uncertainties caused by financial insecurity, leading to negative child-rearing experiences. The reproductive rights of couples should be considered and they have to be supported for safe access to modern medical technologies and contraceptives to achieve planned and positive parenthood. The Basic Law for Child and Maternal Health and Child Development that provides 'seamless support from pregnancy to birth and thereafter' was enacted in 2018, raising high expectations for its application.

Third, it is necessary to support not only the current reproductive generations but also the younger generations of school age, through education, for them to positively engage in reproduction and parenting in adulthood as well as achieving financial independence through employment. The introduction of compulsory education for 'home economics' among junior high and high school students, regardless of gender, in the 1990s contributed to fewer students in favour of conventional norms or gender-typical roles of child-rearing, and enhanced their understanding of the preparation required to be a parent.[40]

However, sex education still lags far behind and discussions of the topic have not been welcomed.[41] At the same time, older generations who were educated within the conventional norms, still have influence over households, work places, and society. In politics, the proportion of members of parliament under age 40 was 8.39% in Japan and ranked 125th, with 90% of seats occupied by men.[42,43] These statistics warrant more younger generations and women to be included in politics, to influence policies prioritizing children and reproductive-aged adults. 'Education' across all age groups could improve the fertility rate in Japan.

References

1. OECD. *OECD Factbook 2013: Economic, Environmental and Social Statistics.* Paris: OECD Publishing 2018. Available at: https://doi.org/10.1787/factbook-2013-en [last accessed 19 February 2020].
2. Baba S, Goto A, Reich MR. Looking for Japan's missing third baby boom. *J Obstet Gynaecol Res* 2018;44(2):199–207.
3. Statistics of Japan. Summary of the results of the National Census 2015 (in Japanese). Available at: http://www.stat.go.jp/data/kokusei/2015/kekka/pdf/gaiyou1.pdf [last accessed 19 February 2020].

4. Matsuda S. Economic recession and low fertility LifeDesign report (in Japanese). 2009. Available at: http://group.dai-ichi-life.co.jp/dlri/ldi/report/rp0907b.pdf [last accessed 19 February 2020].

5. Aoki H. A report of the First Japan Population Conference (in Japanese). *Jinko Mondai Kenkyu.* 1974;132:41–5.

6. Kelley DH. Exploring ancient skies: a survey of ancient and cultural astronomy. *Cram101 Textbook Reviews* 2016: 166.

7. Akabayashi H. After the generation of *Hinoeuma* (in Japanese). *The Monthly Journal of the Japan Institute of Labour* 2007;12:17–28.

8. Kim MJ, Chang JY. Low fertility in Korea (in Japanese). *The Review of Comparative Social Security Research* 2007;160:111–29.

9. World Bank Open Data. Available at: https://data.worldbank.org/ [last accessed 19 February 2020].

10. Nam DW, Ro KK. Population research and population policy in Korea in the 1970s. *Population and Development Review* 1981;74:651–69.

11. Yang JM. An overview of family planning in Korea (1961–1978). *Yonsei Medical Journal* 1979;20(2):184–97.

12. Kim MJ. Comparison of Japan and Korea in fertility (in Japanese). Nissei Basic Research Institute. Available at: https://www.nli-research.co.jp/report/detail/id=42526?site=nli [last accessed 19 February 2020].

13. Statistics Korea. Vital Statistics of Korea. Available at: http://kosis.kr/statHtml/statHtml.do?orgId=101&tblId=DT_1B8000F&language=en [last accessed 19 February 2020].

14. Wang C. Induced abortion patterns and determinants among married women in China: 1979 to 2010. *Reprod Health Matters* 2014;22(43):159–68.

15. RIETI. Available at: https://www.rieti.go.jp/users/china-tr/jp/170404kaikaku.html?ref=rss (in Japanese) [last accessed 19 February 2020].

16. Yip PSF, Lee J, Cheung YB. The influence of the Chinese zodiac on fertility in Hong Kong SAR. *Soc Sci Med* 55;10:1803–12.

17. Wan W. Chinese couples are now rushing to get pregnant, because no one wants their kid to be a sheep. *The Washington Post*. Available at: https://www.washingtonpost.com/world/asia_pacific/chinese-couples-rush-to-get-pregnant-before-dreaded-year-of-the-sheep/2014/05/08/e9f4adbc-d529-11e3-8a78-8fe50322a72c_story.html [last accessed 19 February 2020].

18. Baba S, Tsujita S, Morimoto K. The analysis of trends in induced abortion in Japan: an increasing consequence among adolescents. *Environ Health Prev Med* 2005;10(1):9–15.

19. Japan Federation of Bar Associations. Available at: https://www.nichibenren.or.jp/library/ja/opinion/report/data/2017/opinion_170216_07.pdf (in Japanese) [last accessed 19 February 2020].

20. Ministry of Health, Labour and Welfare. Report on Public Health Administration and Service (in Japanese). Available at: https://www.mhlw.go.jp/toukei/saikin/hw/eisei_houkoku/17/ [last accessed 19 February 2020].

21. Sedgh G, Singh S, Shah IH, Åhman E, Henshaw SK, Bankole A. Induced abortion: incidence and trends worldwide from 1995 to 2008. *Lancet* 2012;379(9816):625–32.

22. Fujime Y. *Sei no rekishi gaku* (in Japanese) (*Historiography of Sex*). Japan: Fuji publication 1997.

23. Ministry of Finance Printing Bureau. White Paper on Population (*Jinko mondai shingikai*) (Population Issue Council) 1959.

24. Sekiguchi, A, Ikeda T, Okamura K, Nakai A. Safety of induced abortions at less than 12 weeks of pregnancy in Japan. *Int J Gynaecol Obstet* 2015;129:54–7.

25. Korea Institute for Health and Social Affairs. Survey on induced abortion (in Korean). Sejong: Ministry of Health and Welfare 2018. Available at: https://www.kihasa.re.kr/web/news/report/view.do?menuId=20&tid=51&bid=79&ano=10778 [last accessed 19 February 2020].

26. Jiang Y, Han J, Donovan C, Ali G, Xu T, Zheng Y, et al. Induced abortion among Chinese women with living child: a national study. *Adv Dis Control Prev* 2017;2(1):10–15.

27. Durex. Global sex survey results [Internet] 2005. Available at: http://www.data360.org/pdf/20070416064139.Global%20Sex%20Survey.pdf [last accessed 19 February 2020].

28. Ghaznavi C, Sakamoto H, Yoneoka D, Nomura S, Shibuya K, Ueda P. Trends in heterosexual inexperience among young adults in Japan: analysis of national surveys, 1987–2015. *BMC Public Health* 2019;18:355. Available at: https://doi.org/10.1186/s12889-019-6677-5

29. Moriki Y, Hayashi K, Matsukura R. Sexless marriages in Japan: prevalence and reasons. In: Ogawa N, Shah IH (eds), *Low Fertility and Reproductive Health in East Asia*. Dordrecht: Springer Netherlands 2015:161–85.

30. United Nations Department of Economic and Social Affairs. World Contraceptive Patterns 2013 [Internet]. Available at: http://www.un.org/en/development/desa/population/publications/family/contraceptive-wallchart-2013.shtml [last accessed 19 February 2020].

31. Japan Society of Obstetrics and Gynaecology. Clinical reports of ARTs in 2016 and the lists of registered institutes in July 2018 (in Japanese) [Internet]. Available at: https://plaza.umin.ac.jp/~jsog-art/) [last accessed 19 February 2020].

32. Qiao J, Feng HL. Assisted reproductive technology in China: compliance and non-compliance. *Transl Pediatr* 2014;3(2):91–7.

33. Cabinet Office, Government of Japan. White Paper on Children and Youth 2015 (in Japanese). Available at: https://www8.cao.go.jp/youth/whitepaper/h27honpen/b1_01_01.html [last accessed 19 February 2020].

34. Tsutsui J. *Work and Family* (in Japanese). Japan: Chuokoro-Shinsha 2015.

35. Sato R, Iwasawa M. The sexual behavior of adolescents and young adults in Japan. In: Ogawa N, Shah IH (eds), *Low Fertility and Reproductive Health in East Asia.* Dordrecht: Springer Netherlands 2015:137–59.

36. Gauthier AH. Social norms, institutions, and policies in low-fertility countries. In: Ogawa N, Shah IH (eds), *Low Fertility and Reproductive Health in East Asia.* Dordrecht: Springer Netherlands 2015:11–30.

37. Cabinet Office, Government of Japan. Urgent policies to realize a society in which all citizens are dynamically engaged. Available at: http://www.kantei.go.jp/jp/topics/2015/ichiokusoukatsuyaku/kinkyujisshitaisaku_en.pdf [last accessed 19 February 2020].

38. Cabinet Office, Government of Japan. Learn about free early childhood education and care. Available at: https://www.youhomushouka.go.jp/about/en/ [last accessed 19 February 2020].

39. BBC. Migrant workers exploited in Japan. Available at: https://www.bbc.com/news/av/world-asia-49448757/migrant-workers-exploited-in-japan [last accessed 19 February 2020].

40. Nakanishi Y. Effects and issues of coeducational home economics (in Japanese). *Journal of Japan Association of Home Economics Education* 2011;53:217–25.

41. Nishioka E. Historical transition of sexuality education in Japan and outline of reproductive health/rights (in Japanese). *Jpn J Hyg* 2018;73:178–84.

42. Inter-Parliamentary Union. Youth participation in national parliaments: 2018. Geneva 2018. Available at: https://www.ipu.org/file/6076/download?token=7Aog71dH [last accessed 19 February 2020].

43. Inter-Parliamentary Union. Women in national parliament: situation as of 1 February 2019. Available at: http://archive.ipu.org/wmn-e/classif.htm [last accessed 19 February 2020].

3

Gender Inequalities in Japan

Gender Division of Labour and Health

Kaori Honjo

3.1 An Overview of Gender Inequalities in Japanese Society

While most measures of gender inequality in Japanese society have shrunk, many important challenges remain. While the gender gap in academic qualification attainment in Japan shrinks with each passing year, still more men achieve higher levels of academic qualifications than women.[1] Moreover, Japan's gender differences in university majors are arguably the greatest of the developed countries, evidenced by fewer Japanese women choosing to do their degree in Science, Technology, Engineering, and Mathematics (STEM) fields, especially in engineering.[1,2]

Gender differences are in employment as well. Japanese women's labour force participation rate (numbers of the labour force participation divided by the total number of population aged 15 and over) is lower than Japanese men (women: 50.3% versus men: 70.5% in 2016) and women in other developed countries: 58% in the UK, 56.8% in the US, and 69.6% in Sweden.[3]

Japanese women's labour force participation patterns by age group show a unique 'M-shaped' curve (Figure 3.1), noting women's departure from the workforce in their late 20s and early 30s due to marriage or childbirth and childcare. Many return to the job market in their 40s when their domestic and parenting duties have somewhat subsided. The magnitude of this marked drop in Japanese women's labour force participation originates in the fact that some 47% of working Japanese women exited into the domestic role after the birth of their first child between 2010 and 2014.[1]

Clear gender differences in occupational position are also evident in Japan: women are overrepresented in service and clerical work, while disproportionally more men occupy managerial positions at firms, conferring them greater prestige and higher incomes (Figure 3.2). Japanese women are

Kaori Honjo, *Gender Inequalities in Japan* In: *Health in Japan*. Edited by: Eric Brunner, Noriko Cable, and Hiroyasu Iso, Oxford University Press (2021). © Oxford University Press. DOI: 10.1093/oso/9780198848134.003.0003

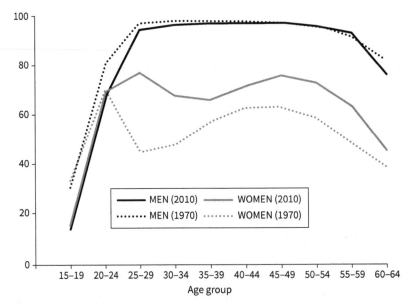

Figure 3.1 Labour force participation rate by age group

Source: data from 19-5 Labour Force and Labour Force Participation Rate by Age Group and Sex (1948--2010). Statistical Survey Department, Statistics Bureau, Ministry of Internal Affairs and Communications. http://www.stat.go.jp/data/chouki/zuhyou/19-05.xls

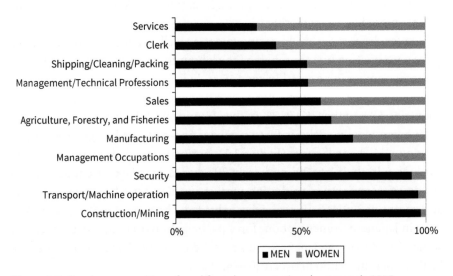

Figure 3.2 Gender composition of workforce by occupational category in 2017

Source: data from Labour Force Survey - Annual Report 2017. Office for National Statistics.

also more likely to engage in non-regular employment status: i.e. as part-time workers, temporary staff, or contract employees: 56.1% of women fell into this category in the 2018 *Labour Force Survey*, compared with just 22.2% of men.[4]

The Global Gender Gap Report, published annually by the World Economic Forum (WEF), confirms women's lower social standing in Japanese society. The report ranks countries of the world based on a composite index, summarizing 14 types of data in four domains of gender equality (economy, education, health, and politics). In 2018, Japan was 110th out of 149 nations examined, and the lowest among the G7. Japan scored especially low in the domains of economic participation and opportunity, and political empowerment.[5]

3.2 Possible Factors for Gender Inequalities in Japan: Gender Division of Labour and its Link with the Male Breadwinner Model

These striking gender inequalities in Japanese society are likely to be attributed to persistent and longstanding preference in gender division of labour, grounded in the male breadwinner model that women are to stay at home, attending domestic chores as opposed to men in employment as the sole breadwinner. Dramatic changes in industrial structures, observed as shifting from primary to secondary industries, have occurred after World War II. These changes were accompanied by an exodus of people from their homes, especially from farming to work at factories or offices,[6] physically cutting people their home from this newly defined 'workplace'. For married couples, this shift of workplace made it more reasonable for one party to pursue employment, while the other stayed at home to do house-work-related chores and take care of their children, i.e. division of labour.

The practices of gender division of labour held strong in Japanese society during the 1960s and 1970s.[7] A 'full-time housewife' was an assumed 'occupation' for millions of Japanese women and guaranteed their standing in Japanese society. Women were expected to take on the role of sole carer for the household. In 1980, the proportion of households with full-time housewives was approximately 65% of all married couple households.[1] Despite their commitment to household and family duties, these full-time housewives could not claim much credit for Japan's rapid economic growth and achievements in the light of their 'corporate warrior' husbands.

However, this traditional framework of the male breadwinner model has recently begun to fall out of favour, as ideas of gender equality spread in the population and women are increasingly empowered.[8] Now, the proportion of double-income households is significantly higher than that of households with full-time housewives (33% in 2018).[1] However, the idea of the male breadwinner model still gains relatively high support in Japanese society, as evidenced by 40.6% of supporters regardless of their gender in the 2016 public opinion survey run by the Gender Equality Bureau of the Cabinet Office.[1]

Evidence highlights that the male breadwinner model is acting as a root cause of gender inequality across a wide variety of socioeconomic metrics.[7] For one, educational attainment for women has been seen as less important than for men, as women are expected to take on a domestic role for the rest of their life after marriage.[1] Even those who pursue higher education have faced an inherently biased curriculum, instilling women with the knowledge and skills necessary to be 'good wives and wise mothers'. After university education, women are expected to leave the workforce following marriage and childbirth; firms neglect to invest in their female staff or mentor them for executive roles, leading to a paucity of women among management-level positions in Japan that persists even today.

If married women do decide to remain in the labour force, it is usually in order to supplement their family income.[1] This makes casual employment more attractive to both firms and married women, channelling them into part-time and precarious employment as a result. Persistent problems due to family and work life of women and employment practices in Japan originate in the gender division of labour firmly grounded within the male breadwinner model.[9] This is arguably one of the most distinctive characteristics of Japanese society which is discussed further in the next section.

3.3 Gender Division of Labour as a Social Determinant of Japanese People's Health

3.3.1 Effects of Marriage and Living Arrangements on Population Health in Japan

In Japan, women have long been expected to play supporting roles in the family unit—as parents, caregivers, and 'nurturers'—thus freeing up men to work long hours outside the home. Men are usually considered to be the head of the family,[9-11] as evidenced by their limited contribution to housework and child care and conventional social norms of household-related work being seen as 'women's work'.

These conservative tendencies are likely to explain many of the striking findings in Japanese studies on the health effects from sociodemographic factors, namely marital status. For example, one longitudinal study of middle-aged and elderly Japanese found greater mortality risk among divorced and widowed men than those who had never experienced either life event, yet no such differences were apparent among women.[12] Another study, this one of elderly married men and women, found mortality risk to be identical between men who lost their spouse during the tracking period and those who did not, yet significantly lower, nearly 70% less likely, among widowed women than their still-married counterparts.[13] Another longitudinal study showed that living arrangements, particularly solitary living, was related to risks for depression among older male adults.[14] Men who lived alone were at greater risk of depressive symptoms than men who lived with a spouse. On the other hand, women in spouse-only households were at similar risk of becoming depressed to their solitary-living counterparts, while women living with a spouse and child(ren), in fact, were at lower risk than both groups.[14]

Collectively, these findings suggest that men and women's health are likely to be affected differently by marital status and living arrangements in Japan, possibly via the assigned role based on long-held social norms cultivated in Japanese society. Given that, we could say that traditional gender norms still permeate Japanese society, and marital status and living arrangements are key drivers of gender differences in health and wellbeing.

3.3.2 Family and Work Life as Social Determinants of Health in Japan

Traditional attitudes towards gender and employment hold great influence over Japanese citizens' health in another respect: the balance between family and work life. Despite increasing numbers working outside the home since the 1970s, women are still, by and large, expected to perform the same domestic roles as before. Japanese husbands spend considerably less time on housework than their counterparts in many Western countries[11] (Figure 3.3). In dual-income families with a child under six years of age, they average just 84 minutes on chores per week, compared with over six hours (370 minutes) for women in 2018.[15]

One nationwide survey on how chores and childcare are divided in two-income households found that the wife is responsible for 85.1% of housework on average.[16] These conditions have made it extremely difficult for working

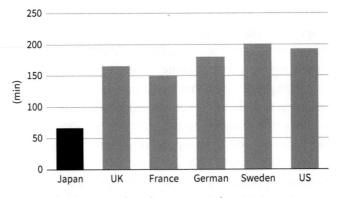

Figure 3.3 Average time consumed on chores per week among men

Source: data from Survey on Time Use and Leisure Activities. Summary of results. Statistics Bureau, Ministry of Internal Affairs and Communications, Government of Japan. 2011; How Europeans Spend Their Time Everyday Life of Women and Men. Eurostat. 2004; American Time-Use Survey Summary. Bureau of Labor Statistics of the U.S. 2006.

women to achieve harmony between their work and home lives, commonly known as *work–life balance.*

In regard to family and work life, 'work–family conflict'—a broad term encompassing situations at home that interfere with one's work, and vice versa—can have deleterious effects on women's health. A cross-sectional study of civil servants in Japan found that female employees experienced greater work–family conflicts and worse mental health than their male counterparts, while the observed gender inequalities in mental health was largely explained by work–family conflict.[17] Findings suggest that Japanese women's greater susceptibility to poor mental health could be due to no relief from the domestic roles and responsibilities that they disproportionately shoulder on top of their work demands. Placed in an impossible situation both at home and work, their work–life balance is likely to suffer, leading to poor overall health status. When this study's findings were subsequently compared with corresponding data for government officials in the UK and Finland, Japanese women had the most severe work–family conflicts and the lowest subjective health status in these three countries.[18]

However, Japanese men and their health are not immune from negative effects from traditional attitudes towards gender and employment. For example, they are much more likely to work long hours compared to Japanese women; overtime rates are even higher than among male workers in Western developed countries.[19] Working long hours is associated with a variety of negative health outcomes, including sleep insufficiency, fatigue, and physical and mental illness, not to mention elevated risk for cardiovascular disease. In addition, Japan was the location of the first documented case of 'death from overwork', a phenomenon so connected with the country that English publications even refer to it by its Japanese name: *karōshi* (see Chapters 6 and 7). These harms men suffer from being forced to work long hours outside the home are just some of the detrimental health effects attributable to the male breadwinner model, and traditional gender division of labour by extension.

3.3.3 Health Effects of Socioeconomic Status Inconsistency

Socioeconomic status inconsistency (or status inconsistency in socioeconomic status) arises when Japanese fail to receive professional work commensurate with the time and effort invested in their education.[20] Lack of respect or prestige one would normally expect of a given occupation or educational level can create role conflicts and have detrimental effects on health. In Section 3.1, it was said that more Japanese women are pursuing a degree in higher education than ever before, whereas their employment patterns maintain this distinctive feature: departure from the workforce around their late 20s and early 30s for marriage, staying out of the labour force during childbirth and childcare, and subsequently returning in their 40s once their caring responsibilities have subsided. Traditionally, job performance and commitment were evaluated via acceptance of long working hours, devaluing women's working patterns.[21] After leaving the labour force, even highly educated women will tend to return to relatively unskilled job sectors such as service and sales and have non-regular employment arrangements that are likely to generate large numbers of women with socioeconomic status inconsistency.

One large-scale cohort study of Japanese community residents[22] found that highly educated (college-equivalent) women in relatively 'low-status' jobs—i.e. sales or service positions, or manual labour—were at unexpectedly higher risk for stroke incidence than any other groups created by both educational level and occupational status. The highly educated women with manual jobs showed approximately 3.5 times higher stroke risk compared to highly educated women with professional or managerial jobs. Consequently, as a group, highly educated women have essentially the same stroke risk as their least-educated (junior high school-equivalent) counterparts compared to the middle group (high school-equivalent). One could conclude that job dissatisfaction and frustration created by socioeconomic status inconsistency could be emotionally distressing, which in turn can be a risk factor for stroke. The disproportionate number of women dealing with socioeconomic status inconsistency is systematic and structured within society, based on social norms and employment practices.

3.4 Why Do Japanese Women Enjoy the World's Longest Life Expectancy, Despite Their Low Social Status? The Gender Paradox Explained

Globally speaking, a society with healthier men and women has smaller gender inequality,[23,24] but there is one notable exception: Japan. Japanese society has greater gender inequalities, including those discussed in previous sections, demonstrating overall lower social standing of women in Japan. However, Japanese people, especially women, enjoy longer life expectancies in the world, a fact recognized around the globe. What could be the explanation for this paradox?

The first potential explanation is the host of positive health behaviours that Japanese women tend to engage in. In one international study aimed at exploring the factors behind Japanese longevity using two cohorts of older adults in Japan and England, Japanese women's low smoking rate was the single greatest contributor to their longer average survival than their British counterparts.[25] Japanese society initially saw the signs of a rise in female smokers in parallel with increased labour force participation,[26] but it soon abated, and today, a mere 7.2% of Japanese women smoke, compared with 29.4% of men.[27] Likewise, obesity ($BMI \geq 30$ kg/m^2) is much less prevalent among women in Japan than in other developed countries: in 2016, a mere 4.0% were classified as obese, compared with 26.6% of British and 41.6% of American women.[28] These trends have led some observers to conclude that positive health behaviours—typified by low rates of smoking and obesity—are one of the key reasons for their remarkable longevity (see Chapter 11).

The second explanation lies in the fact that Japan's social institutions have been founded on traditional ideas about gender division of labour. As explained in Chapters 8 and 10, most of Japan's social welfare regimes were designed in the 1970s, modelled on the 'household' unit at the time when it was essentially defined as a father working full-time, a stay-at-home mother, and two children. Japan's social security programmes assume that the family unit should be the primary benefactor, each member's role defined by conventional gender-based social norms: husbands at work and wives at home.

Given the synonymity between the male breadwinner model and conventional Japanese household composition at that time, social security programmes were designed to protect women as well—the vast majority of whom were full-time homemakers, and if they did work, only part-time—within the framework of the household unit.[7] For example, if a wife earns less than a certain amount per year working part-time (typically ¥1.03 million ≒ US $9,400), not only is she granted a special income tax deduction, but her husband can receive a similar one from his own income as head of the household (called 'marital deduction'), as if she were a full-time housewife. A wife cannot be removed from her husband's social insurance plans (pension, unemployment, etc.) as long as she earns less than a certain amount per year (typically ¥1.30 million ≒ US$12,000).[7] Such protection from the social welfare system might offset negative health outcomes due to Japanese women's lower social standing in society, while it is likely to bind Japanese women to households.

The third potential explanation is women's greater decision-making power over home finance that is unique in Japan. It is undeniable that Japanese women have much less economic power than men in Japanese society. However, one survey of typical salaried families found that household finances were most commonly managed by the wife alone (46.1%), ahead of both husband and wife (31.7%) and the husband alone (20.9%).[29] It is possible that married women in Japan are holding sway over the financial decisions of the home, regardless of their earnings, which in turn could give them authority and self-efficacy, counterbalancing the deleterious effects of low social standing on their health.

3.5 Recent Gender Effects on Health Due to Social Changes

During the 1970s, the Japanese saw the establishment of a multitude of social programmes in Japan of which the contents and practices were largely predicated on the male breadwinner model. This helped to safeguard the countless housewives as discussed in the previous section. Driven by pragmatic demographic changes in Japan, described throughout in this book, the structure of Japanese households has become increasingly diverse, unduly disadvantaging those individuals who deviate from the picture of conventional families, especially those in single-never-married and single-mother households. This trend continues to foster the new and growing social issue of *female poverty* that adds another dimension to the previously discussed Japanese paradox.

Japan's relative poverty rate ('poverty rate' thereafter) has been on the rise in recent years. The 2016 *Comprehensive Survey of Living Conditions* found that 15.6% of adults fell below the poverty line,[27] one of the highest rates among OECD member countries.[26] The poverty rate is higher for women than men in almost all age groups—economic inequalities balloon in elderly demographics—and is remarkably high among single households, especially for divorced and widowed women (Figure 3.4).

The loss of a spouse is especially devastating for women, in financial terms. Their greater risk of a career interruption makes their membership in a low-income bracket more likely: institutional favouritism towards the traditional family household in social security programmes means they receive little financial support following the death of a husband.

Single-parent households have increased noticeably in the last 35 years—single-mother households by 1.7-fold, and single-father households by 1.3-fold—with the former occupying the vast majority (approx. 87% in 2016).[30] Findings from the 2016 *Comprehensive Survey of Living Conditions*[27] showed that more active households consisting of one adult and children (<18 years of age) fell below the poverty line than did two-parent households with children (50.8% versus 12.9%),[30] indicating that poverty affects far more single-mother households in Japan. Moreover, according to the 2017 *Nationwide Survey on Single Parent Households*,[30] single-mother households earned less than half of the mean annual income of all households with young children, just 49.2% on average in 2016. High numbers of single mothers report poor

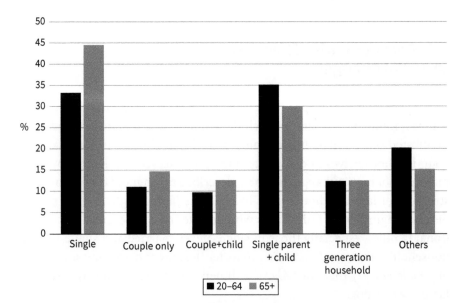

Figure 3.4 Female poverty rate by household type and age group in 2010

Chart created from special statistics collected by the 'Women and the Economy' working group (led by Aya Abe), within the Expert Investigative Committee on Basic Problems and Impacts of Gender Equality.

Source: 2010 Comprehensive Survey of Living Conditions; White Paper on Gender Equality 2012.

subjective health: compared with spouse-only households in which at least one party works full-time, it is especially poorer among single mothers (and single women generally) with only precarious employment.[31]

Most Japanese single mothers participated in the labour force (>80%)[30] with many in precarious and non-regular employment. The underlying cause of Japan's sky-high poverty rate in single-mother households—the highest in the developed world—can be due to current social institutions not being well-equipped to address needs of single parent households. Social institutions, which were designed to protect conventional families, are failing to respond flexibly to current complex family and household structure, contributing to the rise of female poverty and the attendant problems on health and wellbeing.

3.6 Conclusions

In summary, long-held gender division of labour in Japan is arguably one of the most distinctive characteristics of Japanese society, which is grounded by social norms and the male breadwinner model. Japanese gender division of labour directly affects countless other social factors, such as marital status, living arrangements, and family and work life, as well as citizens' health. Many research findings relevant to Japanese society link the cultural norms unique to Japanese society with their practice in gender division of work. Nevertheless, Japanese women enjoy the longest life expectancy in the world. This unexpected paradoxical relationship may be explained by 1) positive health behaviours—typified by low rates of smoking and obesity, 2) Japan's post-war social security programmes and institutions that intended to protect full-time homemakers, and 3) their financial authoritative role in the family.

Predicated on the male breadwinner model, established social programmes in Japan helped to safeguard countless housewives. However, the social institutions have failed to keep up with an increasingly diverse social demography, characterized by greater numbers of single-occupant, single-mother households that are deviating from the conventional household of a breadwinner husband, typically a white collared salary man who works long hours, a full-time housewife, and children. A sharp rise in female poverty, a major social issue in Japan, has been one of the consequences. These demographic changes in family and household composition will only accelerate. Without urgent reform in current social institutions, gender inequalities will increase, and Japanese women's social position will not meet the standards of other developed countries.

References

1. Gender Equality Bureau Cabinet Office, Government of Japan. Women and Men in Japan 2019. Available at: http://www.gender.go.jp/english_contents/pr_act/pub/pamphlet/women-and-men19/index.html [last accessed 19 February 2020].
2. OECD. OECD Education at a Glance 2013. Available at: http://www.oecd.org/education/eag2013%20(eng)--FINAL%2020%20June%202013.pdf [last accessed 19 February 2020].
3. The Japan Institute for Labour Policy and Training. *Databook of International Labour Statistics 2018*. Tokyo: The Japan Institute for Labour Policy and Training 2018.
4. Statistics Bureau, Ministry of Internal Affairs and Communications, Government of Japan. Labour Force Survey 2018. Available at: http://www.stat.go.jp/english/data/roudou/report/2018/index.html [last accessed 19 February 2020].
5. World Economic Forum. The Global Gender Gap Report 2018. Available at: http://www3.weforum.org/docs/WEF_GGGR_2018.pdf [last accessed 19 February 2020].
6. Saitoh O. Historical origin of the male breadwinner model (in Japanese). *Nihon Rodo Kenkyu Zasshi* 2013;638:4–16.
7. Honjo K, Kanbayashi H. Gender and health (in Japanese). In: Kawakami N, Hashimoto H, Kondo N (eds), *Society and Health: Integrated Scientific Approach to Eliminate Health Gaps*. Tokyo: University of Tokyo Press 2015:95–113.
8. NHK Broadcasting Culture Research Institute. *The Structure of Japanese Attitudes Today* 7th ed. (in Japanese). Tokyo: NHK Publishing Inc. 2009.
9. Shirahase S. *Invisible Inequalities in an Aging, Low Fertility Society* (in Japanese). Tokyo: University of Tokyo Press 2005.
10. Murata H, Aramaki H. Does satisfaction with family life depend on how household work is shared? From the ISSP survey on family and changing gender roles. NHK Broadcasting Culture Research Institutes 2019. Available at: https://www.nhk.or.jp/bunken/english/reports/pdf/report_16091501.pdf [last accessed 19 February 2020].
11. Watanabe Y. Why does the gender gap in housework time remain wide? NHK Broadcasting Culture Research Institute. Available at: https://www.nhk.or.jp/bunken/english/reports/pdf/report_17040601.pdf [last accessed 19 February 2020].
12. Ikeda A, Iso H, Toyoshima H, et al. Marital status and mortality among Japanese men and women: the Japan Collaborative Cohort Study. *BMC Public Health* 2007;7:73.

13. Nagata C, Takatsuka N, Shimizu H. The impact of changes in marital status on the mortality of elderly Japanese. *Ann Epidemiol* 2003;13(4):218–22.

14. Honjo K, Tani Y, Saito M, et al. Living alone or with others and depressive symptoms, and effect modification by residential social cohesion among older adults in Japan: the JAGES longitudinal study. *J Epidemiol* 2018;28:315–22.

15. Statistics Bureau, Ministry of Internal Affairs and Communications, Government of Japan. 2016. Survey on Time Use and Leisure Activities. Summary of results (in Japanese). Available at: https://www.stat.go.jp/english/data/shakai/2016/pdf/timeuse-b2016.pdf [last accessed 19 February 2020].

16. National Institute of Population and Social Security Research. The 5th National Survey on Family in Japan, 2013 (in Japanese). Available at: http://www.ipss.go.jp/ps-katei/j/NSFJ5/Mhoukoku/Mhoukoku.pdf [last accessed 19 February 2020].

17. Sekine M, Chandola T, Martikainen P, Marmot M, Kagamimori S. Sex differences in physical and mental functioning of Japanese civil servants: explanations from work and family characteristics. *Soc Sci Med* 2010;71:2091–9.

18. Chandola T, Martikainen P, Bartley M, et al. Does conflict between home and work explain the effect of multiple roles on mental health? A comparative study of Finland, Japan, and the UK. *Int J Epidemiol* 2004;33:884–93.

19. Lee S, McCann D, Messenger JC. *Working Time Around the World: Trends in Working Hours, Laws, and Policies in a Global Comparative Perspective.* Geneva: International Labour Office 2007.

20. Peter R, Gässler H, Geryer S. Socioeconomic status, status inconsistency and risk of ischaemic heart disease: a prospective study among members of a statutory health insurance company. *J Epidemiol Community Health* 2007;61:605–11.

21. Umeda M, McMunn A, Cable N, Hashimoto H, Kawakami N, Marmot M. Does an advantageous occupational position make women happier in contemporary Japan? Findings from the Japanese Study of Health, Occupation, and Psychosocial Factors Related Equity (J-HOPE). *SSM Population Health* 2015;1:8–15.

22. Honjo K, Iso H, Inoue M, Sawada N, Tsugane S, and JPHC Study Group. Socioeconomic status inconsistency and risk of stroke among Japanese middle-aged women. *Stroke* 2014;45:2592–8.

23. Sen G, Ostlin P. Unequal, Unfair, Ineffective and Inefficient. Gender Inequality in Health: Why It Exists and How We Can Change It. Final report to the WHO Commission on Social Determinants of Health 2007. Available here: https://www.who.int/social_determinants/resources/csdh_media/wgekn_final_report_07.pdf [last accessed 19 February 2020].

24. Kawachi I, Kennedy BP, Gupta V, Prothrow-Stith D. Women's status and the health of women and men: a view from the States. *Soc Sci Med* 1999;48:21–32.

25. Aida J, Cable N, Zaninotto P, et al. Social and behavioural determinants of the difference in survival among older adults in Japan and England. *Gerontology* 2018;64:266–77.

26. Marugame T, Kamo K, Sobue T, et al. Trends in smoking by birth cohorts born between 1900 and 1977 in Japan. *Prev Med* 2006;42(2):120–7.

27. Ministry of Health, Labour and Welfare, Government of Japan. Overview of Comprehensive Survey of Living Conditions 2018 (in Japanese). Available at: https://www.mhlw.go.jp/toukei/saikin/hw/k-tyosa/k-tyosa17/dl/10.pdf [last accessed 19 February 2020].

28. OECD. OECD health statistics 2018. Available at: http://www.oecd.org/health/health-statistics.htm [last accessed 19 February 2020].

29. Yamada M. Japanese men who do not use money—pocket money system contributes to consumption stagnation (in Japanese). *Weekly Toyo Keizai*, 7 March 2010.

30. Ministry of Health, Labour and Welfare, Government of Japan. Nationwide Survey on Single-parent Households 2017 (in Japanese). Available at: https://www.mhlw.go.jp/file/04-Houdouhappyou-11923000-Kodomokateikyoku-Kateifukishika/0000190325.pdf [last accessed 19 February 2020].

31. Kachi Y, Inoue M, Nishikitani M, Yano E. Differences in self-rated health by employment contract and household structure among Japanese employees: a nationwide cross-sectional study. *J Occup Health* 2014;56(5):339–46.

4

Child Health in Japan

Takeo Fujiwara, Nobutoshi Nawa, and Yusuke Matsuyama

4.1 Introduction

Japan is known for its population longevity worldwide. Some of the secrets of this longevity among Japanese can be found elsewhere in this book; however, the contribution of child health to Japanese longevity is less well known. For example, the infant mortality rate was more than 150 per 1,000 live births in the mid-1920s, but has been declining since even before the World War II to reach 1.9 per 1,000 live births in 2017—the lowest in the world. In South Korea and China, the infant mortality rate was 3 and 8 per 1,000 live births in 2017, respectively.[1] Children's nutritional status improved after World War II, and consequently the height of Japanese children has increased over the past 50 years. Another important factor for healthy longevity is oral health. Paediatric dental caries have decreased due to the use of fluoride toothpaste and improved socioeconomic conditions. Water fluoridation is not implemented in Japan.

At the same time, there are negative aspects of child health in Japan. Birth weight decreased to around 3,000 g in 2010, while the rate of low birth weight was about 10%. In South Korea and China, the rate of low birth weight was 5.5% in 2013 and 6.1% in 2011, respectively. Vaccination is another unresolved problem in Japan. Due to the prevailing fear of the side effects of vaccination, Measles, Mumps, and Rubella (MMR) vaccination has since been withdrawn, with only MR and individual measles and rubella vaccines being administered now. Recently, the proactive recommendation of HPV vaccination has also been suspended due to several reported cases of side effects, although the causality is questionable. Child maltreatment, defined as physical abuse, sexual abuse, and neglect, is an emerging issue. Notably, over 122,575 cases were recorded by the Child Guidance Centre in 2016—120 times more since 1990 (1,101) cases, although the sharp increase might be

Takeo Fujiwara, Nobutoshi Nawa, and Yusuke Matsuyama, *Child Health in Japan* In: *Health in Japan*. Edited by: Eric Brunner, Noriko Cable, and Hiroyasu Iso, Oxford University Press (2021). © Oxford University Press. DOI: 10.1093/oso/9780198848134.003.0004.

due to reporting issues. In conjunction with child maltreatment, child poverty (defined as earning less than half their country's median income) is another unresolved problem. The prevalence of child poverty in Japan in 2012 stood at 16.3%, which means one in six children was living under poverty, which is above the average of OECD countries. Furthermore, one of the most dire outcomes is child suicide, and the incidence rate is on the rise.

This chapter examines both the positive and negative aspects of child health in Japan, as outlined above. The origins of adult health stem from early life to a large extent. Therefore, it will be interesting to consider how the Japanese achieved their world-record longevity so rapidly after World War II. We postulate this was bolstered by two fundamental policies which contributed to the health of Japanese children: the mother and child health system introduced in 1942, and the school lunch programme which became a nationwide service in 1954.

4.2 Maternal and Child Health Handbook

The distribution of a maternal and child health handbook may explain the sharp decline in the infant mortality rate in Japan, in comparison to the US.[2] It was first distributed in 1942, that is, during World War II, as 'Maternal Handbook' under the national policy to increase population (so-called '*umeyo fuyaseyo*', that is, 'delivery and increase') by preventing maternal mortality, preterm abortion, and infant mortality. Mothers were to register their pregnancy at health centres, and to receive and fill out the maternal handbook. One of the motivations for this was material provision, that is, the mother could receive rice, sugar, or other health-related products, such as cotton cloth, which can be used for babies. The contents of the maternal handbook included the health status of the mother during pregnancy, delivery, and after delivery.

The significance of the maternal handbook can be summarized in four points: 1) establishment of a pregnancy registration system, 2) a self-monitoring system for pregnant women, 3) a data-collection system using a uniform format across the country, and 4) provision of education on disease prevention for mother and child. As a result of this system, the government could provide the necessary interventions for new mothers when appropriate. Furthermore, doctors were required to fill out the blood pressure, proteinuria status, and urine sugar status in the maternal handbook, while mothers filled out the weight and height themselves.

In 1966, the maternal handbook was expanded to the 'Maternal and Child Health Handbook' to record details of development such as height and weight for children, and immunization record. This child health record was an important part of the universal health care system, introduced in 1961. Japanese citizens can attend any hospital, and the maternal and child health handbook is therefore used as a health record by paediatricians and family doctors.

4.3 School Lunch Programme

The Japanese experienced extreme food shortages, which induced malnutrition after the end of World War II.[3,4] To address malnutrition among children, a school lunch programme was launched in elementary schools.[5] A recent study confirmed the impact of the school lunch programme on child health; more specifically, inducing a habit of eating fruit and vegetables. It was reported that older people who had higher socioeconomic status in childhood were more likely to eat fruit and vegetables, but only among the age group of 70–76 years of age who were partially exposed to the school lunch programme. In contrast, among those who were fully exposed to the shool lunch programme (aged 65–69 years old), there were no such gradients.[6]

Another recent study on children living in Greater Tokyo confirmed the effectiveness of the school lunch programme to minimize the gap between rich and poor.[7] That is, it is known that compared with children with high maternal education, children with low maternal education eat less vegetables and fruit; however, fruit and vegetable intakes from school lunch did not vary by maternal education or socioeconomic status among children. Thus, a universal school lunch programme in elementary schools may contribute to better health status as a population approach for children in Japan.

4.4 Secular Growth Trends among Japanese Children

With the recovery from the aftermath of World War II, Japan regained economic security and rebuilt society with universal health care and education systems.[8] The living conditions of Japanese children improved significantly, including nutrition. In parallel, the height and weight of Japanese children increased.[9–11]

Studies assessing the secular trend of child growth in Japan from 1900 to 2000 showed that the height and weight of Japanese children in 2000 were significantly greater than those of children in 1900 in both genders. However, the increase from 1950 to 1960 after the war was catch-up growth to compensate for the poor growth due to malnutrition, poor hygiene, and other precarious living conditions during wartime.[9] The latest school health examination survey in 2018 reported that the average height and weight of children at age 11 was about 1 cm taller and 1 kg heavier than those of children in 1988 in both genders, although the increase reached a plateau around 2000.[11] Similarly, data from the annual nationwide survey (National Nutrition Survey in Japan) conducted from 1976 to 2000 found an increase in the age-adjusted average BMI by 0.32 kg/m^2 and by 0.24 kg/m^2 in a ten-year period among Japanese boys and girls, respectively.[12]

The increase in average weight reflects obesity problems in some Japanese children. Prevalence of obesity in Japanese children is defined as 20% excess body weight compared with standard weight-for-height by sex; in boys aged six to 14 this increased from 6.1% for the period 1976–1980, to 11.1% for the period 1996–2000.[12] Similarly, the prevalence increased from 7.1% to 10.2% among girls aged six to 14. Of note, subgroup analysis, stratifying by size of living area, revealed that the increase in prevalence of obesity was most evident among children living in small towns, for both genders. The increase was not seen in girls living in metropolitan areas.[12]

Regarding the potential reasons behind this, Western lifestyle had an influence on the increasing trend in height and weight among Japanese children.[10] Interestingly, studies have found that an increase in leg length has contributed to the increased height among Japanese children, which could be influenced by the Western diet, especially due to the shift from a rice-based diet to a more diverse diet including dairy foods.[10] Cole et al. examined the growth data of Japanese children between 1950 and 2010 and argued that puberty (the stage when children experience peak height velocity) started at an increasingly younger age and that the duration of puberty became shorter, which may have affected the growth of Japanese children.[10] A similar trend was noted in the latest school health examination survey in 2018.[11]

4.5 Increase of Low Birth Weight

Japan has achieved the lowest infant mortality rate internationally, and maternal mortality is also very low. However, a problem of low birth weight babies has emerged in recent decades. The mean birthweight for singleton live births has decreased from 3,240 g in 1975 to 3,040 g in 2009 for boys, and 3,140 g in 1975 to 2,960 g in 2009 for girls. Furthermore, the prevalence of low birthweight infants (<2.5 kg) has increased from 5.1% in 1975 to 9.6% in 2006.[13] These trends may be related to the changing patterns in Japanese women's nutritional status: a preference for thinness, and the relatively strict recommended limit on weight gain during pregnancy to prevent preeclampsia.

Regarding the weight of Japanese women, surveys show that mean BMI decreased from 20.92 to 20.58, 20.80 to 20.39, and 21.25 to 20.57 between the late 1970s and late 1990s for 15–19, 20–24, and 25–29 years of age, respectively, and that the prevalence of thinness, defined as BMI<17 kg/m^2, increased from 2.4% in the late 1970s to 4.2% in the late 1990s.[14] Several possible explanations for the cause of thinness among Japanese women have been suggested, including the effect of mass media promoting thinness as beautiful or stylish.

The belief that motivates women to control their weight during pregnancy may have an impact on pregnancy outcomes.[15] Among average-weight and underweight women in Japan, the most common reason was 'for ease of delivery and/or her health and wellbeing'. In fact, mothers who considered their gestational weight gain should be lower delivered lower birthweight babies. Thus, one measure to reduce the currently high incidence of low birthweight, is dissemination of information on appropriate gestational weight gain.

In short, while the rate of infant mortality in Japan is very low, which is probably partially due to the advancement of medical technology and neonatology, the rate of low birthweight babies is too high. Factors such as Japanese women's thinness and beliefs about ideal gestational weight gain during pregnancy need to be considered.

4.6 Decline of Dental Caries

In developed countries, dental caries in children have declined dramatically in the last 30 years,[16] although it remains a highly prevalent disease worldwide.[17] In Japan, in the 1950s–1960s, dental caries become more prevalent, presumably due to increased sugar consumption after the end of World War II, peaking in the late 1980s. Since then, the prevalence of dental caries and the average number of decayed teeth among children have been decreasing (Figure 4.1). Nonetheless, it should be noted that despite this remarkable improvement, more than 30% of children have experienced dental caries before the age of 12 years old, and geographical and social inequalities on prevalence

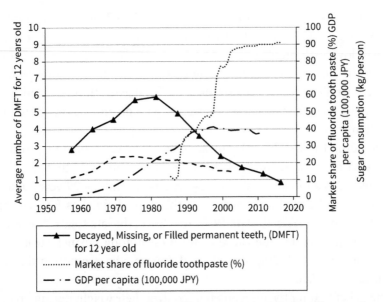

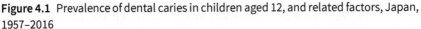

Figure 4.1 Prevalence of dental caries in children aged 12, and related factors, Japan, 1957–2016

Source: DMFT data from Survey of Dental Diseases, Ministry of Health, Labour, and Welfare. 2016; Market share of fluoride toothpaste: Japanese Association of Fluoride for Caries Prevention. List of Fluoride Products in Japan. Oral health association of Japan. Tokyo 2016; GDP: Cabinet Office. System of National Accounts. 2012; Sugar statistics Year book. Seitokougyokaikan. Tokyo. 2002.

of dental caries of children have been reported.[18,19] Accordingly, in 2011, the Japanese government administered a fundamental law to promote oral health,[20] suggesting attention from policy makers on this issue.

The question then is, what factors brought about the marked decline in dental caries? International discussion is still ongoing about the main contributors. Use of fluoride in various forms appears to be one of the main causes of the decline of dental caries in developed countries.[21] In Japan, while water fluoridation has not been introduced (except in US military bases), fluoridated toothpaste has been increasingly used since the 1990s (Figure 4.1). The utilization of fluoride products could be the main reason for the decline in dental caries in Japan in the last 30 years. Some schools adopted a fluoridated mouth rinse programme with an overall coverage of 10.4% in 2016.[22] It has also been reported that the programme worked as a proportional universalism which resulted in the reduction of dental caries on average and its results are differentiated by area.[23]

Although the benefit of fluoride products appears substantial, there could be an additional factor that caused the decrease in dental caries in Japan because the decline started even before the widespread use of fluoridated toothpaste (Figure 4.1). Changes in oral health behaviours and decline in sugar consumption are suggested as causes of decline in dental caries, however the average amount of sugar consumed in Japan has been consistently low compared to other countries. Several determinants, such as diet, as well as social conditions, have been improved during the period of rapid economic development. Similar to other health outcomes, the association between better socioeconomic conditions and lower rates of dental caries in children is evident in Japan[24] and other countries.[16]

4.7 Vaccination Hesitancy

Vaccination is one of the most cost-effective measures to prevent infectious diseases. However, it is estimated that because vaccination rates have remained less than optimal in many populations, 1.5 M preventable deaths per year have occurred globally.[25] The WHO Strategic Advisory Group of Experts on Immunization defined vaccine hesitancy as 'a delay in acceptance or refusal of vaccination despite availability of vaccination services'.[26] In 2019, WHO identified vaccine hesitancy as one of the top ten threats to global health, alongside HIV, Ebola virus, and air pollution.[25]

Vaccine hesitancy is a serious problem in Japan.[27] Highly educated populations are generally more concerned about the safety of vaccines, and this tendency is evident within the Japanese population.[27] Issues surrounding vaccination in Japan are complicated by historical concerns, media treatment of vaccines, and government policy.

The current law for immunization was enacted in 1948. Since then, there have been several important events that may have influenced public opinion and attitudes regarding vaccination in Japan.[28-31] For example, in the late 1980s to the early 1990s, the MMR vaccine was linked to risk of aseptic meningitis, and the MMR vaccination was withdrawn by the government.[28-31] Since then, the MMR vaccine has not been used in Japan, although the combination vaccine of measles and rubella without the mumps component (MR vaccine) and individual measles, mumps, and rubella vaccines are available.[28-31] Currently Japan faces the challenge of the human papilloma virus (HPV) vaccine. The Ministry of Health, Labour and Welfare suspended its recommendation to vaccinate after media reports of adverse events following HPV vaccination.[32-35]

Studies to investigate the determinants of immunization rates have been conducted in Japan, with the aim to develop strategies to improve uptake rates. An area study found that higher social capital, such as social trust or mutual aid, was associated with higher measles immunization rates, while higher income inequality was associated with lower rates.[36] At the level of the individual, the number of social ties and social trust were positively associated with the uptake of the second dose of measles vaccination, whose coverage is suboptimal in Japan.[37]

A study conducted before the period when varicella (chickenpox) vaccination was included in the routine immunization programme found that in a city with no vaccine subsidy, higher household income was associated with a higher immunization rate, whereas in a city with subsidy, there was no association between household income and vaccine uptake. Routine immunization programmes appear to be effective in achieving herd immunity and disease prevention.[38]

The influenza vaccination rate has been suboptimal in Japan. Aiming to understand public concerns and to encourage greater acceptance of the influenza vaccine, Nawa et al. analysed questions regarding influenza vaccination using 'Yahoo! Answers', the largest Japanese online question and answer bulletin board service with over 16 M posts collected over a four-year period.[31,39] They found that public concerns change over time, particularly in relation to seasonal influenza epidemics. Of note, concerns regarding vaccine effectiveness increased abruptly during the seasonal epidemic period, suggesting the value of providing the public with accurate and timely information in response to public concerns, in order to improve vaccination rate.[39]

4.8 Child Poverty and Inequality

Income inequality has been an important issue globally since the late 1980s, and Japan has been affected by this problem. The rate of child poverty in Japan was 16.3% in 2012, which was higher than the OECD average. According to the OECD, in Japan, the Gini coefficient measure of income inequality increased from 0.28 in 1985 to 0.33 in 2006. It is well known that income inequality affects adult health, such as mortality and self-rated health,[40] and it is likely child health is affected too.

A recent study in Japan suggests income inequality may affect child health through its influence on foetal development.[41] It was found that a higher Gini coefficient at prefecture level in Japan was associated with higher rates of small-for-gestational-age babies and pre-term births. These associations were only observed if the father was of a lower educational level, that is, lower than tertiary education. It may be that a lower educated father feels stressed in a community with higher income inequality, and in turn, the stress may resonate to the mother, leading to poor foetal development.

Child poverty is associated with poorer child growth, including weight faltering. A recent study showed that infants in the lowest quartile of household income were 1.29 times in 2001 and 1.27 times in 2010 more likely to experience weight faltering than those in the highest income quartile.[42] Child poverty can be associated with poor development of lung function. Another study among children living in Greater Tokyo revealed that children in a low-income family had lower forced expiratory volume (FEV), which is a marker for asthma.[43] Furthermore, child poverty is associated with child mental development, such as autism spectrum disorder. Although cross-sectional, a recent study revealed a robust association between lower parental socioeconomic status and autism spectrum disorder.[44] Possible explanations of this link include prenatal genetic damage due to toxic exposure, e.g. pesticide, low intake of micronutrients, e.g. zinc, and poor parenting leading to attachment disorder, a phenotype related to autism spectrum disorder.

Global economic shock, such as the great recession in 2008, may affect child health in Japan, resulting in weight-gain and obesity.[45] Using representative longitudinal data, it was shown that children aged eight years or older in the lowest household income quartile (lowest 25%) were more likely to become overweight after the great recession compared with children of the same age in the highest income quartile.

To reduce the problem of child weight-gain and obesity, Adachi City in Tokyo started an 'Eat Vegetables First at Meals' (vegi-first) programme in public primary (elementary) schools in 2013. The intention of this programme was to introduce vegetables as the first dish at every meal in order to increase vegetable intake. A survey conducted two years later confirmed that children aged six to seven years old who ate their vegetables at the start of meals were less likely to be overweight than children who ate meat or fish as the first dish.[46]

4.9 Child Maltreatment: Collapse of Family?

There were 122,575 consulted cases of child maltreatment in Child Guidance Centres in 2016. The actual number of children experiencing abuse or neglect is uncertain. The proportion of cases among children under 18 years old is similar in Japan and the UK (6.1 and 6.9 per 1,000 respectively), according to UK statistics for children in care (96,000 in 2016), defined as a child who has been looked after for 24 hours or more in the child protection system.[47] The main forms of maltreatment in Japan are psychological abuse (51.5%), physical abuse (26.0%), neglect (21.1%), and sexual abuse (1.3%). There are more than 50 child deaths per year recorded due to maltreatment, again similar to the UK figure. Both figures are likely to be underestimates.

The figure for the number of cases of child maltreatment in 2016 is about 120 times higher than reported in 1990. The extent to which the increase in the number of reports of child maltreatment is a consequence of increased reporting and recognition, rather than an actual increase in cases of abuse, is unknown. It has been speculated that the increase in the number of nuclear families and decline in three-generation families may have contributed to the increase. However, recent studies do not support this speculation. Children living with grandparents were not protected from abuse, especially infant abuse in Japan.[48]

Some consider corporal punishment to be embedded in Japanese culture. Due to increased recognition that corporal punishment is a form of child abuse, the number of cases consulted to Child Guidance Centres has increased. In a recent child abuse death case (the 'Yua-chan incident') which took place in Noda, Chiba Prefecture, in 2019, a step-father abused his ten-year-old step-daughter by pulling her hair and spraying cold water on her during winter. The perpetrator argued that this was 'discipline' and not abuse. To address this situation, the Japanese Government considered making corporal punishment a criminal offence. There is substantial health-related evidence to support this ban. For example, even occasional spanking around three years of age is a risk factor for behavioural problems assessed two years later.[49] Similarly, among older children, corporal punishment was linked to later behavioural problems measured by a validated behaviour problems checklist, after accounting for baseline behaviour.[50]

Among the several risk factors for child maltreatment, child poverty is one of the most important determinants. Poverty may lead to lack of time spent with children, which is strongly linked to poor parenting. Parental mental health may deteriorate due to poverty, increasing the probability of child maltreatment. Poverty may also induce social isolation, and parents who face financial difficulties may not receive adequate social support, including information about child education and health. A recent study revealed the pathway of the association between poverty and child maltreatment. That is, poverty leads to a lack of social capital and parental psychological distress, both of which mediated the association between poverty and child maltreatment.[51]

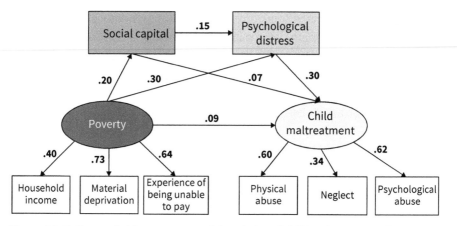

Figure 4.2 Pathways linking poverty, social capital, and child maltreatment; figures represent standardized path coefficients

Questionnaire study of school children (6–7 years old), Adachi City, Tokyo.

Source: Reproduced from Isumi, A., et al., Mediating effects of parental psychological distress and individual-level social capital on the association between child poverty and maltreatment in Japan. Child Abuse & Neglect, 2018;83:142–150.

The impact of social capital at the contextual level for child maltreatment was confirmed,[52] suggesting that boosting community social capital may be a promising intervention for child maltreatment (Figure 4.2).

4.10 Child Suicide and Bullying

Although the number of children is decreasing in Japan (Chapter 2), the number of suicides among children is not. According to the Police Agency, over 300 elementary, junior-high, and high school children committed suicide in 2016 (2.6 per 100,000 of those 19 years or younger). The rate is close to the average among OECD countries. The motive, according to an analysis of suicide notes, was family problems (18.4%), health problems (19.5%), and school problems (40.8%). Notably, when it comes to school problems, most indicated difficulty in achieving good academic performance (9.9%) and worries over what path to take after graduation (9.9%). Interestingly, bullying was not one of the major reasons (1.8%).

To prevent suicide among children, several elementary schools have since launched the 'Education on how to send an SOS' programme to promote self-esteem and to encourage children to send an SOS message to an adult whom they can trust, as well as to cultivate a feeling of the importance of life through videos.[53]

Although there is only a weak direct association between child suicide and bullying, bullying is nonetheless a major problem in Japan. There were 414,378 reported cases of bullying in the Fiscal Year 2016 (April 2016–March 2017), a considerable increase (90,000 cases) over the previous year. Specifically, a higher increase was observed in elementary school children, and the rate of bullying through a personal computer or mobile phone stood at 12,632 (3%), which is the highest on record. Although most of the bullying cases consisted of bantering or verbal abuse (62.3%) or being ignored (14.1%), more serious behaviours, such as beating or kicking (5.8%), and dangerous activities (7.6%) were not unusual.

4.11 Conclusion

Child health in Japan is one of the best in the world in terms of infant mortality rate. Physical health development has improved over the past decades due to public health initiatives. Nonetheless, there remain challenges, such as low vaccination uptake, low birth weight, child maltreatment, bullying, and suicide. Child poverty and inequality appear to be important upstream causes of these negative aspects. In a life-course perspective, adverse childhood experiences such as child maltreatment and poverty are important determinants of adult health in Japan.[4,54] As children are the future, greater investment in policies to promote child health is needed to safeguard the health and well-being of the Japanese population.

References

1. UN Inter-agency Group for Child Mortality Estimation. Child Mortality Estimates 2019. Available at: https://childmortality.org [last accessed 20 February 2020].
2. Kiely M, et al. Infant mortality in Japan and the United States. In: H. Wallace, et al. (eds), *Health and Welfare for Families in the 21st Century*. Massachusetts: Jones and Bartlett Publishers 1999:375–97.
3. Yoshimura T, et al. Poor nutrition in prepubertal Japanese children at the end of World War II suppressed bone development. *Maturitas* 2005;52(1):32–4.
4. Fujiwara T, et al. Associations of childhood socioeconomic status and adulthood height with functional limitations among Japanese older people: results from the JAGES 2010 Project. *J Gerontol A Biol Sci Med Sci* 2014;69(7):852–9.
5. Tanaka N, Miyoshi M. School lunch program for health promotion among children in Japan. *Asia Pac J Clin Nutr* 2012;21(1):155–8.

6. Yanagi N, et al. Association between childhood socioeconomic status and fruit and vegetable intake among older Japanese: The JAGES 2010 study. *Prev Med* 2018;106:130–6.

7. Yamaguchi M, Kondo N, Hashimoto, H. Universal school lunch programme closes a socioeconomic gap in fruit and vegetable intakes among school children in Japan. *Eur J Public Health* 2018;28(4):636–41.

8. Murphy RT. *Japan and the Shackles of the Past.* Oxford: Oxford University Press 2014.

9. Kagawa M, et al. Secular changes in growth among Japanese children over 100 years (1900–2000). *Asia Pac J Clin Nutr* 2011;20(2):180–9.

10. Cole TJ, Mori H. Fifty years of child height and weight in Japan and South Korea: contrasting secular trend patterns analyzed by SITAR. *Am J Hum Biol* 2018;30(1). doi: 10.1002/ajhb.23054

11. Ministry of Education for Culture, Sports, Science, and Technology, Government of Japan. School Health Examination Survey2018 (in Japanese). Available at: http://www.mext.go.jp/b_menu/toukei/chousa05/hoken/kekka/k_detail/1411711.htm [last accessed 20 February 2020].

12. Matsushita Y, et al. Trends in childhood obesity in Japan over the last 25 years from the national nutrition survey. *Obes Res* 2004;12(2):205–14.

13. Ministry of Health, Labour and Welfare, Government of Japan. Vital statistics 2019 (in Japanese). Available at: https://www.mhlw.go.jp/toukei/list/81-1.html [last accessed 20 February 2020].

14. Takimoto H, et al. Thinness among young Japanese women. *Am J Public Health* 2004;94(9):1592–5.

15. Ogawa K, et al. Association between women's perceived ideal gestational weight gain during pregnancy and pregnancy outcomes. *Sci Rep* 2018;8(1):115–74.

16. Nadanovsky P, Sheiham A. Relative contribution of dental services to the changes in caries levels of 12-year-old children in 18 industrialized countries in the 1970s and early 1980s. *Community Dent Oral Epidemiol* 2008;36:1–2.

17. Marcenes W, et al. Global burden of oral conditions in 1990–2010: a systematic analysis. *J Dent Res* 2013;92:592–7.

18. Aida J, et al. An ecological study on the association of public dental health activities and sociodemographic characteristics with caries prevalence in Japanese 3-year-old children. *Caries Res* 2006;40:466–72.

19. Sheiham A, et al. Global oral health inequalities: task group-implementation and delivery of oral health strategies. *Adv Dent Res* 2011;23:259–67.

20. Ministry of Health, Labour and Welfare, Government of Japan. Dental and Oral Health Promotion Law 2011.

21. Petersson GH, Bratthall D. The caries decline: a review of reviews. *Eur J Oral Sci* 2007;104:436–43.

22. Japanese Association of Fluoride for Caries Prevention. Statistics for fluoride mouthrinse program in school 2016 (in Japanese). Available at: http://www.nponitif.jp/index.htm [last accessed 20 February 2020].

23. Matsuyama Y, et al. School-based fluoride mouthrinse program dissemination associated with decreasing dental caries inequalities between Japanese prefectures: an ecological study. *J Epidemiol* 2016;26:563–71.

24. Aida J, et al. Contributions of social context to inequality in dental caries: a multilevel analysis of Japanese 3-year-old children. *Community Dent Oral Epidemiol* 2008;36:149–56.

25. WHO. Ten threats to global health in 2019. Available at: https://www.who.int/emergencies/ten-threats-to-global-health-in-2019 [last accessed 20 February 2020].

26. Larson HJ, et al. Measuring vaccine hesitancy: the development of a survey tool. *Vaccine* 2015;33(34):4165–75.

27. Larson HJ, et al. The state of vaccine confidence 2016: global insights through a 67-country survey. *EBioMedicine* 2016;12:295–301.

28. Saitoh A, Okabe N. Current issues with the immunization program in Japan: can we fill the 'vaccine gap'? *Vaccine* 2012;30(32):4752–6.

29. Kuwabara N, Ching MS. A review of factors affecting vaccine preventable disease in Japan. *Hawaii J Med Public Health* 2014;73(12):376–81.

30. Nakayama T. Vaccine chronicle in Japan. *J Infect Chemother* 2013;19(5):787–98.

31. Nawa N, Kogaki S, Ozono K. Listening to public concerns on vaccinations in order to provide information in a timely manner. *Vaccine* 2017; 35(10):1369.

32. Hanley SJ, et al. HPV vaccination crisis in Japan. *Lancet* 2015;385(9987):2571.

33. Tsuda K, et al. Trends of media coverage on human papillomavirus vaccination in Japanese newspapers. *Clin Infect Dis* 2016;63(12):1634–8.

34. Larson HJ. Japanese media and the HPV vaccine saga. *Clin Infect Dis* 2017;64(4):533–4.

35. Wilson R, Paterson P, Larson HJ. The HPV vaccination in Japan. A report of the CSIS Global Health Policy Center. Washington: Center for Strategic & International Studies 2014.

36. Nagaoka K, Fujiwara T, Ito J. Do income inequality and social capital associate with measles-containing vaccine coverage rate? *Vaccine* 2012;30(52):7481–8.

37. Nawa N, Fujiwara T. Association between social capital and second dose of measles vaccination in Japan: results from the A-CHILD study. *Vaccine* 2019;37(6):877–81.

38. Nagaoka K, Fujiwara T. Impact of subsidies and socioeconomic status on varicella vaccination in Greater Tokyo, Japan. *Front Pediatr* 2016;4:19.

39. Nawa N, et al. Analysis of public concerns about influenza vaccinations by mining a massive online question dataset in Japan. *Vaccine* 2016;34(27):3207–13.

40. Kondo N, et al. Income inequality, mortality, and self-rated health: meta-analysis of multilevel studies. *BMJ* 2009;339:b4471.

41. Fujiwara T, Ito J, Kawachi I. Income inequality, parental socioeconomic status, and birth outcomes in Japan. *Am J Epidemiol* 2013;177(10):1042–52.

42. Kachi Y, et al. Parental socioeconomic status and weight faltering in infants in Japan. *Front Pediatr* 2018;6:127.

43. Amemiya A, Fujiwara T. Association of low family income with lung function among children and adolescents: results of the J-SHINE study. *J Epidemiol* 2019;29(2):50–6.

44. Fujiwara T. Socioeconomic status and the risk of suspected autism spectrum disorders among 18-month-old toddlers in Japan: a population-based study. *J Autism Dev Disord* 2014;44(6):1323–31.

45. Ueda P, Kondo N, Fujiwara T. The global economic crisis, household income and pre-adolescent overweight and underweight: a nationwide birth cohort study in Japan. *Int J Obes* 2015;39(9):1414–20.

46. Tani Y, et al. Does eating vegetables at start of meal prevent childhood overweight in Japan? A-CHILD study. *Front Pediatr* 2018;6:134.

47. NSPCC Knowledge and Information Service. Statistics briefing: Looked After Children, 2019. Available at: https://learning.nspcc.org.uk/media/1622/statistics-briefing-looked-after-children.pdf [last accessed 23 March 2020].

48. Fujiwara T, Yamaoka Y, Morisaki N. Self-reported prevalence and risk factors for shaking and smothering among mothers of 4-month-old infants in Japan. *J Epidemiol* 2016;26(1):4–13.

49. Okuzono S, et al. Spanking and subsequent behavioral problems in toddlers: a propensity score-matched, prospective study in Japan. *Child Abuse Negl* 2017;69:62–71.

50. Miki T, et al. Impact of parenting style on clinically significant behavioral problems among children aged 4–11 years old after disaster: a follow-up study of the Great East Japan Earthquake. *Front Psychiatry* 2019;10:45.

51. Isumi A, et al. Mediating effects of parental psychological distress and individual-level social capital on the association between child poverty and maltreatment in Japan. *Child Abuse Negl* 2018;83:142–50.

52. Nawa N, Isumi A, Fujiwara T. Community-level social capital, parental psychological distress, and child physical abuse: a multilevel mediation analysis. *Soc Psychiatry Psychiatr Epidemiol* 2018;53(11):1221–9.

53. Kaneko Y, et al. Education on how to send an SOS: three practical models for national program. *Jisatsu Sogo Seisaku Kenkyu* 2018;1(1):1–47.

54. Amemiya A, et al. Adverse childhood experiences and higher-level functional limitations among older Japanese people: results from the JAGES study. *J Gerontol A Biol Sci Med Sci* 2018;73(2):261–6.

5

Family, Community, and Mental Wellbeing

Noriko Cable, Michikazu Sekine, and Shinsuke Koike

5.1 Background: An Illustration of Family Composition and Mental Wellbeing in Japan

The profile of Japanese family composition has changed dramatically over the last four decades, with the average size of the household now half what it was in 1980, and with double the number of households including an older person (Figure 5.1).[1] Notably, the proportion of three-generation households (grandparents, parents, and children) declined[2] from 50% in 1980 to 16% in 2010, and even further to 11% in 2017. The primary factors for this decline in multiple generation households in Japan were urbanization and the economic boom during the post-war period,[3] driving young adults to relocate to cities for better employment opportunities and living conditions, leaving their parents and neighbours behind.

Urbanization led to more than doubling of the proportion of solo households. This trend continues, as people in couple-only households lose their spouse.[2] In the post-war period, family-based social ties promoted mental wellbeing[4] and longevity.[5] Today's demography and living arrangements may pose a threat to mental wellbeing among the Japanese.

Suicide statistics in Japan and the UK reveal a contrasting picture of mental wellbeing in the two countries. Overall, though suicide rates have declined in Japan, they remain significantly higher across age groups (Figure 5.2). Although in both countries more men than women committed suicide, Japanese men's suicide mortality rises from adolescence until age 29, and the rate rises again in mid-life.

The dominant reasons for suicide since 1978[6] have been health, and economic and family problems (Chapters 6 and 15). Some suicides are associated with mental disorders (Chapter 15). Given the increased suicide rate during

Noriko Cable, Michikazu Sekine, and Shinsuke Koike, *Family, Community, and Mental Wellbeing* In: *Health in Japan.* Edited by: Eric Brunner, Noriko Cable, and Hiroyasu Iso, Oxford University Press (2021). © Oxford University Press.
DOI: 10.1093/oso/9780198848134.003.0005.

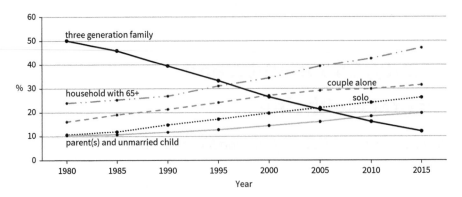

Figure 5.1 Household type (%), Japan, 1980–2017

Source: Annual report on the Ageing Society. Tokyo. Cabinet Office of Japan 2019.

the recent economic recession, the Japanese government introduced new measures in 2006.[7] Since 2010, there has been a modest decline in the rates.

Initiatives have targeted suicide in the shrinking reproductive age group (Chapter 2) and at the same time there has been reform of mental health policies. A large proportion of psychiatric diagnoses in Japan are of schizophrenia.[8]

In respect to common mental disorders such as depression and anxiety, cross-national surveys suggest wellbeing in Japan may be lower on average than in Britain or Finland.[9,10] However, Japan's culture is a 'depressing'

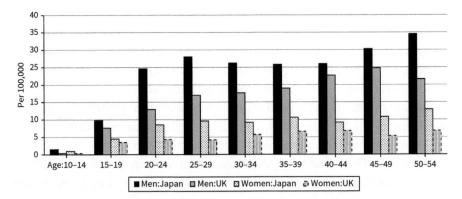

Figure 5.2 Suicide rate per 100,000 by five-year age group, men and women, 2017, Japan and the UK

Source: Japanese data from White paper: implementation for suicide 2018. https://www. mhlw.go.jp/wp/hakusyo/jisatsu/18/index.html; Suicide in the UK 2017, https://www.ons. gov.uk/peoplepopulationandcommunity/birthsdeathsandmarriages/deaths/bulletins/ suicidesintheunitedkingdom/2017registrations#suicide-patterns-by-age

influence on self-evaluation of wellbeing, and therefore statistical comparisons with European countries are tentative (Chapter 1.2.2). This chapter considers how families act as a social determinant of mental health and wellbeing in Japan.

5.1.1 Families as a Social Determinant of Mental Wellbeing

Families have a direct impact on individual mental wellbeing, through influences including emotional, verbal, and practical transactions. The life course approach in epidemiology identifies the family as an 'immediate agent'[11] that determines mental health of the individual from birth to death, through those exchanges.

In the psychosocial dimension, families play a significant role in forming individual thinking and attitudes. The 'mental programme'[12] acts as a prototype for relationships that extend to the community and social levels. Collective beliefs and attitudes through the 'mental programme' tend towards a uniform culture (Chapter 15). Despite the considerable changes in household composition since the 1964 Tokyo Olympics, collective family-based beliefs and norms, referred to as *ie* (Section 5.3), continue to exert substantial influence on the mental wellbeing of family members. In the next section, an historical overview of mental health in Japan examines the links between the *ie* culture and mental wellbeing in Japan through the roles played by family.

5.2 Historical Overview of Caring for the Mentally Ill in Japan

We could say that worldwide, a negative stigma is attached to mental ill health, with some differences in degree according to time and place. At the end of the Edo period, mentally ill patients were neglected, and in general kept in confinement in the family house. This arrangement was quite the opposite of the English system of 'asylums' during the same period, when local government had the duty of care for the mentally ill.[13] Admissions to asylum institutions in England were driven mainly by the needs of families, lacking the physical, emotional, or financial resources to care for their mentally ill relative. Home confinement of people with mental illness in Japan meant the family had to provide for them, even though resources were often in short supply, even for themselves. Chapter 15 provides more detail on the historical treatment and legislation of mentally ill people in Japan.

5.2.1 Roles of the Family in Caring for the Mentally Ill

The Japanese social welfare system during the pre-war period was limited to injured and disabled soldiers,[14] while mentally ill individuals were the responsibility of the police, who were given a monitoring role in 1900.[15] The family was responsible for caring for disabled or mentally ill family members, away from society in house confinement.

Kure,[15] a pioneering psychiatrist, described the care of mentally ill patients around this time. Individuals were registered with local police. (At that time police had statutory oversight for aspects of the health and welfare of the nation.) Kure and his team visited about one-third of the prefectures and met nearly 300 patients in house confinement.

Of these, 81% were men, and many were middle-aged.[15] Half of the families surveyed were rated by the team as poor, based on the living conditions of the family. The poor families often did not have enough food. Half of the cases were forced to live in areas rated poor, based on the level of lighting, ventilation, structure, and size (around 3.3–5m^2). Lighting was usually inadequate because windows were covered with heavy wooden lattices. A hole in the floorboards or a commode served as a toilet. Most places of confinement lacked heating and were not cleaned regularly. In his report, Dr. Kure expressed sadness at the inhumane treatment and care of mentally ill patients and stated: 'Mentally ill patients in Japan had not only the misfortune of suffering from their mental illness, but also of being born in this nation.'

Until the changes implemented in 1950 (Chapter 15), the primary purpose of the regulation of the mentally ill individual was maintenance of civil order and safety.[16] The family was subjected to punishment in the case of disturbance caused by their mentally ill relative. House confinement was a necessity for most families as there was only a handful of state and private mental health hospitals.[15]

The designated responsible person for a mentally ill family member was generally the father or spouse. On the other hand, the primary carer for the mentally ill person was the mother, or the wife of the head of the household, who also took care of other family members. Confined individuals were held for five or more years.[15] Some families made repeated attempts to cure their relative with cleansing rituals or remedies. One folk remedy involved medication made by charcoaling illegally procured human body parts.

The universal social welfare system was introduced with the new post-war constitution when basic rights to healthy living conditions were guaranteed for all.[17] The Mental Health Act of 1950 and national public insurance system set up in 1961 (Chapters 8 and 15) provided long-suffering mentally ill patients with some medical care, and abolition of home confinement. In 1964, Reischauer, the American ambassador, was stabbed by a mentally disturbed person. This incident led to increased institutionalization of the mentally ill. Psychiatric care was not reviewed again until exposure of patient abuse at a large mental institution in 1983 (Chapter 15).

5.2.2 Stigma of Mental Illness and the Role of the Family

Before 1950, individuals with mental illnesses in Japan were isolated from the rest of society. This situation was echoed in the language which differentiated between 'normal' and 'abnormal'. Japanese beliefs about this distinction can be glimpsed in the representation of normal, *seijo* = 'correct', 'default', while abnormal is *ijo*, which represents an alteration of the 'default' state. Similarly, sanity, *shoki*, and insanity, *kyoki*, indicates respectively the norm/correct state of mind, and the abnormal/opposite state. Japanese attitudes towards mental health are likely to have been developed and reflected in this polarized language.

Comparative research has shown that Japanese cultural attitudes tend to be more stigmatizing towards mental illness than Australian, especially schizophrenia.[18] Japanese respondents considered mental ill health as a weakness of the mind and expressed preference for distancing themselves from people with mental illness. Negative attitudes towards schizophrenia were weaker in children than their parents, and correlated with each other.[19] Education to promote mental health literacy in Japan have been introduced recently.[20] It is hoped that these programmes will increase knowledge and reduce prejudice.

The *ie* (family, kin, or clan) is the fundamental blood-based patriarchal unit and the core structure in Japanese society.[21] However, the low fertility rate in Japan (Chapter 2) threatens the continuous family line as the core social structure, particularly if there is no male child. Our question here is how the *ie* culture determines Japanese mental health and wellbeing, both in the past and in today's Japan. The next section addresses these questions in turn.

5.3 The *Ie* Bond: *Uchi* versus *Soto* and the Present Picture

In the *ie* culture, a woman married into a man's family, adopting his family as her own, over her original family.[22] The *ie* line of descent is directly from father to son (biological, or rarely, adopted) with wife and other unmarried children placed in a side-line.[22] The patriarchal *ie* culture placed an expectation that married women care for family members. A multi-generational family was not the default family unit[22] because, apart from the eldest son, children are expected to leave the parental household when they marry. At departure, younger male siblings formed their own households and a new bloodline. Recently, the extended family has become increasingly unusual, as the traditional system gives way to the nuclear family and solo living (Section 5.1).

A unique aspect of Japanese society is that unrelated people can form an *ie*-like bond within a defined or enclosed space such as a village or a company.[21,23,24] This arrangement creates *uchi* (insiders), and *soto* (outsiders), broadly equivalent to 'us versus them'.[12] The settings that bind people are referred to as *ba*, a catalyst in forming a shared entity.[16] The shared common ground provides a unified identity for the group, distinct from others.[21,25]

Within the *uchi* group, the group structure resembles a family with a leader who adopts a father-like role, and takes significant interest in the members.[21] In the case of a company, managers are expected to bond with their subordinates, knowing them at a personal level.[21,23] The strong bond within the *ba* community acts to drive cohesion and reduce the risk of depression among those with disadvantaged social status.[26] The same bond is reflected in an emotional distance from *soto* people.[21] This distance may be perceived as a barrier, increasing the risk of depression among *soto* people.[26] The next section describes the current picture of the *uchi* bond in Japan.

5.3.1 Becoming a *Muen* (Detached) Society: The Current Picture of the *Uchi* Bond in Japan

As described in the previous section, forming an *uchi* bond requires *ba* as a catalyst. Table 5.1 shows differences in the level of social participation by city size,[27] indicating the various opportunities for the shared entity, *ba*. Overall, people living in a small city were more likely to participate in one or more

Table 5.1 Social participation by type and by city size

	Large (459) %	Medium (823) %	Small (493) %
Residents association	20.0	27.2	32.3
Hobby groups	17.6	20.3	18.1
Sports clubs	19.2	17.7	19.7
Senior clubs	6.7	10.0	14.4
Retiree's groups	4.6	5.6	5.9
Volunteer groups	4.4	4.9	6.9
Adult learning groups	5.9	3.6	3.9
Silver recruitment organizations	1.7	3.3	3.2
Women's groups	0.9	2.1	4.1
Business/commerce groups	0.7	1.6	2.2
Non-political organizations	1.7	1.1	2.2
Want to participate, but unable to	29.6	20.4	19.5
Do not wish to participate	20.3	20.9	17.0

Source: Cabinet Office report, Government of Japan, 2014[27]

groups (63.5%). Sport or learning groups were preferred among people living in a large city, while residents associations, senior clubs, volunteering, or women's clubs were the preference for those living in a small city, indicating that smaller cities are more likely to foster community-based ties than larger ones.

Social contact is regarded as a source of mental wellbeing in all cultures.[28] In a recent Japanese survey, more men than women (25.3% versus 19.8%) among older adults (aged 60+) reported having 'no contacts' in their neighbourhood. This group generally reported their primary source of social support to be their spouse or children.[29] If the generations are geographically separated, this situation becomes a social problem (Section 5.4).

Many men in the older age group reported having no one to rely on (35% versus 1.5% of women). Surprisingly, in the same age group, 22.6% of men and 16.4% of women indicated that they 'do not wish to rely on others for practical support'. Across age groups, the proportion reporting 'no contact' in large cities has been considerable in the past.[1] Social isolation appears to have grown in small towns and villages in recent decades, and is converging with the level in cities (5.4% versus 8.0% in 2011). The evidence suggests a trend in loss of social connections in cities and small communities.

Amid fragmenting social connections and large proportions of solo-living of older adults, there is a growth of *kodokushi* (dying alone) in Japan, with double the numbers from the last decade.[30] *Kodokushi* is not limited to older people, but is increasingly also found in men and women of working age. Other manifestations of social detachment are becoming evident in Japan.

5.4 Shrinking Families and Social Detachment

In the *ie* culture, Japanese society places caring responsibilities on family members, but current changes in demographics and individual social preferences challenge the sustainability of this conventional care framework. This section discusses problems arising from the gradual disappearance of the traditional family unit, the declining fertility rate, and social detachment— namely, *ro-ro kaigo*: the old caring for the very old; *kaigo rishoku*: leaving the labour force to become a care giver; and '8050': parents in their eighties caring for socially withdrawn adult children in their fifties.

5.4.1 *Ro-ro Kaigo* and *Kaigo Rishoku*

Fuelled by the growing ageing population (Chapters 1, 2, 8, and 9), the *ro-ro kaigo* pattern of caring in Japan has become more widespread. In the *ie* system, it was assumed that the wife would be the carer of her husband, however children may also be important.[21] With the increased longevity of both genders in recent years, carers also age along with the one for whom they care. Close to 60% of male and female carers are now aged over 60.[31] In some cases, children leave work (*kaigo rishoku*) to care for ageing parents who can no longer live independently.[32] In other cases, individuals still in employment may additionally care for family members.

Over 800,000 working-age adults, of whom 80% were women, left employment to care for a disabled family member in 2011/2012.[33] Care of a dependent family member falls mostly on the spouse (68%), followed by a child (21.8%), or the spouse of the child (11.1%).[29] The proportion of households with one or more parents and an unmarried adult child is growing (Figure 5.1). In such households, the child is likely to take a carer role and exit the labour force when a parent falls ill or loses their independence. In a recent survey, the two most frequent reasons for leaving the labour force to become a carer were that work was not conducive to doing both, followed by the carer's own declining physical and mental health.[31]

Problems related to these two current patterns of caring for the old include the emotional burden on carers. Among ageing carers, 80–90% said they required medical attention, while 50% resented their caring role, and 30% said they wanted to die.[34] Descriptions of emotions included: feeling chronic fatigue, having no fulfilment in life, suffering victimization or financial burden, and long caring hours. Those who had left employment to take up the care giver role may provide a high level of assistance, such as help with hospital visits, toileting, bathing, and housework. The number of hours of caring depended on the level of need.[2] The proportion who spent all day caring has been stable in recent years, at around 20%.

5.4.2 The '8050' Household

The '8050' household is characterized by ageing parent/s, often in their eighties, caring for a *hikikomori* (socially withdrawn) child, approximately in his/her fifties.[35] Prolonged *hikikomori* cases are thought to be due to disorders including major depression, anxiety, panic disorders, social phobia, or alcohol misuse, sometimes requiring the continual support of healthcare professionals (Chapter 15).

Frequently, the '8050' household is impoverished, with the main source of income being the parent's pension. In comparison with solo-living older adult households, the '8050' household is less likely to be supported by existing social care programmes, making it harder for their problems to be addressed. Government-level support for *hikikomori* is relatively new.[36] Seventy-five support centres had been set up nationally by 2019.

The common feature of *ro-ro kaigo*, *kaigo rishoku*, and '8050' is placement of caring responsibility on the family. Culturally inherited feelings about collective self-preservation through the *uchi* bond may drive family members to think unnecessarily that they should manage their responsibilities by themselves, and avoid disclosing their problems to *soto* people.[21] In contrast, the current Japanese health and social care system founded after World War II is based on work- or municipality-based plans.[37] However, such insurance arrangements generally assume traditional family composition consisting of a head of the household/breadwinner, typically a man, and his dependants.[38]

These defaults for the current care system have not been sufficiently re-examined in the context of demographic change, including population ageing and fertility rate decline. With the diminishing size and capacity of the family, the social problems of *ro-ro kaigo*, *kaigo rishoku*, and '8050' are likely to fall below the cracks of the current health and social care system. With the increasing trend toward social detachment, it is likely that these problems will become even harder to address. The next section discusses a Japanese initiative to reconnect people within communities.

5.5 Redrawing the *Uchi* Boundary? Towards Inclusive Society

The strong bond within *ie*-like *uchi* groups is the driving force of social cohesion, which is the source of mental wellbeing to many in Japan. As described in Chapter 2, the Japanese are presented with the task of surviving the demographic crisis due to prolonged low fertility rates, declining younger population growth, and a rapid increase in the ageing population. To do that, the Japanese may be required to shift their cultural paradigm of *uchi* and *soto* to extend their social connections. Two Japanese initiatives, *mimamori* (monitoring) and *chiiki kyosei* (area-based symbiotic society) are examples of initiatives to extend social connections.

5.5.1 *Mimamori* and *Chiiki Kyosei*: Two Initiatives to Reconnect People

After the Kobe-Awaji earthquake, most cases of *kodokushi* (dying alone) were among older people who had been placed in temporary housing.[39] It appeared that moving to temporary housing resulted in a loss of community ties and isolation. Social isolation and disconnection was worsened further by repeated moves, and as a result it was impossible for daily needs to be picked up and supported by community networks.

Learning from negative experiences of *kodokushi* cases in temporary housing settings, Kobe developed a system to look out and care for isolated older people, called *mimamori*, aiming to prevent social detachment. The programme encouraged the interest of volunteers to help vulnerable older people in their community, partly by developing rapport between the older people and the volunteers.[40]

Chiiki kyosei shakai (area-based symbiotic society) is a government initiative which started in 2016, and is due to be implemented across the country by 2020.[41] This initiative aims to restructure local support networks, to reduce cases of social isolation by providing everyone with a role in caring for and accepting others, and supporting one another as needed. The government has acknowledged that the existing vertical social care system was failing to address today's complex and diverse individual needs, to provide care for children, older family members with care needs, and support for those with mental health problems to enter and stay in employment, as well as maintaining their wellbeing. One aim of giving a role to everyone is to reduce the need for *kaigo rishoku* (Section 5.4.1). The initiative also aims to discourage the mentality of 'providers' and 'recipients' and to form bonds of mutual support in the community. The government also wants to utilize 'hidden' community resources such as abandoned fields, forests, empty houses, closed shopping areas, and people who are not in employment, including retirees and disabled people. The plan is to facilitate *ikigai* (meaningful lives) for people in the community.

Before the government's official announcement of *chiiki kyosei*, experts discussed the value of educating citizens about various social problems and individual vulnerabilities, including mental illness, to help prevent those in crisis from falling through the safety net.[42] Related to this discussion, mental health literacy has been introduced into the curriculum (Section 5.2.2) to help modify conventional cultural norms about wellbeing, and to promote community interaction and mutual support. One type of activity is intended to provide better support for individuals with mental health needs.[41]

Mimamori and *chiiki kyosei* are examples of recent initiatives to bring about a paradigm shift in *ie* culture, creating an integrated *ie* at community level, partly by linking individuals with the local administration. As Nakane[21] described it (Section 5.3), the Japanese bond through sharing. These examples develop shared entities to link individuals, who may lack a sense of belonging, into community-based social support networks. This new government initiative asks people to take others' concerns as their own (*wagakoto*). In this way, the new *ie* does not have to be based on blood, but on emotional closeness, including those who were excluded in the past, such as the mentally ill.

5.6 Conclusion

Throughout this chapter, the stigma directed at the mentally ill has been shown to be strong, nurtured to some degree within the family, while the mentally ill have been excluded from society and family members have borne the burden. A similar set of relationships is now seen with *ro-ro kaigo*, *kaigo rishoku*, and '8050'. From house confinement to institutionalization, laws have changed to protect the wellbeing of the mentally ill, yet social care has not developed sufficiently to address family needs adequately. Rapid changes in family composition and a growing trend towards social disconnection has Japanese society in a state of alarm, particularly in respect of the need to handle ageing-related problems effectively.

In an historical context, we can imagine many people with mental illness watching the first Tokyo Olympics on television in a psychiatric ward, isolated from family and home. Moving to the present, initiatives to restructure *ie* by connecting people at community level, to adjust social norms so that mentally ill people can be closer to society, may enable those who were socially excluded 50 years ago to enjoy the second Tokyo Olympics in a more contented state of mind, along with family and friends.

References

1. Ministry of Health, Labour and Welfare, Government of Japan. White Paper: Labour and Welfare. Tokyo 2011:1–374.
2. Cabinet Office, Government of Japan. The Annual Report on the Ageing Society. Tokyo 2019:1–133.
3. Japan Psychology Association. *The Direction of the Society without Social Connection.* Tokyo: Seishin shobo 2015:1–181.
4. Tani Y, Sasaki Y, Haseda M, et al. Eating alone and depression in older men and women by cohabitation status: The JAGES longitudinal survey. *Age Ageing* 2015;44(6):1019–26. doi: 10.1093/ageing/afv145 [published Online First: 28 October 2015].
5. Aida J, Cable N, Zaninotto P, et al. Social and behavioural determinants of the difference in survival among older adults in Japan and England. *Gerontology* 2018;64(3):266–77. doi: 10.1159/000485797 [published Online First: 19 January 2018].
6. Ministry of Health, Labour and Welfare, Government of Japan. White Paper: Measures for Suicide. Tokyo 2019:1–278.
7. Nakanishi M, Endo K, Ando S. The basic act for suicide prevention: effects on longitudinal trend in deliberate self-harm with reference to national suicide data for 1996–2014. *Int J Environ Res Public Health* 2017;14(1):104. doi:10.3390/ijerph14010104 [published Online First: 25 January 2017].
8. Ministry of Health, Labour and Welfare, Government of Japan. Patient Survey. Tokyo 2017:1–33.
9. Cable N, Chandola T, Lallukka T, et al. Country specific associations between social contact and mental health: evidence from civil servant studies across Great Britain, Japan and Finland. *Public Health* 2016;137:139–46. doi: 10.1016/j.puhe.2015.10.013 [published Online First: 5 April 2016].

10. Sekine M, Chandola T, Martikainen P, et al. Socioeconomic inequalities in physical and mental functioning of British, Finnish, and Japanese civil servants: role of job demand, control, and work hours. *Soc Sci Med* 2009;69(10):1417–25. doi: 10.1016/j.socscimed.2009.08.022 [published Online First: 22 September 2009].

11. WHO. *Social Determinants of Mental Health*. Geneva 2014:1–54.

12. Hofstede G, Hofstede G, Minkov M. *Cultures and Organizations. Softwares of the Mind: Intercultural Cooperation and Its Importance for Survival* (3rd edn.). New York: McGraw Hill 2010:1–561.

13. Wright D. Getting out of the asylum: understanding the insane in the nineteenth century. *Soc Hist Med* 1997;10(1):137–55. doi: https://doi.org/10.1093/shm/10.1.137

14. Ministry of Education, Sports, Science, and Technology, Japan. The history of disability policies in Japan. Tokyo 2010. Available at: http://www.mext.go.jp/b_menu/shingi/chukyo/chukyo3/siryo/attach/1295934.htm [last accessed 6 August 2019].

15. Kanekawa H. *The Profiles of House Confinement of the Mentally Ill by Shuzo Kure and Goro Kashiwada* (translated into modern Japanese). Tokyo: Igakushoin 2012:1–151.

16. Kuroki M. The foundation of mental care in the Meiji Era. *Taisei Gakuin Daigaku Kiyo* 2017;19(26):87–91.

17. The Constitution of Japan. 3 May 1947.

18. Griffiths KM, Nakane Y, Christensen H, et al. Stigma in response to mental disorders: a comparison of Australia and Japan. *BMC Psychiatry* 2006;6:21. doi: 10.1186/1471-244x-6-21 [published Online First: 24 May 2006].

19. Koike S, Yamaguchi S, Ohta K, et al. Mental-health-related stigma among Japanese children and their parents and impact of renaming of schizophrenia. *Psychiatry Clin Neurosci* 2017;71:170–9.

20. Yamada H, Nakatogawa S, Kasuya K, et al. Family's hope on a mentally disturbed individual and early mental health education. *Aichi Kenritsu Daigaku Kango gakubu Kiyo (Bulletin of Aichi Prefectural University School of Nursing & Health)* 2016;22:17–26.

21. Nakane C. *Japanese Society*. Harmondsworth: Penguin Books 1970:1–162.

22. Nakane C. *Family-centered Human Relationships*. Tokyo: Kodansha 1977:1–176.

23. Aida Y. *Japanese Mentality*. Tokyo: Kodansha 1970:1–216.

24. Kawai H. *Examination of Family Relationships*. Tokyo: Kondansha 1980:1–188.

25. Araki H. *Japanese Behavior Patterns*. Tokyo: Kodansha 1973:1–185.

26. Takagi D, Kondo K, Kondo N, et al. Social disorganization/social fragmentation and risk of depression among older people in Japan: multilevel investigation of indices of social distance. *Soc Sci Med* 2013;83:81–9. doi: 10.1016/j.socscimed.2013.01.001 [published Online First: 22 January 2013].

27. Cabinet Office, Government of Japan. A report on older people's attitudes towards social participation. Tokyo 2014:1–102.

28. Cable N, Bartley M, Chandola T, et al. Friends are equally important to men and women, but family matters more for men's well-being. *J Epidemiol Community Health* 2013;67(2):166–71. doi: 10.1136/jech-2012-201113 [published Online First: 25 August 2012].

29. Ministry of Health, Labour and Welfare, Government of Japan. Annual Report on the Aging Society. Tokyo 2017:1–138.

30. Kanawaku K. *Koritsu-shi* (solitary death) and its actual situation. *Nichiidai kaishi* 2016;14(2):100–12.

31. Cabinet Office, Government of Japan. Annual Report on the Aging Society. Tokyo 2017:1–160.

32. Ministry of Health, Labour and Welfare, Government of Japan. A report on working women in 2003 (*H15 Hataraku josei no jitsujo* (in Japanese)). Tokyo 2003.

33. Cabinet Office, Government of Japan. Annual Report on the Aging Society. Tokyo 2018.

34. Hanyu M. An analysis of current conditions of care by the elderly for the elderly (*Ro-ro kaigo no genjo bunseki* in Japanese). *Yamaguchi Keizaigaku Zasshi* 2010;59(4):303–41.

35. KHJ National Family Association of Social Withdrawals. A survey of social isolation problems. Tokyo 2018:1–117.

36. Ministry of Health, Labour and Welfare, Government of Japan. Implementations for social withdrawn individuals 2019. Available at: https://www.mhlw.go.jp/stf/seisakunitsuite/bunya/hukushi_kaigo/seikatsuhogo/hikikomori/index.html [last accessed 26 February 2020].

37. Ikegami N, Yoo B-K, Hashimoto H, et al. Japanese universal health coverage: evolution, achievements, and challenges. *Lancet* 2011;378(9796):1106–15. doi: 10.1016/S0140-6736(11)60828-3

38. Tamiya N, Noguchi H, Nishi A, et al. Population ageing and wellbeing: lessons from Japan's long-term care insurance policy. *Lancet* 2011;378(9797):1183–92. doi: 10.1016/s0140-6736(11)61176-8 [published Online First: 3 September 2011].

39. Cabinet Office, Government of Japan. Annual Report on the Ageing Society. Tokyo 2012:1–133.

40. Kanetani S, Kawano A. Development and evaluation of a 'mimamori' programme for older people involving community residents. *Nihon Chiiki Kangogaku Kaishi* 2015;18(1):12–19.

41. Ministry of Health, Labour and Welfare, Government of Japan. Towards delivery of area-based symbiotic society 2016. Available at: https://www.mhlw.go.jp/stf/seisakunitsuite/bunya/0000184346.html [last accessed 26 February 2020].

42. Science Council of Japan. Suggestion: how to support socially vulnerable individuals from social care perspectives. Tokyo 2018:1–20.

43. Ministry of Health, Labour and Welfare, Government of Japan. White Paper: Implementation for Suicide 2018. Available at: https://www.mhlw.go.jp/wp/hakusyo/jisatsu/18/index.html [last accessed 26 February 2020].

44. Office for National Statistics. Suicides in the UK: 2017 Registrations. Available at: https://www.ons.gov.uk/peoplepopulationandcommunity/birthsdeathsandmarriages/deaths/bulletins/suicidesintheunitedkingdom/2017registrations#suicide-patterns-by-age [last accessed 26 February 2020].

6

Japan's Miracle Decades

Harmony, Hard Work, and Health

Akizumi Tsutsumi

6.1 Historical Background

Table 6.1 summarizes historical movements of economy and employment systems in Japan from the post-World War II era to 2000.

6.1.1 Summary of Pre-war Economy and Industrialization

Japan's industrialization outpaced that of other newly industrialized nations. This rapid industrialization was reflected in the economy's 'dual structure'. Japan's post-war economy consisted of lower and upper levels. Many activities, including small handicraft industries, service industries, retailing, and agriculture, continued from the Tokugawa Shogunate (1600–1868), as domestic industries formed the lower level of the economy. New large enterprises were constructed upon this foundation as an upper level of highly mechanized industry. The two levels differed in scale of productivity, wages, and profitability.

In the pre-war period, the *zaibatsu* (financial cliques) controlled a great part of the upper level of the economy. *Zaibatsu* involved huge financial, commercial, and industrial syndicates, and they represented big business. This came about because numerous government enterprises were sold off to a relatively small number of individuals prior to 1900, contributing to monopolistic wealth and economic power. Close cooperation between government and business continued through the pre- and post-war periods.[1]

After World War II, *zaibatsu* was dissolved, and stock owned by the parent companies was sold. Individual companies within *zaibatsu* were freed from the control of parental companies. Then many companies were more loosely organized around the leading companies or major banks (forming enterprise

Akizumi Tsutsumi, *Japan's Miracle Decades* In: *Health in Japan.* Edited by: Eric Brunner, Noriko Cable, and Hiroyasu Iso, Oxford University Press (2021). © Oxford University Press. DOI: 10.1093/oso/9780198848134.003.0006.

Table 6.1 Trajectories of Japan's economy and related legislation along with emergence of health problems among the Japanese population: post-World War II period to 2000

Years	Economy	Legislation	Health issues	Indices on economy and labour force, social phenomena
1945	- High economic growth (1955–1973)	- *Zaibatsu* dissolution - Introduction of minimum wage system and national pension programme (1958)	- For the whole Japanese population, 14-year rise in life expectancy (1947–1955) prior to high economic growth period (as a result of decreased mortality rates for communicable diseases in children and young adults owing to improved hygiene)[26]	- By around 1950, Japan is a hierarchical society (family-run conglomerates versus poor and needy)
1960	- High economic growth (1955–1973)	- National health coverage and pension system (1961)	- Additional rise in life expectancy (1955–1973) during high economic growth period (owing to screening, referral, and treatment for cardiovascular disease and cancer as well as lifestyle improvements) (Chapters 11 and 12)	- Unemployment rate (male) ~1% (late 1960s to early 1970s) GINI (initial income) 0.3749 (1967) - Buzzwords (e.g. 'company soldier') (late 1960s to early 1970s)
1970	- High economic growth (1955–1973) - Oil shock (1973, 1979)		- Disparities in health across occupational groups reduced along with high economic growth	- All-Japanese-are-middle-class mentality (1970s to the first half of the 1980s) - Annual average working hours for male employees = 2,501 hours (1975) - GINI (initial income) 0.3747 (1975) - *Japan as Number One: Lessons for America* (Ezra Vogel, 1979) - Oil shock considerably slowed economic growth in Japan

	Economic context	Labour market policy	Health	Indicators
1980	- Stable growth (1974–1990) - Bubble economy (1986–1991)	- Easing of regulations (1980–) - Worker Dispatch Law (1985) - Equal Employment Opportunity Act for Men and Women (1985) - Introduction of discretionary labour system into Labour Standards Act (1988)	- Prevalence of poor health declined in the late 1980s (until the early/mid-1990s) (Comprehensive Survey of Living Conditions) - *Karōshi* recognized as a social problem in the late 1980s	- GINI (initial income) 0.3491 (1981) - GINI (initial income) 0.4049 (1987) - Freeter (part-time worker, 1987) - Annual average working hours for male employees = 2,673 hours (1988)
1990	- *Lost decade* - Bubble economy burst (1991–1993) - Post-bubble (1990–) - Advance of new economy or neoliberalism	- Revision of large-scale retail store law (1992) - Easing of employment contract regulations (late 1990s)	- Deterioration of self-reported health in the late 1990s (Comprehensive Survey of Living Conditions) - Surge in suicide numbers (1998) - Increased suicide rate among male managers	- Unemployment rate 2.0% (1991) - Jobs-to-applicants ratio of 1.4 (1991) - Buzzwords: *Kachi-gumi* versus *Make-gumi* (winners versus losers) - "Japanese style in the new era" by Nikkeiren (Japan Federation of Employers' Associations 1995) - Introduction of merit system (late 1990s) - GINI (initial income) 0.4412 (1996)
2000		- Industrial Revitalization Corporation of Japan (2003–2007)	- The health status of employed workers in Japan deteriorates, especially in 2004–2007 (Comprehensive Survey of Living Conditions)	- Unemployment rate (male) 5.5% (2002) - GINI (initial income) 0.4983 (2002) - NEET (Not in Education, Employment, or Training, 2004–) - Increased irregular employment (late 2000s)

groups (*keiretsu*)). They differed from *zaibatsu* in terms of the character of each group's policy coordination and the limited degree of financial inter-dependency between the member companies. Japan's rapid post-war economic growth was largely due to these groups' cooperative nature. They were able to invest the pooling of resources in developing industries to make them globally competitive.

Large enterprises had a primary financing ('main') bank, and co-financing with this bank was important in providing working capital. Traditionally, Japanese enterprises could count on borrowing from re-lated banks to raise the great majority of their funds, rather than relying on the market. The Japanese banks were interested in enterprises' long-term growth and were willing to accommodate them financially in return for guaranteed interest payments. Fostering an excellent company ensured the banks' long-term development and prosperity, and Japanese enter-prises were thus able to make business decisions using a long-term per-spective. Namely, it was a give-and-take relationship between the banks and industries.[2] That system contrasted substantially with the dominant profit motive in Western countries, where enterprises raised capital by is-suing stock, whereupon shareholders pressured them to generate short-term profits.

6.1.2 Emphasis on Post-war Development of the Salaryman System

Many Japanese employment/wage systems were established during the pe-riod of high economic growth from the 1960s to the 1970s. They included career-long employment, seniority-based pay, and the formulation of enter-prise unions. Most Japanese companies hired new graduates, and these em-ployees worked there until retirement. Salary and rank rose commensurate with the individual length of service, at least in large companies. It was highly unusual for employees to have to serve either under colleagues who had en-tered the company at the same time, or junior colleagues. This system helped to reduce internal frictions and nurtured employees' loyalty to their company. Employees who enjoyed secure employment and rising wages over a long pe-riod could support/coach each other using their skills. Career-long employ-ment fostered an integral and lasting commitment between the employee and employer.

High economic growth brought an acute increase in labour demand and mobility. This period was hailed as a time of 'full employment', with the unemployment rate at around 1% for men. To secure labour, even small- and medium-sized enterprises needed to guarantee employees a well-paid job. The high wages these enterprises offered provided the basis for wage standardization.

The spring labour offensive (*Shuntō*), a characteristic activity of labour unions, was a feature set in Japanese industrial relations by the mid-1950s. *Shuntō* is a horizontal wage-determination system based on general market rates. The system sets a specific target for annual wage increases to aid the collective bargaining process. Each spring, all enterprise unions in an industry announce similar wage demands (a 'base-up' target) and on the same day they begin their bargaining with a strike. Each union bargains with its own company management, though industry-wide coordination enables them to set similar wage goals across an industry. The General Council of Trade Unions of Japan (*Sōhyō*) coordinated the days on which each industry strikes.

From the 1960s to the 1970s, both the amounts and rates of annual wage increase raised, while the dispersion of the amounts contracted, resulting in reduced disparities of both wage for workers and household income. Around this period, wage inequality in Japan was less than in the US; in fiscal 1970, the ratio of mean incomes for the top-earning 20% to the bottom 20% of all Japanese workers was 4.3, while the corresponding ratio in the US was 7.1.[2] People had an egalitarian mentality of 'all-Japanese-are-middle-class', and generally believed that their efforts were being rewarded.

Japan achieved universal health coverage in 1961, just before its rapid economic growth began. The social security system pursued equitable service and equities in rates of copayments and contributions. Such equity was achieved by joint efforts of the public and private sectors. These included the subsidies from general revenues to plans that enabled enrolment of people with low incomes, and the cross-subsidization among plans to finance health-care costs for older people. The stable employment situation of the day—full and lifetime employment—helped in establishing the social security system. High economic growth and cost containment allowed the system to be maintained.[3]

6.1.3 The Economic Bubble, Recession, and Decline of Lifetime Job Security

Japanese real estate and stock market prices were substantially inflated during the so-called bubble economy of 1986–1991. Skyrocketing economic and business expansion induced a serious shortage of workers, and extremely long working hours became the norm. Employees hired during this period had considerable numbers of colleagues of the same generation and faced intense competition within their companies. They had a smaller number of subordinates because of the slowed adoption rate of the next generation, and many worked as front-line staff and gave up promotion opportunities (see Section 6.3.2).

Japan's economy tumbled into a prolonged recession—the 'two lost decades'—in the post-bubble early 1990s. The Japanese salaryman system—career-long employment and seniority-based pay system—started to disintegrate. Japan's economy underwent several changes during this recession. Middle-aged and older white-collar workers in large companies, including top manufacturers, became targets of corporate downsizing. From the late 1980s through to the 1990s, many large companies introduced annual salary reviews and merit-based pay, and began to abandon the seniority-based pay system.

The Worker Dispatch Law, enacted in 1985, partially opened the door (through the Employment Security Act) to previously prohibited labour supply businesses. The worker dispatch facilitated liberalization of employment contracts from the late 1990s to the early 2000s, and the number of workers with temporary status grew markedly. In 1995, the Japan Federation of Employers' Associations (*Nikkeiren*) declared it was time for 'Japanese-style management in the new era', following a comprehensive review of the career-long employment system. This declaration marked a watershed between the career-long employment and more fluid employment. Along with these political measures, the 1992 revision of large-scale retail store laws eliminated numerous family-type operations. Meanwhile, the government slashed social welfare spending. Japan's Gini coefficient had been gradually increasing since the 1980s, and the Organisation for Economic Co-operation and Development (OECD) report noted that the inequality in Japan had risen steadily since that time.[4]

Shuntō functioned well until the breakup of *Sōhyō* in 1989, and increasing numbers of non-regular employees, who were ineligible to participate in labour unions, led to labour union shrinkage. The long recession, with declining union membership, shifted the focus of union demands to protection of existing pay structures and jobs. Major unions in key Japanese industries sometimes even accepted zero wage rises from employers. Moreover, increasing income disparity due to changing employment patterns threatened the sustainability of health insurance for employees.[3]

6.2 The Japanese Work Ethic

Japanese work culture is characterized by solidarity; a sort of 'family' and reciprocal commitment between companies and employees. This involves not only strong social capital but also great commitment to work, such as working long hours. Recession and globalization have, however, affected Japan's economic and labour policies, and spurred changes in employment patterns as well as employees' and employers' mindsets.

6.2.1 Collective Spirit

It has often been noted that Japanese people are highly conscious of differences between inside and outside (*uchi* and *soto*, or part of the group versus outside the group). They have strong mutually understood communication and there is a deep-rooted sense of fellowship within a group. Conversely, they tend to maintain a certain distance between themselves and members of other groups. Even when they belong to several groups, Japanese people depend on a basic group, a so-called *marugakae* (completely enveloped) group, and highly value their relationship with this group. There is an understanding that group members take good care of each other, regardless of whether issues are business-related or personal. There is a strong mutual sense of obligation, and admission to and withdrawal from the group are difficult.[2]

Japanese society generally works on the principle of group consensus in which people value the importance of fitting in with others and harmonious interdependence.[5] Coworkers are the most important source of social support for work-oriented Japanese men, as they spend extended time together (even more than with their families on a typical working day). After work, a Japanese salaryman often goes out with coworkers for drinking get-togethers (*enkai*). This is a means of social integration and fosters promotion opportunities in Japanese business society.[6] The traditional employment system of Japanese companies builds up a sense of fellowship. New graduates hired at the same time are generally provided with on-the-job training to acquire business skills and knowledge, while learning about the corporate culture. Amid this, they tend to establish an informal social network.

6.2.2 Two-way Commitment Between Companies and Employees

Japanese companies have a strong mutual sense of loyalty between employers and employees. This relationship is not purely contractual; rather, the employee is seen as a member of the employer's own family. To strengthen their companies, Japanese employers have emphasized a cohesive sense of group unity and solidarity. Accordingly, employers do not merely employ someone for labour, but rather for their complete emotional participation in the community. The saying that 'the enterprise is the people' embodies this. Characteristics as a social group pervaded the private lives of employees at least until the high economic growth period[7] (the characteristics persist among small- and medium-sized enterprises). That is to say, strong social capital was inherent in the company.

Since that period, Japanese people have been characterized as workaholics. Just before the bubble economy burst, a popular advertisement for an energy drink asked, 'Can you fight (keep on working) for 24 hours?' Meanwhile, terms that derided the situation, such as 'company-first person' and 'company soldier', also emerged. In fact, Japanese regular workers do work longer than their counterparts in OECD member countries. Traditionally, the Japanese find virtue in diligence. In the high economic growth period, everyone believed in an equal chance of climbing to the top of the corporate ladder after joining the company. One had to have sufficient intelligence and ability, but he (in that male-dominated society) also had to display dedication by working long hours.

6.2.3 The Changing Japanese Work Ethic

Easing of employment contract regulations, together with the late-1990s recession, increased unemployment and numbers of lower-paid 'precarious' workers. Another type of economic dual structure for wages and benefits increased income disparity. While some high earners have emerged from adoption of a merit-based system, downsizing has resulted in more involuntarily unemployed people. Under these circumstances, various occupational disparities have emerged, as reflected in recently coined terms, *kachi-gumi* (winners) and *make-gumi* (losers).

Meanwhile, employers' mindsets have changed amid the lengthy recession.[8] Increasing globalization requires them to pursue short-term profits, and 'shareholder primacy' has replaced 'employee primacy' in management approaches. Employee mindsets have also changed. Analyses of the Social Stratification and Mobility survey revealed that Japanese society became increasingly rigid and closed in the 1990s.[9] The previous Japanese sense of an open society in which people's efforts were rewarded was replaced by resignation, wherein people received nothing meaningful for that effort.[9] During the bubble economy, employees worked long hours striving for success. However, since then, they have had to continue working long hours in efforts to avoid falling victim to restructuring.[10]

6.3 *Karōshi*, Work Stress, and Occupational Health Inequalities

The bubble economy inflated long working hours that already pervaded the Japanese working climate. In the middle of the bubble economy, *Karōshi* (death from overwork) became recognized as a social problem. Job insecurity accompanying the post-bubble recession seemed a cause of increased suicides among workers and job strain was found to be associated with health problems in Japanese workers. Occupational health inequalities exist, though the pattern is not consistent, as in the West.

6.3.1 Long Working Hours, Cardiovascular Disease, and Mental Health (*Karōshi*)

Annual average working hours for male employees in Japan increased from 2,501 hours in 1975, just after the oil shock, to 2,673 hours in 1988, when the bubble economy was nearing its peak. In 1988, 7,770,000 (6,850,000 men, a quarter of the male workforce, and 920,000 women) worked more than 60 hours/week. Trade friction with Western countries often increased criticism for Japanese long working hours. Accordingly, the Labour Standards Act was amended several times to reduce working hours, but there was no official limit on overtime work until a legal amendment in April 2019.

Karōshi from physical and mental exhaustion was first recognized as a social problem in Japan as early as the late 1980s. Although scientific evidence behind the phenomenon has been accumulated quite recently, *Karōshi* has become a legal issue whereby victims' families seek compensation.[11]

Suicides among employees increased from about 6,000/year in 1997 to about 9,000/year in 1998, remaining stable in the early 2000s. The 1998 surge is considered to be related to the economic recession after the bubble economy burst. Middle-aged male employees, expected to be breadwinners, were major victims.

A cohort study of community residents during the 1990s found that occupational stress was associated with increased risk of stroke incidence, mortality from cardiovascular diseases, and suicide, at least among male employees.[12–14] An analysis of 6,553 male and female Japanese workers showed an association between job strain (a combination of high psychological demands and low job control) and elevated risk of incident stroke[13] (Figure 6.1).

6.3.2 Occupational Class and Health Outcomes

Around 1980, male employees in the lower employment grade suffered higher total mortality rates from all causes.[15] With only limited exceptions, professional and managerial workers had the lowest mortality rates for several

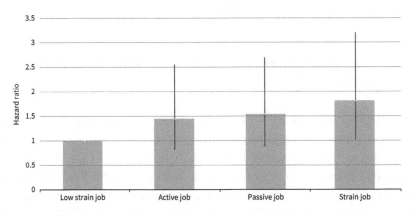

Figure 6.1 Associations of psychosocial job characteristics with risk of incident stroke in a prospective study of 6,553 male and female Japanese workers

Stroke incidence was diagnosed based on ICD-10 codes I60 (subarachnoid haemorrhage) and I61- I62 (intracerebral haemorrhage) and non- haemorrhagic stroke I63 (ischaemic stroke) using standardized criteria. Cross classification of the job control and job demand scales according to their sex- specific median values produced a quadrant scheme with four exposure categories, with low job demand and high job control representing a low- strain job (reference category), high job demand and high job control representing an active job, low job demand and low job control representing a passive job, and high job demand and low job control representing a strain job. Hazard ratios are adjusted for age, sex, smoking status, alcohol drinking, body mass index, educational attainment, occupation, and studied area.

Source: data from Tsutsumi A., Kayaba K., and Ishikawa S. Arch Intern Med. 2009;169:56-61.

diseases across age categories. These trends continued in the decades following, but gradually changed. Age-standardized mortality rates from all causes and some leading causes of death, decreased among all occupations except for professional and managerial workers, among whom mortality rates rose in the late 1990s.[16] From 2000 onwards, professional and managerial workers had the highest suicide rates.[16]

The pattern of occupational inequalities contrasted with what is often observed in the West,[17] where low control at work substantially influences workers' health.[18] Japanese managers tend towards greater job involvement, organizational commitment,[19] and working longer hours than their counterparts in Western countries.[20] Stressful work environments with increased job demands and responsibilities played a role amid the recession because managerial employees in the labour market decreased.[16] Another study suggests that Japanese men in a higher occupational position are more vulnerable to interpersonal conflicts at work, developing depression, than those in lower positions.[21]

Temporal trends in inequality based on self-reported health related to a newly developed theory-based social classification gave another perspective.[22] The trends were tested by using eight triennial waves of large nationally representative surveys between 1986 and 2007 (N = 398,303). The classification was derived from basic occupational and employment status (executives, self-employed with or without employees, employees, and limited contract workers),[23] which reflected changing employment patterns in Japan. The age-standardized prevalence of poor health declined until the early/mid-1990s, and then increased yearly for both genders. The relative and slope indices of inequality for social class remained constant for both genders over the study period.

6.4 Gender-based Division of Labour

The male-breadwinner model deeply permeated twentieth-century Japanese society. Trends in female participation in Japan's labour force (the proportion of women in the labour force versus total female working-age population) by age group shows an M-curve, as many women quit their jobs upon marriage or childbirth (Chapter 3). Although this curve has been gradually flattening, the M shape remains evident. Another unfavourable feature is the wide gap in average wages between male and female ordinary workers, albeit that gap has been narrowing over the long term. The main reason for this disparity is that women still work shorter periods than men; thus, the proportion of women who climb to high positions on the career ladder remains very low.

Before significant numbers of women began to be employed as regular workers following enactment of the Equal Employment Opportunity Act, the advance of the 'new economy', or neoliberalism, had led to employment polarization: core workers with specialized knowledge and skills versus un-skilled labour workers. In this situation, companies tend to hire core workers for their permanent workforce and unskilled labour as a temporary work-force. The economic recession, which occurred simultaneously with this trend's development, led to Japanese companies hiring numerous part-time or temporary workers. Since then, the proportion of non-regular employees has been increasing among both genders, but is particularly high for women. A significant level of commitment (long working hours and frequent reloca-tion) is expected for permanent/core workers and, thus, women (whose ability to commit to long working hours and frequent relocation is limited compared with men) remain more likely than men to have less-secure work. Since the 1990s, the number of women remaining unmarried has increased, along with a denormalization of female labour, resulting in a large increase in the number of female working poor.

Gender-based discrimination and family responsibilities are significant sources of stress among working women, and women who are core workers bear multiple burdens (i.e. domestic responsibilities, including care for chil-dren and older people, in addition to work responsibilities). Age-adjusted occupational trends based on Vital Statistics in Japan suggested that among the female occupational groups, clerical employees had the lowest mortality rate of all causes whereas managers had the highest.[24] Women in higher oc-cupational positions may be more likely to experience stress and/or work-place discrimination than women in lower-level positions.[25] According to a community-based cohort study, a significantly higher risk of incident stroke was observed in men with high job strain in low occupational classes (blue-collar and non-managerial work), but not in those in high occupational classes (white-collar and managerial work). The opposite trends were ob-served in women, i.e. significant elevated risks in high occupational classes, but not in low occupational classes.[25]

6.5 Post-war Economic Miracle and Health

From the post-war era, Japanese people (including working people) have en-joyed good health[26] (Chapters 11 and 12). Nationwide health inequalities also decreased until 1995, but this trend reversed from 1995 to 2000.[27] Increases and decreases in health inequality among various occupational groups coincided with the changes in economic environment, labour policies, and the employment system during this period (Table 6.1).

The traditional employment system and high economic growth in the post-war period had a substantial impact. Japanese employees displayed an egalitarian outlook, and hoped their efforts would be rewarded. During the periods of economic growth and at least before the bubble economy burst, job security and the salaryman system enabled employees to enjoy their work free from anxiety, and nurtured committed relationships among them (i.e. social capital) (Figure 6.2). *Shuntō*, based on enterprise unions, functioned as a type of horizontal wage-determination system.

The limited wage inequality in Japan during this period, evidenced by the culture of employees and employers having a common interest in the company's success, was a special feature of the Japanese work ethic. This supports Wilkinson's view of income inequality as a key determinant of aspects such as social cohesion, health inequalities, and crime rates.[28] An alternative interpretation is that the strong work ethic and limited income inequality were elements of a more general cultural aspect of the 'Japanese family' sticking together.

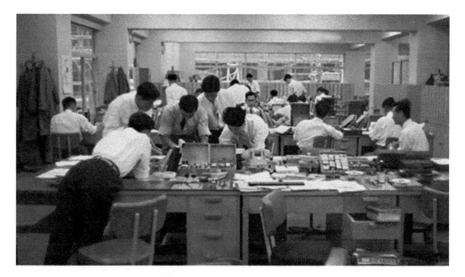

一企業戦士としてがむしゃらに働いた

Figure 6.2 Japanese salarymen in the high economic growth period
Copyright@http://kazuyoshiimuro.jp/chapter2/story_02_01.html

6.6 Policy Implications

The economic recession of the early 1990s, and subsequent economy-related policies, may have worsened health status in the Japanese working population. Disintegration of the career-long employment system, and the accompanying increase in unstable employment, together with increasing social security costs, may have also aggravated concerns about increasing occupational disparities. Analyses based on a national survey support a hypothesis that increased precarious non-regular work is the main factor underlying this effect, and the potential cause of workers' deteriorating health during this period.[29] Several health problems emerged for Japanese workers in the 2000s (Chapter 7).

The trajectories of Japan's economy and the related legislation from the post-World War II period to the year 2000 suggest the rebuilding of social capital in the workplace warrants the highest priority. Recently, at the micro-level, numerous Japanese companies have started to (re)adopt the management style that once produced family-like solidarity. At the macro-level, it is necessary to change economy-first policy. A preferable system lets employees devote themselves in their work without fearing for their livelihood. This may include the strengthening of employment measures, especially for non-regular and female workers.

In 1999, an economic strategy council under the Cabinet published a report titled 'The strategy of rebirth of the Japanese economy'. This recommended the adoption of a US-style 'shareholder primacy' model to help rebuild the crisis-hit Japanese management culture, both regarding finance and employment. The report recommended Japan make a clean break from 'the traditional excessive equitable society based on extreme regulation and protection' and shift to US-style management based on 'individual responsibility and self-help efforts'. Modern-day Japan's rapidly ageing society and contracting labour force are additional factors. The next chapter explores what happened after the year 2000.

Acknowledgements

This work was supported by KAKEN Challenging Research (Exploratory): Exploration of methods of measurement and analyses of theory-based social class classification for health research in Japan (Project/Area Number 18K19699). The author thanks the Edanz Group (www.edanzediting.com/ac) for editing a draft of this manuscript.

References

1. Reischauer EO. *The Japanese Today: Change and Continuity*. Tokyo: Charles E. Tuttle Company 1988.

2. Vogel EF. *Japan as Number One*. Cambridge, Massachusetts: Harvard University Press 1979.

3. Ikegami N, Yoo BK, Hashimoto H, Matsumoto M, Ogata H, Babazono A, et al. Japanese universal health coverage: evolution, achievements, and challenges. *Lancet* 2011;378:1106–15.

4. OECD. *OECD Economic Survey of Japan*. Paris: OECD Publications 2006.

5. Markus HR, Kitayama S. Culture and the self: implications for cognition, emotion, and motivation. *Psychological Review* 1991;98:224–53.

6. Ikeda A, Kawachi I, Iso H, Inoue M, Tsugane S. Gender difference in the association between social support and metabolic syndrome in Japan: the 'enkai' effect? *J Epidemiol Community Health* 2011;65:71–7.

7. Nakane C. *Japanese Society*. Berkeley: University of California Press 1970.

8. Dore RP. New forms and meanings of work in an increasingly globalized world. International Institute for Labour Studies, International Labour Office 2004.

9. Sato T. *Unequal Society Japan—Goodbye Total Midstream* (in Japanese). Tokyo: Chuokoron-Shinsha 2000.

10. Kawahito H. *Karō Jisatsu (Suicide from Over Work)*. Tokyo: Iwanami 1998.

11. Tsutsumi A. Preventing overwork-related deaths and disorders—need of continuous and multi-faceted efforts. *J Occup Health* 2019;61:265–6.

12. Tsutsumi A, Kayaba K, Hirokawa K, Ishikawa S. Psychosocial job characteristics and risk of mortality in a Japanese community-based working population: The Jichi Medical School Cohort Study. *Soc Sci Med* 2006;63:1276–88.

13. Tsutsumi A, Kayaba K, Kario K, Ishikawa S. Prospective study on occupational stress and risk of stroke. *Arch Int Med* 2009;169:56–61.

14. Tsutsumi A, Kayaba K, Ojima T, Ishikawa S, Kawakami N. Low control at work and the risk of suicide in Japanese men: a prospective cohort study. *Psychother Psychosom* 2007;76:177–85.

15. Kagamimori S, Matsubara I, Sokejima S, Sekine M, Matsukura T, Nakagawa H, et al. The comparative study on occupational mortality, 1980 between Japan and Great Britain. *Ind Health* 1998;36:252–7.

16. Wada K, Kondo N, Gilmour S, Ichida Y, Fujino Y, Satoh T, et al. Trends in cause-specific mortality across occupations in Japanese men of working age during a period of economic stagnation, 1980–2005: retrospective cohort study. *BMJ* 2012;344:e1191.

17. Drever F, Whitehead M, Roden M. Current patterns and trends in male mortality by social class (based on occupation). *Population Trends* 1996;86:15–20.

18. Marmot MG, Bosma H, Hemingway H, Brunner E, Stansfeld S. Contribution of job control and other risk factors to social variations in coronary heart disease incidence. *Lancet* 1997;350:235–9.

19. Lincoln JR, Kalleberg AL. Work organization and workforce commitment: a study of plants and employees in the US and Japan. *ASR* 1985;50:738–60.

20. Maruyama S, Morimoto K. Effects of long work-hours on life-style, stress and quality of life among intermediate Japanese managers. *Scand J Work Environ Health* 1996;22:353–9.

21. Inoue A, Kawakami N. Interpersonal conflict and depression among Japanese workers with high or low socioeconomic status: findings from the Japan Work Stress and Health Cohort Study. *Soc Sci Med* 2010;71:173–80.

22. Hiyoshi A, Fukuda Y, Shipley MJ, Brunner EJ. Inequalities in self-rated health in Japan 1986–2007 according to household income and a novel occupational classification: national sampling survey series. *J Epidemiol Community Health* 2013;67:960–5.

23. Hiyoshi A, Fukuda Y, Shipley MJ, Bartley M, Brunner EJ. A new theory-based social classification in Japan and its validation using historically collected information. *Soc Sci Med* 2013;87:84–92.

24. Hasegawa T. Japan: historical and current dimensions of health and health equity. In: Evans T, Whitehead M, Diderichsen F, Bhuiya A, Wirth M (eds), *Challenging Inequities in Health: From Ethics to Action*. New York: Oxford University Press 2001:90–103.

25. Tsutsumi A, Kayaba K, Ishikawa S. Impact of occupational stress on stroke across occupational classes and genders. *Soc Sci Med* 2011;72:1652–8.

26. Ikeda N, Saito E, Kondo N, Inoue M, Ikeda S, Satoh T, et al. What has made the population of Japan healthy? *Lancet* 378;9796:1094–105.

27. Fukuda Y, Nakao H, Yahata Y, Imai H. Are health inequalities increasing in Japan? The trends of 1955 to 2000. *Biosci Trends* 2007;1:38–42.

28. Wilkinson RG. *The Impact of Inequality: How to Make Sick Societies Healthier*. New York and London: The New Press 2005.

29. Nishikitani M, Tsurugano S, Inoue M, Yano E. Effect of unequal employment status on workers' health: results from a Japanese national survey. *Soc Sci Med* 2012;75:439–51.

7

Work and Health in a Diverse and Disparate Labour Market

Mariko Inoue, Yoshiharu Fukuda, and Eric Brunner

7.1 Introduction

Japan experienced fast-rising economic development during the 1960s, 1970s, and 1980s. However, a long period of slow growth since 1990, the 'lost decades', gradually transformed occupational culture away from the lifetime salaryman system.

This chapter focuses on social changes in an era of increasingly diverse employment arrangements, collapse of the lifetime, seniority-based employment system, and a large rise in non-standard employment. We review Japan's labour market trends and discuss the impact on workers' health across different employment arrangements.

7.2 Changes in Society and Employment Arrangements in the Lost Decades

7.2.1 The Lost Decades

After years of growth, Japan experienced economic stagnation during the Heisei era that extended from 1989 to 2019. In 1993, the country officially went into recession as Gross Domestic Product (GDP) declined, wages fell, and income inequality increased (Table 7.1). Japan's economic growth did not return to the level seen in 1990. Internationally, Japan has faced many external challenges, including stiff competition from the Asian Tigers (the highly developed economies of Hong Kong, Singapore, South Korea, and Taiwan) and recession at the beginning of the new millennium. Domestically, it continued to face difficulties such as a rapidly ageing population, a significantly declining

Mariko Inoue, Yoshiharu Fukuda, and Eric Brunner, *Work and Health in a Diverse and Disparate Labour Market* In: *Health in Japan*. Edited by: Eric Brunner, Noriko Cable, and Hiroyasu Iso, Oxford University Press (2021). © Oxford University Press. DOI: 10.1093/oso/9780198848134.003.0007.

Table 7.1 Chronology of Japanese economy, employment legislation, and health, 2000–2019

Year	Economy	Legislation	Workers' health issues	Economic and social indices
2000	- 2000–2002 Internet bubble - Third Heisei recession	- 2003 Agency Workers Act - Improved working conditions for agency workers	- Increasing all-cause mortality and suicide rates among male managers[19]	- Unemployment rate more than 5% (2001–2003) - Increasingly diverse working patterns
2005	- Global Financial Crisis (2007–2009)	- 2006 Revised Industrial Safety and Health Act to regulate long working hours - Equal Opportunity Act for men and women in work - 2007 Employment Act prohibits discrimination against part-time workers	- 2004–2007 Health of workers deteriorates, regardless of type of employment[21]	- GINI (income before tax) 0.526 (2005), 0.532 (2008) - Unemployment rate more than 5% (2009–2010) - Women continue to face dismissal after pregnancy or delivery, despite new Equal Opportunity Act
2010	- 2013 *Abenomics* reforms to stimulate economy and society	- 2010 Insurance Act extends coverage for non-standard employment - 2013 Elderly Employment Act; retirement age raised to 65 - 2014 Prevention of Death and Injury from Overwork Act - 2015 Labour Contract Act where organizations are obliged to offer a permanent contract after five years of satisfactory employment		- Unemployment rate 5.1% (2010) - GINI 0.554 (2011) - Great East Japan Earthquake (2011)
2015	- 2013–2019 Low growth in 13 financial quarters since January 2015, the economy contracted in 4 quarters	- 2015 Promotion of Women's Workplace Participation and Advancement Act - 2016 Pension Insurance and Health Insurance Acts extended to part-time work (20+ hours/week) - 2019 Labour law revised to limit overtime; revised Immigration and Refugee Act	- Part-time workers have higher mortality rate than permanent workers[31] - Non-standard employees more likely change job after pregnancy[40]	- Unemployment rate 3.5% (2015) - GINI 0.570 (2014) - Unemployment rate less than 3.0% (2017–2018) - More migrant worker visas to meet labour shortages
2019			- Employment law reforms (*Hatarakikata Kaikaku*)	

birth rate, and major natural disasters. These multiple factors led to an increase in social expenditure. Instead of an increase in productivity, continued deflation fuelled the accumulation of the largest governmental debt of any country, amounting to 237% of GDP in 2015 as compared to the UK's 109%.[1]

The Japanese have long struggled with the hardships of recession, economic stagnation, and expanding social disparity. Restoration of the Japanese economy and reduction in economic disparity became the main policy agenda in the 2015 radical reforms. The current policy aims to improve productivity by enhancing labour conditions and diversifying work opportunities for the population.

Although the government encouraged flexible working arrangements, the system continued to be biased in favour of regular workers, in terms of labour conditions and compensation schemes. Japanese social security, workers' pay, and the occupational health system were based on the social designs of the salaryman era and remain largely unchanged, with minor exceptions (Table 7.1). Non-standard employment is associated with fewer career prospects and less job security than regular employment, and this may translate into poorer health over working life.

7.2.2 A Shift Towards Diverse Working Arrangements

Japan's conventional lifelong employment culture of the second half of the twentieth century was disrupted by economic problems and deregulation in working arrangements. The percentage of workers with stable and lifelong employment, categorized as 'permanent' or 'regular' workers, decreased rapidly through the lost decades, whereas non-standard (part-time, contract, temporary agency) workers increased. Non-standard employment accounted for 37.9% of the workforce in 2018, as compared to the earliest statistic of 5.3% in 1984. There was an increase in non-standard employment over these three decades, and a difference between men and women (Figure 7.1).[2]

In the context of gender, more than half of working women in Japan were in non-standard employment after 2002. Because more women in their twenties to forties keep working through their child-rearing period, the Japanese M-shaped curve of the labour force participation rate, by age group, has been increasing for the last three decades. However, the majority of women engage in non-standard work, while men in the same age group work in regular jobs.

Flexible patterns of work help to make diverse lifestyle choices possible and encourage people to join the workforce. However, non-standard employment may not be a voluntary choice. Increasingly, there is a dearth of regular jobs in the labour market. The proportion of involuntary non-standard workers

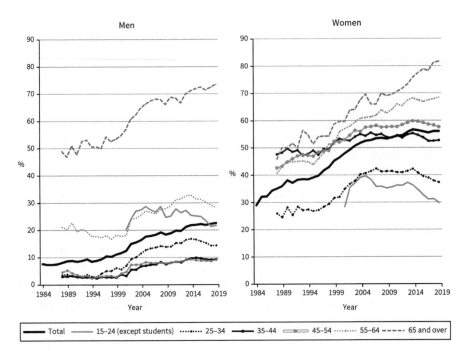

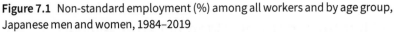

Figure 7.1 Non-standard employment (%) among all workers and by age group, Japanese men and women, 1984–2019

Data for 2019 based on January–June average.

Source: data from Ministry of Internal Affairs and Communication. Labour Force Survey. 2019. Date accessed 30 July 2019.

in 2014, in their current job due to shortage of regular positions, was 38% among temporary agency workers, 32% among fixed-term workers, and 12% among part-time workers.[3] Non-standard employment poses seven potential threats to existing work conditions according to the International Labour Organization (ILO): (1) instability of employment, (2) lower earnings, (3) less flexible hours of work, (4) less occupational safety and healthcare, (5) lower social security protection, (6) fewer opportunities for training, and (7) under-representation of rights at work.[4] All seven of these insecurities apply to Japanese non-standard workers. For instance, an official estimate for 2018 shows the average monthly income of regular workers was 323,900 yen (£2,500, US$3,050), while non-standard workers made 209,400 yen (£1,620, US$1,970),[5] indicating a considerable gap in lifetime incomes.

Differences between regular and non-standard employment rights continue. Some employment-related conditions have been equalized. Part-time workers putting in at least 30 hours/week are entitled to the same amount of annual leave as full-time workers and the number of days of leave for those who work less than 30 hours/week is regulated. Involuntary non-standard employment, in particular, may result in lower life satisfaction, while those who choose part-time and temporary work may be satisfied with their work-life balance.

7.2.3 Social Change During the Lost Decade

Three factors are linked to the decline of the Japanese lifelong employment system:

1) deregulation of work arrangements to offset high unemployment rates and the economic slowdown;
2) attempts to promote women's participation in the labour market; and
3) encouraging continued paid work among the elderly.

Economic stagnation is a key contributory factor for the shift towards diverse working arrangements. Employers and unions recognized non-standard employment as a buffer for those with permanent regular contracts, and the employment rights which go along with them. Non-standard workers accepted lower wages, reduced social security, and could easily be laid off. After 2000, revision of labour regulations tended to allow more flexible work structures. Deregulation of the Temporary Agency Workers Act (1986), which limited the number of temporary agency workers in 13 occupations, was a significant step. After 1999, as new industries developed, the government expanded the number of occupations that allow temporary agency workers. Agency workers are just one example; intermittent and part-time employment has become more widely accepted in Japanese society.

The same period saw higher unemployment rates than before 1990, and college and university graduates were finding it increasingly difficult to obtain regular employment. Between 1993 and 2005, fresh graduates failed to secure a first job that ensured lifelong employment and thus, took up initial jobs as non-standard workers, ushering in the era of the 'ice age for job seekers'(*Shushoku Hyogaki*). Between 1999 and 2004, 61% of high school graduates and 44% of college graduates started working as non-standard workers.[6] In the conservative Japanese job market, young adults in non-standard employment struggled to become regular workers. Late into their thirties and forties, many in the *Shushoku Hyogaki* generation remain in non-standard employment with weaker employment rights.

The second factor relates to women in the labour market. As compared to the past, women today have more options. Conventionally, women quit their jobs after marriage to pursue childrearing and housekeeping. The current

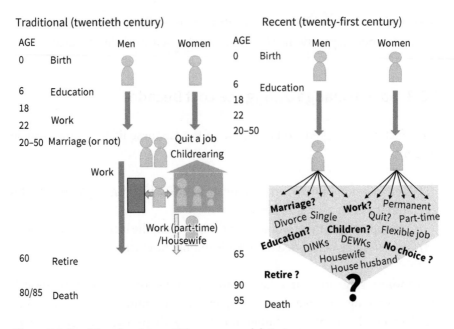

Figure 7.2 Traditional and recent life course models in Japan
DINK: double income no kids; DEWK: dually employed with kids

model of women's career paths is diverse (Figure 7.2). A marked change in attitudes encourages women to continue working after marriage, and resume work after childbirth (Chapter 2). Flexible patterns of work may be welcomed by those who value work-life balance (Chapter 3).

The third factor driving changing employment patterns is delayed retirement and moves to encourage paid work among the elderly. In 2017, 12.2% of people 65 or older continued working.[2] This proportion is expected to increase because of revision to the law in 2013 that stabilizes employment of older people. In a national survey, when asked, 'Until what age would you like to continue working?', 42% of the general older population answered, 'As long as I can'.[7]

Changes in working arrangements progress against the backdrop of these aforementioned factors. In relation to health and wellbeing, there are favourable consequences through the diversification of working arrangements, and some undesirable aspects also, such as growing social disparities.

7.2.4 People Left Behind During the Lost Decades

Disadvantaged and vulnerable groups have increased in size during the lost decades. Two groups are discussed here, workers in poverty, and people living in a state of social withdrawal.

7.2.5 Working Poor

Japan's poverty level has increased since the year 2000. The relative poverty rate (percentage of people with income below 50% of median income) rose from 12.0% in 1985 to 15.6% in 2015.[8] Growing numbers of citizens were forced to live on welfare. Japan, once regarded as an equal society, became one of the countries with the highest relative poverty rates among member countries of the OECD in 2015.[9] The child poverty rate in single working parent families was the highest among OECD countries, in 2008. Around 50% of single working parent families were categorized as poor households, even though the parent was working (Chapter 3).[10]

One of the main causes of poverty is low income. In the past, many non-standard workers were supplemental earners, e.g. a wife working part-time while her husband was the main earner. Low wages often do not support living circumstances today. Lower marriage rates and higher divorce rates have led to an increase in the number of people who need to support themselves on a non-standard income. The unmarried rate among 35–39 year olds is 35% in men and 23% in women in 2015, whereas the rates were 14% and 7% respectively in 1985.[11] Unmarried persons and single mothers limited to non-standard work suffer the consequences of being the sole low wage earner, and are at risk of falling below the poverty line. Losing a job may mean losing the home. At the time of the 2008 recession, workers with a fixed-term contract and company housing had to move out when they were made redundant. Structural changes in the employment system must reflect current realities and be required to secure a reasonable standard of living regardless of working arrangements. A rise in minimum wage levels and reform of employment rights could reduce the burden of working poor.

7.2.6 NEET and *Hikikomori*

Social withdrawal among the younger generation is an important concern. In 2018, some 2.1% (N = 710,000) of people aged 15–39 years, identified as 'Not in Education, Employment, or Training' (NEET), and an estimated 1.6% of this age group (N = 541,000) were *Hikikomori*.[12] The government considered both NEET and *Hikikomori* to be mainly a problem among younger adults. However, the 2018 survey found the prevalence of *Hikikomori* in adults aged 40–64 years was similar (1.5%) to that in younger adults, and 77% were men (Chapter 5.4.2).[12]

Box 7.1   Otaku

Otaku is a general term that refers to someone who possesses deep knowledge of one subject. The term began to be used in the 1980s among subculture enthusiasts to refer to each other, as the word *otaku* is a polite way of saying 'you' in Japanese. *Otaku* is typically used to refer to a person who is obsessed with a particular aspect of popular culture such as animation, manga, video games, and young female pop stars. *Otaku* is sometimes confused with *hikikomori*, in the sense of staying at home and being isolated from society. However, *hikikomori* does not necessarily refer to a subculture enthusiast.

The term *Otaku* has become accepted to describe someone who knows one topic very well. For example, *Kenko* (health) *Otaku* is a phrase used to describe a person who pays excessive attention to his or her health and lifestyle, perhaps taking many nutrient supplements and over-exercising. One recent survey showed a change in Japanese perceptions. Although the most common answer still captured the typical image of someone obsessed with a hobby (62%), 38% answered that *Otaku* is someone who knows a lot about one thing.

Widely regarded as social withdrawal, hikikomori is defined as 'abnormal avoidance of social contact'.[13] People affected by *Hikikomori* often spend their days in their bedroom. In some cases, the family has poor communication with the *Hikikomori*, and abandon them instead of protecting them. Several reasons for developing *Hikikomori* seem to be important, including social and psychological risk factors,[14] and unemployment. *Otaku* can be misunderstood as *Hikikomori*, but it is entirely distinct (Box 7.1).

Hikikomori are widely considered to have a psychological disorder. Diagnoses of schizophrenia, mood disorder, or anxiety disorders are common.[15,16] An alternative view is that *Hikikomori* is a social phenomenon and speculatively a sign of a sick population in need of treatment. The populations of working poor, NEET, and *Hikikomori* are said to be products of societal inequality and broken social ties. A related phenomenon in super-ageing Japan is *Kodokushi*, dying alone and undiscovered at home (Chapter 5.5.1). For the future, social withdrawal and isolation may continue as a vicious cycle down succeeding generations, particularly if the poverty rate is not reduced.

7.3   Health and Wellbeing

7.3.1   Health and the Economic Slowdown

Economic stagnation may be an important influence on the health of Japanese workers. Depression and psychological distress have been shown to increase during economic crises.[17] During the lost decades, self-rated health in the general Japanese population tended to decline (Chapter 1). Another negative health consequence of the stagnant economy appears to be the particular impact of work pressures on the health of company executives and managers. Higher all-cause mortality rates, including suicide, in this group compared to manual workers have resulted in reduced health inequality, measured in terms of relative mortality rates.[18,19] Nevertheless, low income and unemployment have been shown to be key determinants of inequalities in self-rated health in this period.[20]

The social and economic disparity between regular and non-standard workers led the ILO in its 2016 global report on employment conditions to state that 'Japan has a highly dualistic labour market'. [4] The labour market situation is particularly challenging for Japanese women and can ultimately affect the wellbeing of the entire population.[21] Exposure to the 'ice age for job seekers' (*Shushoku Hyogaki*) was likely to have affected their subjective health thereafter.[22]

7.3.2 Long Working Hours and *Karōshi*

In post-war Japanese culture, long working hours were standard. The Japanese had the longest hours when compared to other OECD countries.[23] However, average annual working hours decreased from 2,052 in 1990 to 1,846 in 2017–2018.[23] This decrease could be related to the growing number of part-time and flexible contracts. A change in working patterns may result in shorter working hours for full-time workers.

Lengthy working hours are known to be associated with health risks such as depression, sleeplessness, and coronary heart disease.[24] The phenomenon of *Karōshi*, death by overwork, is well known. Major causes of *Karōshi* include heart attack, stroke, and suicide. *Karōshi* statistics are based on reports and approved cases of workers' compensation. In 2017, workers' compensation was paid for 92 cases of stroke or heart disease deaths and 98 cases of death due to mental illness.[25] Due to the lack of statistics on *Karōshi*, reported and approved cases of *Karōshi* might just be the tip of the iceberg. Protecting the health of an overworked population is thus a major challenge for the government.

Efficiency will improve Japanese productivity if working hours are limited and companies try to support the change. Despite long working hours among full-time workers, Japanese economic productivity and GDP per hour were found to be slightly below the OECD average.[26] Shorter working hours and increased efficiency could reduce the risk of *Karoshi* and improve work-life balance in the working population.

7.3.3 Working Arrangements and Health: Focus on Non-standard Employees

In principle, flexible working arrangements support a sustainable work-life balance for people with differing personal circumstances. The challenge is that globally, non-standard employment has tended to be associated with inferior labour conditions, compared to regular employment, and a risk of psychological distress [27] and increased mortality rate.[28]

Evidence is accumulating for the health effects of non-standard employment in Japan. Men and unmarried women working part-time or for an employment agency had almost double the risk of developing serious psychological distress than regular workers over four years of follow-up.[29] In a Japanese research institute, fixed-term compared to permanent contracts were associated with poorer mental health, indexed by the number of visits to company clinics for mental health concerns over one year.[30] Among middle-aged Japanese women, part-time working and self-employment was associated with higher mortality rates, compared to regular employment.[31] The occupational injury rate has risen congruently with the percentage of non-standard workers.[32] Cross-sectional studies have conflicting results. Some suggest that non-standard workers have lower physical and mental health problems,[33,34] while others found the opposite.[35,36] Causal relationships are uncertain, as some individuals may take up non-standard employment as a result of poor physical or mental health. Complicating factors include job insecurity among fixed-term and temporary workers, and overwork among regular workers. Regular workers in Japan may be exposed to greater job stress, such as excessive overtime, than non-standard workers.[37]

7.3.4 The Problem of Healthcare Insurance

The reasons for health disparities between regular and non-standard workers may be difficult to establish. Ill health may have developed before signing a non-standard contract. The consequences of this problem include reduced access to insurance and health checkups. In 2014 almost all permanent workers had insurance cover: health insurance: 99.3%, pension: 99.1%, and unemployment insurance: 92.5%. The respective benefits were held by 37.6%, 35.3%, and 60.6% of part-time workers and 81.8%, 76.5%, and 83.8% of temporary agency workers. Some part-time and temporary workers were covered through a full-time employed or self-employed family member.[3] Compared to full-time workers, temporary and part-time workers have poorer access to health checkups.[38]

The work environment may be discouraging or even hostile for temporary workers. Workplace bullying may be experienced more often than by regular employees.[39] Non-standard workers change jobs more frequently following pregnancy or childbirth.[40] Adverse lifestyle, such as smoking and poor diet, have been linked to non-standard employment in Japan.[41,42] The extent to which such differences are due to working conditions rather than socioeconomic and educational background is likely to depend on employer and employee.

In summary, there are few large-scale, long-term follow-up studies of associations between working arrangements and health during the Japanese 'lost decades', however existing evidence does suggest that improvement of employment conditions for non-standard workers is needed to support health equity across Japan's disparate labour market.

7.4 Recent Policy Developments

In 2019, employment law reforms (*Hatarakikata Kaikaku*) were introduced in response to the continuing transformation in working arrangements. The reforms aim to secure fair treatment, equal wages, and to reduce working hours for all employees, regardless of employment contract. Overtime working is now restricted to 45 hours/month and 360 hours/year, however these limits are subject to several exemptions and the company fine for violation was set at a low level (¥300,000, £2,300, US$2,800).[43] The principle of equal pay for equal work will take time to be achieved, however Japan's work culture is changing.

The government hopes these changes will stimulate productivity. New assistance provides support for NEETs and *Hikikomori* to find work. Support is also extended for older graduates (40+ years) in non-standard employment who wish to move into regular work. The Immigration Control and Refugees Recognition Act (2019) relaxed visa controls on migrant workers in 14 areas of the economy, including social care, agriculture, construction, and food services. This development is an important response to the labour shortage in many occupations.

Technological innovation will provide opportunities for new businesses and jobs. Industry 4.0, the fourth industrial revolution of artificial intelligence, cyber systems, and the Internet of Things will lead to innovation in working arrangements. Working online at home, in the cloud, instead of an office or in a factory, has positive and negative implications: time flexibility is increased, but so too is social isolation. Regulations and occupational health protection will be needed for workers in these novel settings.

Over the next decade, pressure for changes in work culture will come from two distinct sources. Japan has the economic challenge of China and the Asian Tigers, and the public health challenge to provide healthy work and fair pay for men and women, Japanese and foreign, regardless of employment arrangements and working hours.

7.5 Conclusion

Japanese social transitions throughout the lost decades have had both a positive and negative impact on health and wellbeing. More flexible employment opportunities contributed to the enlarged set of possibilities that life now offers, especially to women and the elderly. On the flipside, social and economic disparities between regular and non-standard workers, including wages and employment conditions, indicate that Japan has a dualistic labour market that needs to be harmonized. Currently, over one third of Japanese workers have a non-standard contract. Equally, problems of poverty and social isolation including *Hikikomori* have emerged as major public health and governmental concerns for the population's continuing high quality of life and health. Monitoring health inequalities, and the health of all these vulnerable groups, by means of population surveys and epidemiological studies has never been so important.

Technological innovation has and will continue to impact the labour market and health. Industrial innovation adds economic growth, but it will substitute for many jobs and change others. As work changes, occupational health hazards from new technology and industries will be identified, needing careful research and policy development. Based on this evidence, support can be provided for the diverse working population.

The 2019 reform of employment law targets Japan's long working hours culture to promote work-life balance and provide fair working conditions to all workers regardless of their employment arrangement. This reform confirms the principle of equal pay for equal work, and is designed to reduce the disparities between regular and non-standard workers in terms of labour conditions and work-related health outcomes. Continuing policy analysis and development is necessary for the success of recent and future reforms for decent work and a fairer society.

References

1. Shibuya K, Hashimoto H, Ikegami N, et al. Future of Japan's system of good health at low cost with equity: beyond universal coverage. *Lancet* 2011;378:1265–73.
2. Ministry of Internal Affairs and Communication. Labour Force Survey 2019 (in Japanese). Available at: https://www.stat.go.jp/data/roudou/longtime/03roudou. html#hyo_2 [last accessed 28 February 2020].
3. Ministry of Health, Labour and Welfare, Government of Japan. General Survey on Diversified Types of Employment 2014 (in Japanese). Available at: https://www.mhlw.go.jp/toukei/itiran/roudou/koyou/keitai/14/ [last accessed 28 February 2020].
4. International Labour Organization. What is non-standard employment? In: *Non-standard Employment Around the World: Understanding Challenges, Shaping Prospects*. Geneva: International Labour Office 2016: 7–45.
5. Ministry of Health, Labour and Welfare, Government of Japan. Basic Survey on Wage Structure 2018. Available at: https://www.mhlw.go.jp/english/database/db-l/wage-structure.html [last accessed 28 February 2020].
6. Hori Y. Current status of 'the ice age for job seekers' (in Japanese). *Nihon Rodo Kenkyu Zasshi* 2019; 706:17–27.
7. Cabinet Office, Government of Japan. Annual Report on the Ageing Society 2018. Available at: https://www8.cao.go.jp/kourei/english/annualreport/2018/2018pdf_e.html [last accessed 28 February 2020].
8. Ministry of Health, Labour and Welfare, Government of Japan. Comprehensive Survey of Living Conditions. Available at: https://www.mhlw.go.jp/toukei/saikin/hw/k-tyosa/k-tyosa17/index.html [last accessed 28 February 2020].
9. OECD. Poverty rate. Available at: https://data.oecd.org/inequality/poverty-rate. htm [last accessed 28 February 2020].
10. OECD. *Policy Brief on Child Well-being. Poor Children in Rich Countries: Why We Need Policy Action.* Paris: OECD Publishing 2018.
11. Cabinet Office, Government of Japan. Annual Report on the Declining Birthrate 2018. Chapter 1. Current status of low birth rate (*Shoshi ka wo meguru genjo*) (in Japanese). Available at: https://www8.cao.go.jp/shoushi/shoushika/whitepaper/measures/w-2018/30pdfgaiyoh/30gaiyoh.html [last accessed 28 February 2020].
12. Cabinet Office, Government of Japan. White Paper on Children and Young People 2019 (in Japanese). Available at: https://www8.cao.go.jp/youth/whitepaper/r01honpen/pdf_index.html [last accessed 28 February 2020].
13. Oxford English Dictionary. Available at: https://www.oed.com/viewdictionaryentry/Entry/276284 [last accessed 28 February 2020].

14. Horiguchi S. Chapter 6. *Hikikomori*: how private isolation caught the public eye. In: Goodman R, Imoto Y, Toivonen T (eds.). *A Sociology of Japanese Youth from Returnees to NEETs.* London: Routledge 2012:122–38.

15. Kondo N, Sakai M, Kuroda Y, et al. General condition of *hikikomori* in Japan: psychiatric diagnosis and outcome in mental health welfare centres. *Int J Soc Psychiatry* 2013;59:79–86.

16. Koyama A, Miyake Y, Kawakami N, et al. Lifetime prevalence, psychiatric comorbidity and demographic correlates of 'hikikomori' in a community population in Japan. *Psychiatry Res* 2010;176:69–74.

17. Avendano M, Berkman LF. Chapter 6. Labor markets, employment policies, and health. In: Berkman LF, Kawachi I, Glymour MM (eds.). *Social Epidemiology* (2nd ed.) New York: Oxford University Press 2014:182–233.

18. Tanaka H, Toyokawa S, Tamiya N, et al. Changes in mortality inequalities across occupations in Japan: a national register based study of absolute and relative measures, 1980–2010. *BMJ Open* 2017;7:e015764.

19. Wada K, Kondo N, Gilmour S, et al. Trends in cause specific mortality across occupations in Japanese men of working age during period of economic stagnation, 1980–2005: retrospective cohort study. *BMJ* 2012;344:e1191.

20. Kachi Y, Inoue M, Nishikitani M, et al. Determinants of changes in income-related health inequalities among working-age adults in Japan, 1986–2007: time-trend study. *Soc Sci Med* 2013;81:94–101.

21. Nishikitani M, Tsurugano S, Inoue M, Yano E. Effect of unequal employment status on workers' health: results from a Japanese national survey. *Soc Sci Med* 2012;75:439–51.

22. Oshio T. Lingering impact of starting working life during a recession: health outcomes of survivors of the 'employment ice age' (1993–2004) in Japan. *J Epidemiol* 2019. doi: 10.2188/jea.JE20190121

23. OECD. Hours worked. Available at: https://data.oecd.org/emp/hours-worked.htm [last accessed 28 February 2020].

24. Bannai A, Tamakoshi A. The association between long working hours and health: a systematic review of epidemiological evidence. *Scand J Work Environ Health* 2014;40:5–18.

25. Ministry of Health, Labour and Welfare, Government of Japan. White Paper on Prevention of *Karoshi* 2018 (in Japanese). Available at: https://www.mhlw.go.jp/toukei_hakusho/hakusho/ [last accessed 28 February 2020].

26. OECD. GDP per hour worked. Available at: https://data.oecd.org/lprdty/gdp-per-hour-worked.htm [last accessed 28 February 2020].

27. Virtanen M, Kivimäki M, Joensuu M, et al. Temporary employment and health: a review. *Int J Epidemiol* 2005;34:610–22.

28. Kivimäki M, Vahtera J, Virtanen M, et al. Temporary employment and risk of overall and cause-specific mortality. *Am J Epidemiol* 2003;158(7):663–8.

29. Kachi Y, Otsuka T, Kawada T. Precarious employment and the risk of serious psychological distress: a population-based cohort study in Japan. *Scand J Work Environ Health* 2014;40:465–7.

30. Inoue M, Tsurugano S, Yano E. Job stress and mental health of permanent and fixed-term workers measured by effort-reward imbalance model, depressive complaints, and clinic utilization. *J Occup Health* 2011;53:93–101.

31. Honjo K, Iso H, Ikeda A, et al. Employment situation and risk of death among middle-aged Japanese women. *J Epidemiol Community Health* 2015;69:1012–17.

32. Ministry of Health, Labour and Welfare, Government of Japan. Report on occupational injury in 2017. Available at: https://www.mhlw.go.jp/bunya/roudoukijun/anzeneisei11/rousai-hassei/ [last accessed 28 February 2020].

33. Inoue A, Kawakami N, Tsuchiya M, Sakurai K, Hashimoto H. Association of occupation, employment contract, and company size with mental health in a national representative sample of employees in Japan. *J Occup Health* 2010;52:227–40.

34. Uchimura K, Ngamvithayapong-Yanai J, Kawatsu L, et al. Permanent employment or public assistance may increase tuberculosis survival among working-age patients in Japan. *Int J Tuberc Lung Dis* 2015;19:312–18.

35. Tanaka O, Maeda E, Fushimi M, et al. Precarious employment is not associated with increased depressive symptoms: a cross-sectional study in care service workers of Japan. *Tohoku J Exp Med* 2017;243:19–26.

36. Sugawara N, Yasui-Furukori N, Sasaki G, et al. Gender differences in factors associated with suicidal ideation and depressive symptoms among middle-aged workers in Japan. *Ind Health* 2013;51:202–13.

37. Inoue M, Tsurugano S, Nishikitani M, Yano E. Effort-reward imbalance and its association with health among permanent and fixed-term workers. *Biopsychosoc Med* 2010;4:16.

38. Inoue M, Tsurugano S, Nishikitani M, Yano E. Full-time workers with precarious employment face lower protection for receiving annual health check-ups. *Am J Ind Med* 2012;55:884–92.

39. Tsuno K, Kawakami N, Tsutsumi A, et al. Socioeconomic determinants of bullying in the workplace: a national representative sample in Japan. *PLoS One* 2015;10:e0119435.

40. Suga R, Tsuji M, Tanaka R, et al. Factors associated with occupation changes after pregnancy/delivery: results from Japan Environment & Children's pilot study. *BMC Womens Health* 2018;18:86.

41. Inoue M, Minami M, Yano E. Body mass index, blood pressure, and glucose and lipid metabolism among permanent and fixed-term workers in the manufacturing industry: a cross-sectional study. *BMC Public Health* 2014;14:207.

42. Tsurugano S, Inoue M, Yano E. Precarious employment and health: analysis of the Comprehensive National Survey in Japan. *Ind Health* 2012;50:223–35.

43. Ministry of Health, Labour and Welfare, Government of Japan. Outline of the 'Act on the Arrangement of Related Acts to Promote Work Style Reform' (Act No. 71 of 2018). Available at: https://www.mhlw.go.jp/english/policy/employ-labour/labour-standards/index.html [last accessed 28 February 2020].

8

Health and Financial Sustainability in Ageing Japan

Hideki Hashimoto

8.1 Introduction

The 2020 Olympic Games are coming back to Tokyo after 56 years. Tokyo has changed dramatically since the last Olympics, economically and technologically, but the most drastic change we can see is change in the demographics. When the Tokyo Olympic Games were held in 1964, the Japanese population was still young, with only 6% aged 65 and over. Today, the proportion has reached 28%, compared to 19% in the UK (Table 1.1). The pace of population ageing in Japan far exceeds that in European countries, while more rapid change is expected in China and other Asian countries in the next decades (Chapter 2). Japan's experience is a new model for the demographic ageing challenge era.

8.2 Health and Health Inequality in the Past Half Century in Japan

After World War II, Japan's life expectancy started its recovery from around 60 years old in the 1950s. By 1970, it reached the average of OECD countries, mainly owing to child mortality reduction through improved hygiene and economic conditions.[1] Since 1970, it exceeded the OECD average, specifically by improved survivorship among the middle- to old-aged populations through dramatic reduction in stroke mortality, as described in detail in Chapter 11.

What brought this drastic population health improvement? Marmot and Davey Smith[2] listed possible reasons, e.g. improved access to medical services through universal health coverage since 1961, improved diet behaviours through mass health education, etc. However, they specifically focused

Hideki Hashimoto, *Health and Financial Sustainability in Ageing Japan* In: *Health in Japan*. Edited by: Eric Brunner, Noriko Cable, and Hiroyasu Iso, Oxford University Press (2021). © Oxford University Press. DOI: 10.1093/oso/9780198848134.003.0008.

on Japan's normative attitude towards socioeconomic equality. In respect of health equity, a World Bank report in 2014 endorsed the view that Japan's universal health coverage policy helped to equalize national income distribution, particularly by increasing the resilience of economically vulnerable older people to maintain their health.[3]

Whether Japan is a more equal country than the UK is a matter of debate. In Japan, improvement of life expectancy was accompanied by a closing gap in life expectancy at prefectural level. There was almost six years difference in life expectancy during the 1960s, which was reduced to about two years in the late 1970s. In other words, equality and longevity in population health were simultaneously achieved in a relatively short period in Japan. Since 2000, the within-country gap in life expectancy across prefectures has enlarged. This reversal in health equity is not explained by local availability of medical and healthcare resources.[4,5] The next section explores the health gap in Japan in terms of cause of death.

8.2.1 Population Ageing and the Changing Trend in Causes of Death

The major causes of death in Japan were once stroke, followed by cancer, then heart disease, until 1979. Afterwards, cancer came to the top, followed by stroke and heart disease, and most recently by pneumonia.[6]

Besides this, a large disease burden of non-life-threatening disability conditions were derived mainly from low back and neck pain, sensory loss e.g. hearing and vision, and depression, of which contribution has been constantly observed in the past three decades.[5] With population ageing, some other conditions are expected to be further added to the nation's burden of disease and disability. They are frailty and dementia, which are discussed in the next section.

8.2.2 Prevalence and Risk Factors for Frailty in the UK, US, Japan, and Other Countries

Frailty is defined as 'a clinical syndrome in which three or more of the following criteria are present; unintentional weight loss (10 lbs in the past year), self-reported exhaustion, weakness (grip strength), slow walking speed, and low physical activity'.[7] Frailty is not uncommon among older people.

A community-based study of people aged 65 years and older in the US reported that the overall prevalence of frailty was 6.9%. A large community-based study in Japan showed a similar prevalence of 5.6%.[8] However, a recent Japanese community-based study in a city near Kyoto reported the prevalence of frailty (using the same criteria) to be about 10% in both men and women.[9]

Frailty poses a risk of physical function decline, loss of independence, need for long-term care, and mortality, which is also thought to be related to other ageing-related chronic conditions such as osteoporosis, sarcopenia (or reduction in muscle strength and mass), depression, and malnutrition.[8] Ongoing discussion places frailty as a consequence of biological conditions (e.g. genetic properties determining muscle volume, malnutrition, and/or chronic diseases), as well as of ongoing interactions with socioeconomic conditions such as poor education, economic deprivation, and social isolation. Given the prevalence and impact of bio-socio-psychological consequences of ageing, frailty becomes a major public health issue in Japan. Public health issues related to ageing are concerns of other countries as well as Japan, including the UK and US, that are explored further in the next section.

8.2.3 Prevalence and Risk Factors for Dementia in the UK, US, Japan, and Other Countries

Dementia is another threat to population health in ageing/aged society. Dementia is basically characterized by the loss of short-term memory function that deters orientation of time and space, contextual understanding, and subsequently social interaction, with other dysfunction in emotional and physical control. The pathological causes of dementia are diverse; vascular dementia by lacunar stroke was the major one, but has been replaced with Alzheimer's disease, or a degeneration of nerve cells in parts of the brain related to cognition.

A unique study on dementia has been conducted in a suburban town in Southern Japan, Hisayama Town, located about five miles away from Hakata City, the largest city in Kyushu district. Since 1985, a research team at Kyushu University has periodically tracked the cognitive function of the majority of community dwellers aged over 65, through health checkups, screening interviews, and brain imaging tests with a specially equipped mobile brain scanner. In addition to this, the majority of residents provided informed consent to allow post-mortem examination after their death, which allowed researchers to confirm the pathological basis of dementia status.[10,11]

The Hisayama study revealed that the prevalence and incidence rate of dementia has been increasing in Japan beyond the pace of population ageing from 1985 until 2012. The crude prevalence (without adjustment for age composition) among those aged 65 and over in 1985 was 5.7%, then went up to 7.1% (1992), 12.5% (2005), and 17.9% (2012).[10] Currently, the best available estimate of dementia prevalence in Japan, at 15% among those aged 65 and over,[12,13] comes from a survey undertaken in eight rural cities including Hisayama in 2009–2012.

The prevalence in Japan seems considerably higher, compared to existing reports from the UK, US, and even China.[14–16] A large nation-wide social survey of older people in the US identified that the prevalence of dementia was 11.6% among those aged 65 and over as of 2000, and the number has slightly declined to 8.8% in 2012.[14] This decreasing trend of incident rates and age-specific morbidity rates in the past few decades was also observed in the Netherlands[17] and the UK.[15,18,19] Studies have argued that this decreasing trend can be attributed to improved education levels of older people and better treatment and prevention of cardiovascular risk factors, despite increasing prevalence of obesity and diabetes. The reason why the prevalence in Japan is higher and increasing until recently is not known.[NB1]

Previous studies in the US, UK, and Japan consistently found that prevalence of dementia is higher among older old age (aged over 75), and women.[14,20–22] Hypertension and subsequent cerebrovascular diseases were a significant predictor for vascular dementia, while it had no clear association with Alzheimer's disease. Instead, diabetes is a significant risk factor for Alzheimer's disease.[21,22] There have been no associations observed between serum cholesterol level and dementia incidence in Japan. In addition, socioeconomic conditions (lower educational attainment and low income/wealth), and psychiatric conditions (e.g. depression and other major psychiatric diseases) are also known to be associated with dementia.[20]

8.2.4 Future Projection of Dementia Prevalence in the UK, US, and Japan

A group of government sponsored researchers estimated that the number of dementia patients in Japan will increase from 4.7 M (15.0%) in 2012 to 8 M,

---

[1] Most recent unpublished data show that dementia prevalence starts decreasing even in Japan (personal communication with Dr. Toba at the National Institute of Ageing Japan).

or 21% of those aged 65 and over, in 2040.[23] The researchers projected the number could reach 9.5 M in the worst scenario if the increasing trend of diabetes was taken into consideration. The chapter author and his colleague re-estimated the number with the most recently available microsimulation.[24] According to the simulation, the decreasing trend of stroke and increasing trend of diabetes will cancel out each other, resulting in the future estimation of the number of people with dementia to be around 6 M or less. Since reliable estimates of dementia prevalence are not available after 2012, the future projection of dementia prevalence requires further scientific investigation in Japan.

Compared to the projection in Japan, a recent study in the UK estimated the number of people with dementia to be approximately 0.8 M as of 2016, or about 7% of those aged over 65. Despite decreasing trends in incidence and age-specific morbidity rates, the absolute number of people affected by dementia is expected to increase by up to 1.2 M in 2040 in the UK due to improved longevity.[15]

In the US, Hurd et al[20] projected, based on their estimated age-specific prevalence of dementia as of 2010, that the future prevalence of dementia amongst those aged 70 and over would be 16% as of 2040. The authors re-estimated the number under various scenarios of future trend change in the prevalence of dementia, diabetes, and obesity that ranged between 9–16%.[25]

8.3 Policy Response to Social Challenge by Population Ageing in Japan

Japan's frontier position in population ageing as shown earlier in this chapter invokes unique social, economic, and cultural challenges to Japanese society. Ageing population requires increasing demand and larger fiscal space for health and social care, while the productivity of the nation's economy is threatened by decreasing proportion of working age population.

8.3.1 Social and Nursing Care for Older People through Long-Term Care Insurance (LTCI) in Japan

Caregiving for older people in need has relied exclusively on informal care by female family members in many countries. In Japan and other East Asian countries, a traditional family system bound to Confucianism-based seniority culture is still prevalent, which often requires the first son of the family to be responsible for the provision of care for frail older parents, and related gender-role norms forces his wife to be a primary caregiver. Due to demographic change, the size and care capacity of the household has been decreased, and the burden of informal care provision can be overwhelming to such an extent that occasionally it can result in abuse or homicide/suicide of frail elderly by family caregivers even today in Japan.[26,27]

To release the family caregiver from this overwhelming burden of informal care provision, and to provide choice in healthcare options for frail older people, the Japanese government launched the universal coverage of public LTCI for those aged over 65 since 2000.[28] The public LTCI was driven by municipality local government but under a nationwide standardized protocol and fee schedule that covers domiciliary and nursing homecare, community-based formal care including respite care, and institutionalized social and nursing care in this country.

Following a request to the local office, the beneficiary older person is assessed by a municipality board on his/her functional capacity, following the nationally standardized eligibility assessment protocol. Once certified as eligible, the beneficiaries are allowed to use any combination of formal services of social and nursing care under a monthly upper limit of utilization according to their eligibility levels, with 10% copayment and protection from catastrophic copayment, without means test and regardless of household composition.[26] The Japanese system does not provide cash benefit, and all benefits are provided as in-kind services, while the German system allows cash benefit which enables the recipients to pay for family caregivers.[29]

Eligibility criteria is composed of six categories according to the severity of physical and cognitive functional impairment and estimated length of time needed for personal care based on a pilot time study; two support levels (functionally independent but needing attention) and five care levels (moderately to severely disabled) exist. The highest level corresponds to bed-ridden dependent conditions requiring personal support for meals, toileting, clothing, and bathing. Beneficiaries of support levels were eligible to use 'preventive care', or a package of home nurse visits, supportive personal care at home, and respite services. Beneficiaries of care levels were free to choose any combination of 'preventive', social, and nursing care. Compared to the public long-term care system in Germany, the Japanese system is generously open to those with mild disability, totalling about 30% of the eligible beneficiaries.[29]

8.3.2 Financing and Performance of LTCI in Japan

Japanese public LTCI is operationally managed by local municipality-based government insurers. Currently, more than 1,830 municipality insurers provide the services. The LTCI is financed by premiums (50%) and tax subsidies from local municipalities themselves (12.5%), prefectures (12.5%), and the central government (25%). The premium price is amended every three years by each insurer based on the balance of local utilization and cost. In the 2015–2017 period, monthly premium prices ranged widely from 12 GBP to 41 GBP across insurers. Otherwise, the LTCI is allowed to collect copayments from the benefit recipient of 10% of total utilization. More recently, beneficiaries with higher incomes (about 1–2% of beneficiaries) have been asked to pay 20–30% of the copayment rate.

Payment to service providers is based on fee-for-service schemes, with the single nationwide fee schedule priced on a service-per-unit basis. Every three years the fee schedule is amended by the central pricing committee of the Ministry of Health, Labour, and Welfare. The price is universally applied to providers across Japan, without local adjustment. No extra- or under-charge to the standardized fee schedule is allowed.

Since its introduction, the number of eligible beneficiaries has been rapidly growing from 2.2 M older persons in 2000 to 6.3 M in 2017, and the amount of service utilization from 3,600 billion JPY (or 24.8 billion GBP) in 2000 to 74.4 billion GBP in 2017, or 6.7% annual growth rate on average, far exceeding the growth rate of medical care expenditure. About half of the expenditure is spent on social care at home and preventive care.

Several empirical assessments on the effect of these long-term systems of care revealed that it did increase the labour participation rate of women, suggesting it has somehow emancipated women from the normative obligation of informal caregiving at home.[30] However, the increase was only observable among women in high-medium income families,[26] while women with low socioeconomic status remain responsible for informal caregiving, especially for frail elderly relatives with severe disabilities. Otherwise, there is no clear evidence suggesting that the public LTCI reduced the burden on family caregivers. Furthermore, there is no sound evidence indicating that the introduction of public LTCI prevents elderly from frailty, or facilitates their functional recovery.[26]

Even after the introduction of this public care system, informal caregiving by family members remains the major source of social care for frail elderly as it is culturally expected in Japan, and formal care provision by the public system has been regarded solely as a complementary resource.[31] The types of formal care chosen by beneficiaries is determined not only by their functional disability types and levels, but also by the characteristics of family caregivers; e.g. those taken care of by daughters-in-law are more likely to use respite day care services, while those cared for by male spouses and sons are more likely to use house-keeping services.[27] As such, social care for older people in Japan relies heavily on the private domain of family, in line with societal norms, even though it has been two decades since the introduction of the public LTCI system.

8.3.3 'New Orange Plan' and 'Community-based Integrated Care' Programme

In anticipation of the increasing burden of senile dementia, the Japanese government launched a social programme called 'Orange Plan' to prepare medical, technological, and social countermeasures to prevent dementia and to enhance social inclusion of dementia patients through a cross-sectorial collaborative programme led by the Cabinet Office since 2010. The plan has been revised as the 'New Orange Plan'(see https://www.mhlw.go.jp/stf/seisakunitsuite/bunya/0000064084.html) and since 2015 the policy goals have been:

- to provide clinical specialty training for physicians specialized in dementia care and coordination of local institutions to support patients with dementia and their family ('Support Doctor' programme);
- to provide educational programmes to raise understanding and informed choice about dementia care, treatment, and end-of-life care among citizen volunteers ('Supporter' programme);
- to invest in research so as to accumulate evidence to prevent dementia, and to develop innovative treatment and care technology for patients with dementia;
- to involve the labour market to build supportive work environments and provide employment support for people with dementia;
- to establish consumer right protection mechanisms to protect people with dementia from unfair treatment, maltreatment, and deception;
- to enhance public transport systems and universal design of public space and housing for safety and social participation of people with dementia and frailty.

As of February 2019, reportedly 8,000 support doctors and 11 M support volunteers have joined training and/or educational programmes, the numbers far larger than originally planned in 2015. However, when these figures are examined in more detail, we can see that roughly a quarter of support volunteers are school children, and about a third are community participants aged 60 and older. The effectiveness of the plan on the prevention of dementia and improvement in quality of life for people with dementia and their caregivers remains to be seen, even nine years after the original Orange Plan was put into practice.

The government has also put forward a policy agenda called the 'Community-based Integrated Care system', that proposes the involvement and integration of public and private institutions available in the local region to efficiently produce resources for social and health care for older people in need (see also https://www.mhlw.go.jp/english/policy/care-welfare/care-welfare-elderly/dl/establish_e.pdf). Community-based Integrated Care aims at more than a coordinated healthcare system, benefitting from volunteer involvement and community support based on community solidarity. Although ambitious, the concept is starting to be translated into action, but currently suffers from ambiguous job descriptions, conflict of interest between parties, and lack of a clear governance system. See Chapter 9 for details about recent discussion, local examples, and remaining challenges.

8.3.4 Medical Care for Older People in Japan

The Japanese public healthcare system generously covers outpatient, inpatient, prescription, and dental services under universal healthcare coverage based on a social insurance scheme and tax transfer since 1961.[32] Thanks to a free access policy without gatekeeping, reduced copayment rates for older people aged above 70, and public subsidy protection against catastrophic copayment, Japanese older people face fewer challenges in accessing healthcare for economic reasons, compared to their counterparts in other high-income countries in Europe and the US,[33] and equity in healthcare access between the rich and the poor is highly secured specifically for older people.[34,35]

Although the policy design of Japan's public healthcare system is accessible specifically for older people, it poses a challenge to the financial sustainability of the healthcare system due to rapidly increasing expenditure as a result of population ageing, and the fact that the Japanese economy has been stagnant in the past few decades. The total expenditure covered by public health insurance amounts to 41,000 billion JPY, or 283 billion GBP in 2018, with an annual growth rate of 2.6% on average in the past two decades. The expenditure on those aged 65 and over accounts for more than half of total healthcare spending. In the last few decades, the increase in healthcare expenditure has been attributed mainly to the increased care needs for patients in this older age segment[36] (Figure 8.1). Increased expenditure on older people's care is affected by the high frequency of service use, despite a relatively low unit price per visit.

Since 2008, the government has increased the copayment rate from 10% to 20% for older people with relatively high income, in order to increase financial viability and discourage use of non-essential services.[33] However, the growth rate of healthcare expenditure has not been diminished. The government also introduced the national health checkup programme in 2008, following a rationale that preventive services for cardiovascular diseases and obesity would save money in the long run. However, the cost-saving benefit of the health checkup programme has not been empirically proven, and the most recent policy review by OECD questioned its efficiency.[37]

Further plans to manage healthcare finance include institutional regulation in local healthcare systems. The newly amended Medical Service Act (*Iryo-ho* in Japanese) in 2016 mandates prefectural governors to manage excess supply of in-patient services by leading a local negotiation table inviting public and

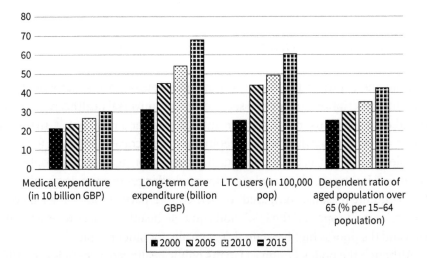

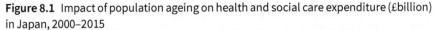

Figure 8.1 Impact of population ageing on health and social care expenditure (£billion) in Japan, 2000–2015

Source: data from National Medical Expenditure, and Long-term Care Insurance Reports. Ministry of Health, Labour and Welfare. 2017.

private healthcare stakeholders, although an effective governance mechanism for resource reallocation between providers has not been established until recently.

8.4 Future Projection and Future Challenge for Japan in 2035

What is the future of Japan as the front-line aged society on the globe? Currently, prevailing projections are very pessimistic (e.g. World Economic Forum[87]); the increasing demand of medical and long-term care for older people, combined with the decreasing working-age population to support the burden of population ageing, threatens the financial sustainability of the Japanese future economy. However, most recent projections developed by the chapter author and his colleague suggest a slightly different story. First, population ageing is not necessarily leading to an unhealthier population. The incidence rate and case fatality rate of stroke, heart disease, and cancer, three major killers in Japan, are constantly decreasing. With continued improvement in the health of older people, it is likely there will be fewer patients suffering from stroke or heart disease in the future compared to now.[24] (Figure 8.2)

Improved longevity would result in new challenges of frailty, dementia, and other chronic conditions, however, expected savings by reduced morbidity would be cancelled out by additional costs for emerging morbidity, with the result that the total expected medical expenditure would only marginally change in spite of population ageing. If the medical expenditure were to exponentially rise, this would mainly be caused by technology innovation and subsequent price inflation. To put it in other words, medical expenditure will not necessarily be an unavoidable burden of population ageing if cost control over technology innovation becomes effective.

However, expenditure for social and nursing care will increase due to two major reasons. One is the increased prevalence of dementia and frailty. The other is the increased demand for formal care due to decreasing capacity for informal care in households. In 2035, metropolitan Tokyo estimates that about half of those aged 65 and over will live alone.[39] Thus, informal care provision by family will no longer be expected as the default source for social care in households, and demand for formal care provision will be accelerated in the near future in Japan (Visionary Future Health; https://visionary.future-health.jp/).

(a)

Top left

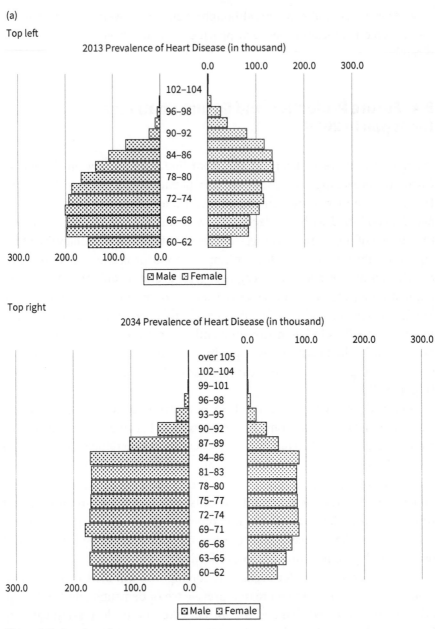

Figure 8.2 Continued.

(b)

Bottom left

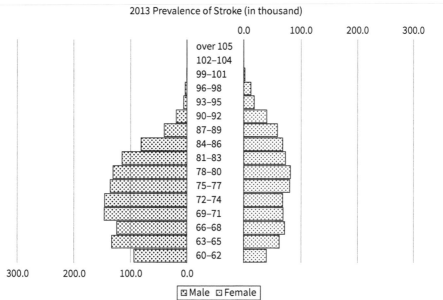

Bottom right

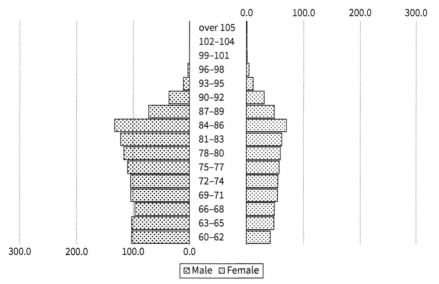

Figure 8.2 Future projection of prevalence (in thousands) of heart disease and stroke among Japanese aged 60+ in 2034 from 2013 by sex.

Men on left (dark bars), women on right (light bars).

Source: adapted from Kasajima et al. Stanford University APARC Working Paper Series #55, 2019.

8.5 Lessons Learnt from the Challenge of Population Ageing in Japan

As discussed in this chapter, Japan, as a front runner of population ageing, faces a future that the human species has never experienced. The good news is that population ageing does not necessarily mean more diseases and higher medical expenditure, thanks to improved longevity and health status among older people. However, improved longevity has brought another challenge of increased demand for social and nursing care due to the increase in numbers of men and women with frailty and dementia. Most prominently, demographic change by population ageing will also require reform in Japanese social norms around family caregiving, social participation, and the role of individuals and the government.

Indeed, our real challenge is not population ageing and the subsequent disease/disability burden. Instead, it is our norms and culture in regard to ageing. Importantly, ageing is no longer about 'weakness' and 'burden'. Older people are not the marginalized exception; ageing is part of social reality. Population ageing requires a new culture of social inclusion. Technology may help us better cope with disease treatment and disability support. However, what society really has to face is the reform of culture around 'being old'. Can Japan successfully face this challenge? We are already witnessing the answer to this question.

References

1. Ikeda N, Saito E, Kondo N, et al. What has made the population of Japan healthy? *Lancet* 2011;378(9796):1094–105. doi: 10.1016/S0140-6736(11)61055-6
2. Marmot MG, Davey Smith G. Why are the Japanese living longer? *BMJ* 1989;23–30;299(6715):1547–51.
3. Oshio T, Miake N, Ikegami N. Macroeconomic context and challenges for maintaining universal health coverage in Japan. In: Ikegami N (ed.). *Universal Health Coverage for Inclusive and Sustainable Development: Lessons from Japan.* Washington, DC: The World Bank 2014. Report 91163:27–40. doi: 10.1596/978-1-4648-0408-3
4. Nomura S, Sakamoto H, Glenn S, et al. Population health and regional variations of disease burden in Japan, 1990–2015: a systematic subnational analysis for the Global Burden of Disease Study 2015. *Lancet* 2017;390(10101):1521–38. doi: 10.1016/S0140-6736(17)31544-1

5. Ministry of Health, Labour and Welfare. Special report of vital statistics 2017 on prefectural mortality trend 2015 (*Jinkodotai tokei tokushuhokoku 2015 Todofukenbetu shiboritsuno gaikyo*). Available at: https://www.mhlw.go.jp/toukei/saikin/hw/jinkou/other/15sibou/index.html [last accessed 5 March 2020].

6. Ministry of Health, Labour and Welfare. Yearly summary of monthly vital statistics report for 2017. Available at: https://www.mhlw.go.jp/toukei/saikin/hw/jinkou/geppo/nengai17/dl/gaikyou29-190626.pdf [last accessed 5 March 2020].

7. Fried LP, Tangen CM, Walston J, et al. Frailty in older adults: evidence for a phenotype. *J Gerontol A Biol Sci Med Sci* 2001;56(3):M146–56.

8. Yoshimura N, Muraki S, Oka H, et al. Do sarcopenia and/or osteoporosis increase the risk of frailty? A 4-year observation of the second and third ROAD study surveys. *Osteoporos Int* 2018;29(10):2181–90. doi: 10.1007/s00198-018-4596-4

9. Yamada Y, Nanri H, Watanabe Y, et al. Prevalence of frailty assessed by Fried and Kihon Checklist Indexes in a prospective cohort study: design and demographics of the Kyoto-Kameoka longitudinal study. *J Am Med Dir Assoc* 2017;18(8):733.e7–733.e15. doi: 10.1016/j.jamda.2017.02.022

10. Ohara T, Kiyohara Y, Kamba S. Epidemiology of dementia in the community-dwelling elderly: the Hisayama study. *Kyushu Shinkei Seishin Igaku (Kyushu Psychiatrics and Neurological Medicine)* 2013;60(2):83–91.

11. Sekita A, Ninomiya T, Tanizaki Y, et al. Trends in prevalence of Alzheimer's disease and vascular dementia in a Japanese community: the Hisayama study. *Acta Psychiatr Scand* 2010;122:319–25.

12. Asada T (ed.). Toshibu ni okeru ninchisho yubyouritsu to ninchisho no seikatu kinoushougai heno taiou (Prevalence of dementia in urban settings, and countermeasures to disabled daily life activities) (in Japanese). Research report by the Research in Aid of Comprehensive Treatment of Dementia team, Ministry of Health, Welfare and Labour, Government of Japan. March 2013.

13. Ikejima C, Hisanaga A, Meguro K, et al. Multicentre population-based dementia prevalence survey in Japan: a preliminary report. *Psychogeriatrics* 2012;12:120–3. doi: 10.1111/j.1479-8301.2012.00415x

14. Langa KM, Larson EB, Crimmins EM, et al. A comparison of the prevalence of dementia in the United States in 2000 and 2013. *JAMA Intern Med* 2017;177(1):51–8. doi: 10.10001/jamainternmed.2016.6807

15. Ahmadi-Abhari S, Guzman-Castillo M, Bandosz P, et al. Temporal trend in dementia incidence since 2002 and projections for prevalence in England and Wales to 2040: modelling study. *BMJ* 2017;358:2856. doi: 10.1136/bmj.j2856

16. Wu YT, Lee HY, Norton S, et al. Prevalence studies of dementia in mainland china, Hong Kong and Taiwan: a systematic review and meta-analysis. *PLoS One* 2013;8(6):e66252.

17. Schrijvers EMC, Verhaaren BFJ, Koudstaal PJ, et al. Is dementia incidence declining? Trends in dementia incidence since 1990 in the Rotterdam study. *Neurology* 2012;78(19):1456–63.

18. Matthews F, Arthur A, Barnes LE, et al. A two-decade comparison of prevalence of dementia in individuals aged 65 years and older from three geographical areas of England: results of the Cognitive Function and Ageing Study I and II. *Lancet* 2013;382:1405–12.

19. Matthews FE, Stephan BC, Robinson L, et al. Cognitive Function and Ageing Studies (CFAS) Collaboration. A two decade dementia incidence comparison from the Cognitive Function and Ageing Studies I and II. *Nat Commun* 2016;7:11398. doi: 10.1038/ncomms11398

20. Hurd MD, Martorell P, Delanvande A, et al. Monetary cost of dementia in the United States. *N Engl J Med* 2013;368(14):1326–34. doi: 10.1056/NEJMsa1204629

21. Ninomiya T, Ohara T, Hirakawa Y, et al. Midlife and late-life blood pressure and dementia in Japanese elderly: the Hisayama study. *Hypertension* 2011;58;22–8.

22. Ohara T, Doi Y, Ninomiya T, et al. Glucose tolerance status and risk of dementia in the community: the Hisayama study. *Neurology* 2011;77:1126–34.

23. Ninomiya T (ed.). Nihon ni okeru ninchisho no koureishajinko no shouraisuikei ni kansuru kenkyuu (Future projection of dementia prevalence among the old Japanese) (in Japanese). Research report by the Research in Aid of Special Research Program by the Ministry of Health, Labour and Welfare, Government of Japan. March 2015.

24. Kasajima M, Hashimoto H, Suen SC, et al. Future projection of the health and functional status of older people in Japan: a pseudo-panel microsimulation model. Stanford University APARC Working Paper Series #55, 2019.

25. Hurd M, Langa K. Future monetary cost of dementia in the United States under alternative dementia prevalence scenarios. *J Popul Ageing* 2015;8(1–2):101–12. doi: 10.1007/s12062-015-9112-4

26. Tamiya N, Noguchi H, Nishi A, et al. Population ageing and wellbeing: lessons from Japan's long-term care insurance policy. *Lancet* 2011;378 (9797):1183–92.

27. Tokunaga M, Hashimoto H, Tamiya N. A gap in formal long-term care use related to characteristics of caregivers and households, under the public universal system in Japan: 2001–2010. *Health Policy* 2015;119(6):840–9. doi: 10.1016/j.healthpol.2014.10.015

28. Ikegami N. Public long-term care insurance in Japan. *JAMA* 1997;278(16):1310–14.

29. Campbell JC, Ikegami N, Gibson MJ. Lessons from public long-term care insurance in Germany and Japan. *Health Aff (Millwood)* 2010;29(1):87–95. doi: 10.1377/hlthaff.2009.0548

30. Fu R, Noguchi H, Kawamura A, et al. Spillover effect of Japanese long-term care insurance as an employment promotion policy for family caregivers. *J Health Econ Dev* 2017;56:103–12. Available at: https://doi.org/10.1016/j.jhealeco.2017.09.011 [last accessed 5 March 2020].

31. Tokunaga M, Hashimoto H. The socioeconomic within-gender gap in informal caregiving among middle-aged women: evidence from a Japanese nation-wide survey. *Soc Sci Med* 2017;173:48–53. Available at: https://doi.org/10.1016/j.socscimed.2016.11.037 [last accessed 5 March 2020].

32. Ikegami N, Yoo BK, Hashimoto H, et al. Japanese universal health coverage: evolution, achievements, and challenges. *Lancet* 2011;378(9796):1106–15. doi: 10.1016/S0140-6736(11)60828-3

33. Sakamoto H, Rahman M, Nomura S, et al. Japan Health System Review 8(1). New Delhi: WHO Regional Office for South-East Asia 2018.

34. Watanabe R, Hashimoto H. Horizontal inequity in healthcare access under the universal coverage in Japan: 1986–2007. *Soc Sci Med* 2012;75(8):1372–8. doi: 10.1016/j.socscimed.2012.06.006

35. Shigeoka H. The effect of patient cost sharing on utilization, health, and risk protection. *American Economic Review*;104(7):2152–84. doi: 10.1257/aer.104.7.2152

36. Ministry of Health, Labour and Welfare. Health Expenditure Report 2016. Tokyo: MHLW 2018.

37. OECD. *OECD Reviews of Public Health: Japan: A Healthier Tomorrow.* Paris: OECD Publishing. Available at: https://doi.org/10.1787/9789264311602-en [last accessed 5 March 2020].

38. World Economic Forum. Japan's population is shrinking: what does it mean for the economy? Available at: https://www.weforum.org/agenda/2016/02/japans-population-is-shrinking-what-does-it-mean-for-the-economy/ [last accessed 5 March 2020].

39. Tokyo Metropolitan Government. Available at: http://www.metro.tokyo.jp/tosei/hodohappyo/press/2019/03/28/33.html [last accessed 5 March 2020].

9

Dementia and Healthy Ageing in Older People

Katsunori Kondo

9.1 Introduction

Japan has been the top runner of ageing societies globally since the 1980s.[1] Japan has worked hard to adapt to social change and to tackle the social problems which arise in its ageing society, such as promoting healthy ageing and the need for an increasing volume of long-term care, especially dementia care. This chapter describes and discusses the following issues based on Japanese experiences: changes in society and family structure from the end of World War II to the present; responses to the increasing number of older people with impairments and disabilities including dementia; caregiving problems; healthy ageing policy to reduce the care burden; establishing the 'Community-based Integrated Care System'; policy emphasis on dementia care policy; prevention policy reform from high risk strategy to population strategy; and implications for other countries.

9.1.1 Changes in Society and Family Structure from the End of World War II to the Present

Japanese society and population changed profoundly after World War II (Chapter 1). Average longevity increased from 59.6 years for men and 63.0 years for women in 1950 to 81.1 years for men and 87.3 years for women in 2018. The industrial structure has evolved from primary industry to secondary and tertiary industries. As a result, there was a large population movement from rural to urban areas, particularly in the younger generation. The proportion of the population engaging in primary industries has decreased from 19.3% in 1945 to 3.5% in 2015.[2] Also, the self-employment rate decreased substantially from 57.6% in 1953 to 12.3% in 2010, whereas the proportion

Katsunori Kondo, *Dementia and Healthy Ageing in Older People* In: *Health in Japan.* Edited by: Eric Brunner, Noriko Cable, and Hiroyasu Iso, Oxford University Press (2021). © Oxford University Press. DOI: 10.1093/oso/9780198848134.003.0009.

employed increased. It has long been recognized that ageing of the population means the number of retired older people, and the time spent with low income after retirement, is increasing.

To respond to those predicted social changes, the universal pension system was introduced in 1961 (Table 6.1). Matured pensions have made it possible for older people to live independently from their children's families. Together with population movement to urban areas, these developments caused changes in traditional family structure. Three-generation-family households and male breadwinner households are declining even among households containing one or more people aged 65 and over (Figure 5.1).[3] Couple-only and solo (one person) households are increasing. These widespread demographic changes mean that older people who need daily support often cannot be cared for by family care givers such as a daughter-in-law, as was the tradition. The necessity for social care provision as an alternative to family care giving was recognized in the 1990s.

9.2 Policy Responses to Increasing Need for Social Care in Older People

The number of people affected by disability, including dementia, has increased rapidly since the 1960s. About 60% of older people with a disability have cognitive decline or dementia, and the prevalence of dementia is around 5% for 65–69 year olds to 60–80% for 95–99 year olds.[4] As family care giving capacity is decreased by social changes after WW II, demands for social care have been increasing. In general Japanese people tend to dislike increasing taxes, while they accept an increase in their health insurance premium payment. Table 9.1 reflects general preference, following the ongoing shortage of tax-funded long-term care facilities and increase in hospital beds subsequent to the expansion of healthcare expenditure for older people during the 1970s.[5]

Hospitals, instead of long-term facilities, admit many older people with a disability. This causes the longest length of hospital stay among developed countries[1] and inappropriate medical-care focused treatment instead of comprehensive care during the 1980s, referred to as 'social hospitalization' or 'bedridden older people'.

After establishing the Gold Plan (a ten-year strategy for the promotion of the health and welfare of older people) and urgent preparation of facilities and in-home welfare services for older people, the Japanese government introduced public long-term care insurance (LTCI) in 2000.

Table 9.1 Historical development of welfare policies for older people in Japan since 1960

	Over 65 years old/ total population (in thousands) Ageing rate per year	Major policies
1960s: Beginning of welfare policies for older people	5,398/94,302 5.7% (1960)	1963: Enactment of the Act on Social Welfare Services for older people • Intensive care homes for the elderly created • Legislation on home helpers for the elderly
1970s: Expansion of healthcare expenditures for older people	7,393/104,665 7.1% (1970)	1973: Free healthcare for the elderly
1980s: Social hospitalization and bedridden elderly people seen as social problems	10,647/117,060 9.1% (1980)	1982: Enactment of the Health and Medical Services Act for the Aged • Adoption of the payment of copayments for elderly healthcare, etc. 1989: Establishment of the Gold Plan (ten-year strategy for the promotion of health and welfare for the elderly) • Promotion of the urgent preparation of facilities and in-home welfare services
1990s: Promotion of the Gold Plan	14,895/123,611 12.0% (1990)	1994: Establishment of the New Gold Plan (new ten-year strategy for the promotion of health and welfare for the elderly) • Improvement of in-home long-term care
Preparation for adoption of the Long-Term Care Insurance System	18,261/125,570 14.5% (1995)	1997: Enactment of the Long-Term Care Insurance Act
2000s: Introduction of the Long-Term Care Insurance System	22,005/126,926 17.3% (2000)	2000: Enforcement of the Long-Term Care Insurance System
2010s: Introduction of the Community-based Care System (CBICS) and promotion of the Orange Plan	29,246/128,057 23.0% (2010)	2012: Establishment of the Orange Plan (Five-year plan for Promotion of Measures against Dementia) 2013: Introduction of the Community-based Care System (CBICS) 2015: Establishment of the New Orange Plan (Comprehensive Strategy to Accelerate Dementia Measures)

The number of people eligible for public long-term care insurance increased.[5] The speed of growth was faster than estimated in 1996 by the Ministry of Health, Labour, and Welfare (MHLW)[6] before the introduction of LTCI. Compared to estimates of 2.8 M, 3.9 M, and 5.2 M in 2000, 2010, and 2025 respectively, in real terms 2.18 M in 2000 was rather lower, but 4.87 M in 2010 was higher, and had already climbed to 5.33 M in 2012, 13 years earlier than estimated.

This growth did not correlate with number of care givers, causing a shortage. MHLW estimated the shortage of human resources for social care at 377,000 in 2025.[7] Colleges and technical schools for care worker education increased their capacity, but these places were not taken up, possibly because the Japanese public regard care work as the so-called '3Ks', i.e. *Kitsui* (hard), *Kitanai* (dirty), and *Kyuryo yasui* (low-paid). The government raised LTCI benefits, providing the financial resources necessary in order to award a pay rise for care workers.

As other countermeasures for the shortage of care workers, the government have started permitting care workers from overseas and have invested to develop care robots as a substitute for human care. These measures are not proving effective to-date. The number of non-Japanese who passed the national qualifying examination for care work lies far behind targets, and a case of an older person drowning during bathing when using a machine has been reported.[8]

9.3 Healthy Ageing Policy as an Instrument to Reduce Need for Social Care

Another countermeasure to eliminate the care burden and the demand-supply gap in social care workers is to strengthen the healthy ageing policy. When 'healthy ageing' is realized, the quality of life of older people increases, demand for care giving is reduced, the family no longer needs to take on the care giver role, and the demand-supply gap of care workers can be moderated.

In 2005, policy reviews of the first five years following the introduction of LTCI in 2000 highlighted that the proportion of older people with a severe disability (care level 3–5) had not dramatically increased, but those with a mild disability (support level to care level 1) increased remarkably from 2000 to 2005.[5] Reducing the proportion of older people with a mild disability was expected to be achieved by an enhanced prevention policy from 2006, called 'care prevention'. This preventions policy for older people with mild disability was based on a high-risk approach, in which older people with frailty were screened and invited to exercise classes.

9.3.1 Establishing the 'Community-based Integrated Care System'

From 2008, MHLW started the discussion on the Community-based Integrated Care System (CBICS) and introduced it into the law from 2013. The aim of CBICS is to make it possible for older people to age in a place familiar to them, in their own way, even if they later become heavily reliant on long-term care. The background to the discussion around CBICS was a shortage and fragmentation of resources including health care, nursing care, prevention, housing, and livelihood support, which need to be integrated in order to achieve their aim. Other factors include the wide discrepancy between people in the speed of ageing, and population shrinkage between municipalities which are insurers of LTCI. Large cities have witnessed rapidly growing older populations with an increase of whole population overall, while on the other hand, the total population of towns and villages has been decreasing, with a gradual increase in the population aged over 75. It is necessary for municipalities as LTC insurers to establish and manage the CBICS based on care needs, because future goals and issues to be confronted among communities will differ from each other.

By 2025, when the baby boomers will be aged 75 and over, a system called CBICS should be established. It is a community-based integrated system that should ensure the provision of healthcare, long-term nursing care, prevention, housing, and livelihood support.[5] Through the CBICS, it is envisioned that older people should be able to grow old in a place familiar to them, even if they develop a disabling health condition such as dementia, until the end of life.

9.4 Dementia Care Policy: A Staged System

In 2012, one year before the G8 dementia summit held in London, the Japanese government published its 'Orange Plan', a five-year plan for accelerating measures for dementia, from prevention to the final stage of the disease. In November 2014, with the Global Dementia Legacy Event in Japan, this was revised to the 'New Orange Plan' (2015–2020).[5]

The clinical journey of the person with dementia depends on the severity of their disability including Behavioural and Psychological Symptoms of Dementia (BPSD), medical complications, and the family care giving capacity. For relatively early stages of dementia with mild disability, the care manager makes a care plan including home-visit services and day services covered by LTCI. Informal services such as cafés for people with dementia and their family care givers, managed by non-profit organizations, are also available. It was reported by MHLW that the number of cafés for people with dementia and their family care givers was 2,253 in 2015, with a growing trend. A survey to all municipalities (N = 1,741, 959 responded, 57.2%) reported more than half (52.4%) of municipalities support and promote cafés. Of those, 76.8% of services are held once a month, with 17.6 people being the average number of participants. The breakdown of participants is: persons with dementia 4.4 people, family members 3.5 people, local residents 8.8 people, and professionals 3.9 people.

For moderate stage, short stay services or residential services are added into the care plan (see Table 9.1).[5] After reaching the final stages where severe disability is experienced and family members can't provide the level of care needed, people with dementia are admitted to long-term in-facility services. Such facilities include private residential homes with public LTCI-covered long-term care and public LTCI-covered nursing home and hospital care for chronic conditions needing medical care. These facilities are registered and supervised by local government to ensure regulation of care quality. Shortage of care workers is often a primary reason for a partial closure of beds and some scandals surrounding care, such as accidents, abuses, and suspicion of murder.

9.4.1 Prevention Policy Reform from High-risk Strategy to Population Strategy

Frailty in older people is linked with declining physical, cognitive, and social functions (see Chapter 8). Frailty is a risk factor for disability, but is potentially reversible, which led to it being viewed as a focus for prevention. Prevention policy introduced in 2006 was based on a high-risk approach following a screening process of those at high risk through annual health checkup in early years or postal self-administered questionnaire in later years. The prevention programme was aimed at older people with frailty who were at high risk of requiring long-term care in the near future but not yet certified as eligible for receiving benefit of long-term care insurance. The Ministry of Health,

Labour and Welfare (MHLW) targeted about 5% of the older population aged over 65 years as participants in the care prevention programme. Screened older people with frailty were encouraged to participate in a care prevention programme.

The limitations of this strategy based on a high-risk approach were gradually revealed through nine years' experience. The cost for screening was larger than the cost of providing the preventive exercise class. Only 0.8% (2013) of older people participated in the exercise programme against a target of 5%. The function of some participants was improved by the end of the programme, but this function level decreased to baseline after one year. Then, the policy was revised in 2014.

Inequalities in health and behaviours were also found. A higher proportion of high-risk people were found among those with lower income and lower educational attainment.[9] Those with lower socioeconomic status were less likely to attend health services such as health checkups or prevention programmes. Therefore, efforts to identify high-risk older people through screening of health checkups or a mail survey and encouraging them to participate in a prevention programme were ineffective.[10,11] Then, prevention policy was reformed from high-risk strategy to population strategy as follows.

9.4.1.1 Japan Gerontological Evaluation Study (JAGES) Initiative

The Japan Gerontological Evaluation Study (JAGES) initiative, which developed from its precedent, the Aichi Gerontological Evaluation Study (AGES), implemented in 1999, provided scientific evidence and knowledge translation into healthy ageing policy in Japan.[11,12,13] JAGES collaborated with about 30–60 municipalities across the country and obtained responses from about 100,000–250,000 older people in 2010, 2013, 2016, and 2019. Their responses were systematically analysed by municipalities for evaluation of social care plans and activities, and were compared across the participating municipalities using key factors for social determinants of health. Using this data, JAGES reported that communities with higher participant rates of older people in community groups such as sports groups or hobby clubs showed a lower prevalence of risks for functional decline (Figure 9.1).[14] Further longitudinal studies confirmed that older people participating in social activity groups or taking a leading role within their social networks showed better health status and were less likely to experience functional decline[15] or develop dementia[16,17] at follow-up.

From 2006, when the new preventive care system was introduced by the MHLW, JAGES started a community intervention study promoting preventive

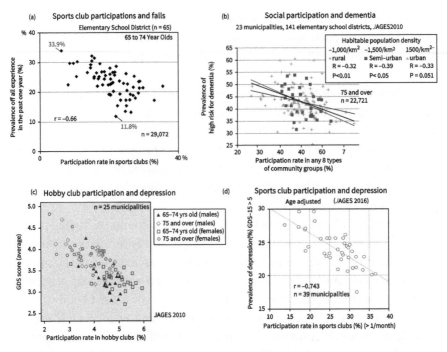

Figure 9.1 Social participation and health among older people

Source: (a, b, c) 47th National council for social security, The Long-Term care Insurance sectional meeting paper. https://www.mhlw.go.jp/file/05-Shingikai-12601000-Seisakutoukatsukan-Sanjikanshitsu_Shakaihoshoutantou/0000021717.pdf

Source: (d) JAGES (Japan Gerontological Evaluation Study), 2016. https://www.jages.net/cdss/jages/2016/municipality/mask/core/double/atlas.html

care through community buildings—a research example of the population approach to reduce health inequalities as an alternative/complementary measure to the high-risk approach.

In Taketoyo town in Aichi Prefecture, with a population of about 10,000 older people, a 'community salon' was established as a place for social exchange, volunteering, gatherings, and for local older residents to enjoy exercise and hobbies together. The number of 'salons' increased to 13 in 2016, with the volunteers organizing activities approximately one to three times a month. On average, approximately 60 older people participated in each activity and more than 10% of all older people participated in the programme.[18] Those who participated in the programme reported increases in both receiving and providing social support, protective factors for functional decline. After eight months and five years follow-up, we confirmed preventive effects on self-rated health[19] and functional decline[20] using advanced statistical analysis, i.e. instrumental variable methods equivalent to a quasi-randomized controlled trial (RCT). Distance from home or the density of salon, correlated with participating rate but not with health status, were used as instrumental variables. In addition, after a seven-year follow-up, we found that the cognitive function of those who participated in the programme was better than non-participants.[21]

Citing these scientific findings from the JAGES initiative, the MHLW reformed prevention policy from 2015, moving from high-risk strategy to community building, based on a population approach and the concept of social capital. The number of salons and exercise groups operated by local residents that are known by municipalities increased from 43,154 locations in 2013 to 106,766 locations in 2018, and the participation rate of older residents in the salons increased from 2.7% to 5.7%.

There are also a substantial number of older residents participating in informal activities, private golf clubs, and fitness clubs, which are not fully known by government administrative organizations. According to the JAGES FY2016 survey, which had 200,000 respondents from 39 cities and towns, 34.8% of older residents participated in hobbies and 28% participated in sporting activities one or more times a month. There is a negative correlation ($r = -0.743$, after adjustment for age) between participation rates in sporting activities at least once a month and the prevalence of depression scoring five or more on the Geriatric Depression Scale (GDS-15) (Figure 9.1d). The increase in the percentage of sports group participation was significantly associated with the decrease in the prevalence of depressive symptoms after adjusting for potential confounding variables in a five-year repeated cross-sectional study.[22]

9.5 Implications for Other Countries

Adapting responses to changes in society, population, and family structure need two or three decades. A strategic approach from an earlier stage is important. Policy responses for increasing disability, including dementia and care-giving problems, need to be comprehensive. Healthy ageing policies should be given high priority from an earlier stage to eliminate the care burden on family and society. The Community-based Integrated Care System, including prevention for long-term care, are needed to support ageing for older people in places familiar to them, even after experiencing severely disabling health conditions such as dementia. As dementia care policy is still in the development stage, many clinical trials and clinical evaluation are needed. Given the scientific evidence in Japan, we suggest that a prevention policy for frailty of older people should be emphasized through community-building based on a population strategy rather than a high-risk approach, together with addressing the social determinants of health.[12,23,24]

References

1. OECD. OECD statistics 2019. Available at: http://stats.oecd.org/ [last accessed 5 March 2020].
2. Statistics Bureau, Ministry of Internal Affairs and Communications. Population census of Japan: overview of population and households of Japan 2018:1–185. Available at: https://www.stat.go.jp/data/kokusei/2015/pdf/wagakuni.pdf [last accessed 5 March 2020].
3. Statistics and Information Department, Minister's Secretariat. Graphical review of Japanese household—from the comprehensive Survey of Living Conditions 2013. Ministry of Health, Labour and Welfare 2014 Available at: https://www.mhlw.go.jp/toukei/list/dl/20-21-h25.pdf [last accessed 5 March 2020].
4. Asada T. Prevalence of dementia in Japan: past, present and future (in Japanese). *Rinsho Shinkeigaku* 2012;52:962–4.
5. Health and Welfare Bureau for the Elderly. Long-term Care Insurance System of Japan. Ministry of Health, Labour and Welfare 2016. Available at: https://www.mhlw.go.jp/english/policy/care-welfare/care-welfare-elderly/dl/ltcisj_e.pdf [last accessed 5 March 2020].
6. Ministry of Health, Labour and Welfare. White Paper—Annual report on Health and Welfare Gyousei 1996.
7. Nihon sogou kenkyujo. Kaigo jinzai no jukyu suikei ni kakawaru tyousa kennkyu jigyo houkokusyo. Nihon sogou kenkyujo 2016. Available at: https://www.mhlw.go.jp/file/06-Seisakujouhou-12300000-Roukenkyoku/0000136696.pdf [last accessed 5 March 2020].
8. Tachibana N. The current state and issues of the special bathtub use in welfare institutions. *Kansai University of Welfare Sciences* 2009;13:49–64.
9. Kondo K. *Health Inequalities in Japan: An Empirical Study of Older People.* Melbourne: Trans Pacific Press 2010.
10. Ministry of Health, Labour and Welfare. Future directions for preventing disabilities 2014 (in Japanese). Available at: http://www.mhlw.go.jp/file/06-Seisakujouhou-12300000-Roukenkyoku/0000075982.pdf [last accessed 5 March 2020].

11. Kondo K. *Prescriptions for Health Gap Society* (in Japanese). Tokyo: Igaku-shoin Publishers 2017.

12. Kondo K, Rosenberg M. *Advancing universal health coverage through knowledge translation for healthy ageing: lessons learnt from the Japan Gerontological Evaluation Study.* Geneva: WHO 2018.

13. Kondo K. Progress in aging epidemiology in Japan. The JAGES Project. *J Epidemiol* 2016;26:331–6.

14. Health and Welfare Bureau for the Elderly. 47th National council for social security document. Ministry of Health, Labour and Welfare 2014.

15. Kanamori S, et al. Social participation and the prevention of functional disability in older Japanese: the JAGES cohort study. *PloS one* 2014;9:e99638–e99647.

16. Saito T, et al. Influence of social relationship domains and their combinations on incident dementia: a prospective cohort study. *J Epidemiol Community Health* 2018;72:7–12.

17. Nemoto Y, et al. An additive effect of leading role in the organization between social participation and dementia onset among Japanese older adults: the AGES cohort study. *BMC Geriatrics* 2017;17:297.

18. Murayama H, et al. Social capital interventions to promote healthy aging. In: Ichiro Kawachi, et al. *Global Perspectives on Social Capital and Health.* New York: Springer Science+Business Media 2013:205–38.

19. Ichida Y, et al. Does social participation improve self-rated health in the older population? A quasi-experimental intervention study. *Soc Sci Med* 2013;94:83–90.

20. Hikichi H, et al. Effect of a community intervention programme promoting social interactions on functional disability prevention for older adults: propensity score matching and instrumental variable analyses, JAGES Taketoyo study. *J Epidemiol Community Health* 2015;69:905–10.

21. Hikichi H, et al. Social interaction and cognitive decline: results of a 7-year community intervention. *Alzheimer's & Dementia: Translational Research & Clinical Interventions* 2017;3:23–32.

22. Watanabe R, et al. Change in municipality-level health-related social capital and depressive symptoms: ecological and 5-year repeated cross-sectional study from the JAGES. *Int J Environ Res Public Health* 2019;16:2038. doi: 10.3390/ijerph16112038

23. Saito J, et al. Community-based care for healthy ageing: lessons from Japan. *Bull World Health Organ* 2019;97:570–4.

24. Kondo K (ed.). *Social Determinants of Health in Non-communicable Diseases: Case Studies from Japan.* Singapore: Springer 2020.

10

Historical Overview of Japanese Society, Health, and Health Inequalities from the Nineteenth to the Twenty-first Century

Ayako Hiyoshi and Naoki Kondo

10.1 The Rise of Life Expectancy

10.1.1 Before World War II

At the beginning of the twentieth century, living standards, estimated by wages of labourers[1] and the supply of purified water[2], were much lower in Japan than the UK, the then wealthiest country in the world. But Japanese life expectancy, on the other hand, was remarkably good and lower only by a few years (Figure 10.1 Panel A).[3–5] The key to such success appeared to be Japan's social and cultural characteristics and the use of public health measures developed in Western countries.

After the Meiji restoration in 1868, the new legal and social systems were structured according to the German system, which created emperor-centred absolutism and cultivated a submissive and compliant population that expected the state to have an active role in the nation's life. The government introduced smallpox quarantine and vaccination and campaigned to improve individual hygiene to prevent infectious disease.

Literacy was initially high in Japan because children from lower social classes were taught to write and, to a lesser extent, arithmetic was also taught in schools run by local lords and villages.[6] Education was extended after the Meiji restoration, and by 1909 the illiteracy rate was less than 10%,[6] lower than in England.[7] Literacy contributed to the success of the new public health measures, as did a general willingness to comply with national policy.[8] These population characteristics, together with an adoption

Ayako Hiyoshi and Naoki Kondo, *Historical Overview of Japanese Society, Health, and Health Inequalities from the Nineteenth to the Twenty-first Century* In: *Health in Japan.* Edited by: Eric Brunner, Noriko Cable, and Hiroyasu Iso, Oxford University Press (2021). © Oxford University Press. DOI: 10.1093/oso/9780198848134.003.0010.

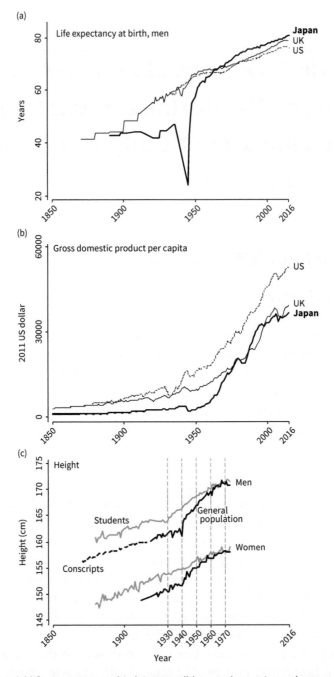

Figure 10.1 (a) life expectancy at birth in men; (b) gross domestic product per capita; (c) height at age 20 by birth year, Japan 1850–2016

Sources: (a) 22nd Life Tables. Japanese Ministry of Health, Labour and Welfare. 2015; How has life expectancy changed over time? UK Office for National Statistics. 2015; Human Mortality Database. University of California, Berkeley, Max Planck Institute for Demographic Research. **B:** Bolt J, et al. Rebasing 'Maddison': new income comparisons and the shape of long-run economic development. Maddison Project Database, 2018. **C:** Kouchi M. Anthropological Science. 1996;104:325-40.

of technologies developed in the West and a reduction of food transportation costs due to the new railway network, reduced the risk of periodic food shortages[9] and helped to offset the higher health risks posed by the low standard of living.

Despite the steady growth of incomes between 1900 and World War II,[10] the life expectancy trend was static and the gap with the UK gradually widened (Figure 10.1a and b). During this period, there was a large height gap between students who were from affluent families and generally poorer conscripts, probably indicating widespread suboptimal nutrition in childhood (Figure 10.1c).[11] At that time, the government's priority was military build-up. Public health measures relied mainly on self-help measures which were limited in potential, while continuing urbanization increased exposure to infectious disease risk, the largest cause of death at that time.[2]

10.1.2 After World War II

Changes followed the defeat. The new constitution of 1947 assured demilitarization, reduction in the status attached to the pre-war ruling class, and equal rights for the people. Demilitarization redirected resources toward public investment, and numerous public health, social, and welfare measures were implemented. The pre-war health and pension insurance systems that had been introduced with limited coverage for maintenance of military strength and serving and retired soldiers, were expanded and made universal in 1961 (Chapter 8).

Although it is not possible to link these specific societal changes directly to changes in population health, life expectancy improved with astounding rapidity. Major causes of death shifted from the dominance of infectious diseases to degenerative diseases characteristic of old age. Japan was the first non-Western country to make this epidemiological transition.[12]

As non-communicable disease deaths increased, stroke (cerebrovascular disease) became a serious problem in Japan in the 1960s, but a salt reduction campaign and dietary education was actively conducted across local communities in Japan.[13] It is likely the deeply-embedded cooperative culture helped to reduce dietary salt intake and subsequently stroke rates. In the 1980s, just a few decades after Japanese life expectancy was much lower than in European countries, Japan recorded the longest life expectancy in the world.

10.2 Social Inequalities in Japan

In any society, social inequalities exist (Box 10.1). The stepwise social gradient in health, that the higher the social position, the better the health status, is generally evident. The current theory of health inequalities predicts that a society with more equity in power, control, and distribution of resource would have relatively smaller health inequalities.

Box 10.1 What Is Social Stratification?

Social stratification is the product of differentiation of people into groups. Social epidemiologists use social classification systems to assess whether different social position results in an unequal distribution of health, i.e. health inequalities.[14] The theoretical origin of several stratification systems goes back to Marx and Weber.

With the development of machine technologies and large-scale production during European industrialization, Marx considered that class conflict would become inherent between people who sell their labour power, and people who control and exploit labour along with accumulation of capital, such as ownership of houses, factories, and other means of wealth production. Marx considered that class was a fundamental determinant of the patterns of people's daily lives.

While Weber also recognized the social divisions generated by productive activities to be an important factor, he focused on the distribution of goods, economic opportunities, knowledge, assets, and skills by which individuals negotiate the labour market and earn income.[14] Differences in the level of possession of these resources are generated by an individual's relation to the means of production. The process generates, in turn, various groups to which people belong, with shared beliefs, values, circumstances, lifestyles (such as clothing, marriage patterns, eating habits) and eventually 'life chances'. Weber saw such factors as indicators of structural mechanisms generating unequal social standing. Social epidemiology has a link to Weberian type thinking because cultural factors are used as indicators of socioeconomic position in society.

10.2.1 Changes around World War II

Substantial social inequalities that had characterized pre-war Japan were dramatically changed by reforms implemented in post-war Japan. Before the end of World War II, around 90% of people were poor and lived in rented accommodation.[15] Income distribution was highly unequal, with an estimated GINI coefficient of 0.4–0.6.[16] The GINI coefficient measures inequality on a scale of 0 to 1, with 0 perfect equality and 1 perfect inequality, i.e. one person receives 100% of national income.

During the decades following World War II, the boundaries of social position were blurred and distinctions between socioeconomic groups were reduced because living conditions became increasingly homogeneous.[17] The unemployment rate was low (around 2%),[18] housing quality improved, homeownership increased to about 60%,[19] enrolment in higher education expanded, the language was standardized, and income was the most equally distributed in Japan's modern history (1960–1990).[16] Japan became the second-largest economy in the world in 1968, and in the 1970s about 90% of people identified their living standard as in the middle, according to a government opinion survey. This 'middle-ness' was considered a symbolic representation of unstratified Japan.[17] Some sociologists challenged such assertions, showing large differences in material and non-material resources within the 'middle class'.[20] Nevertheless, the belief in Japanese classlessness was so widespread that research on social stratification and inequalities was sparse at this time.[21]

10.2.2 Recent Years

Since the late 1990s, academic literature and mass media took a distinct turn, to recognize society as increasingly fragmented and unequal.[22] The economic downturn continued, large companies went bankrupt, the unemployment rate surged, precarious employment expanded, suicide rates increased, and two influential books on social inequalities and stratifications were published.[23,24] Income inequalities measured by the GINI coefficient increased and become comparable to Western countries.[25] Although the GINI coefficient is technically difficult to compare across populations, other indices of inequality were consistent (Table 1.2). Relative poverty, defined as the proportion of people with below half of the national median household-size standardized income after tax, increased from 12% in 1985 to 16% in 2016, well above that of the UK (11%) and the Organization for Economic Co-operation and Development (OECD) average (11%).[26,27] The percentage of children living in a family with less than 50% of the national median income reached around 14%, similar to the OECD average of 13% in the 2010s.[28] The proportion of people living within absolute poverty, defined as an income level that is eligible for welfare assistance, was estimated to have increased from 6% in 1980 to 13% in 2002.[29] Contrary to the earlier high-growth period characterized by belief in classless Japan, discussion of inequalities became salient.[22]

10.3 Trends in Health Inequalities

Health inequalities took a particular form in pre-World-War-II Japan, along with industrial development. Age-standardized death rates were higher in urban areas than rural areas at the beginning of industrialization in the early twentieth century. Regional inequalities reversed by 1930, with higher death rates in the countryside.[8] Differences in the average height of adult men by prefecture-level per capita income have narrowed across Japan since the late nineteenth century,[9] but socioeconomic inequalities in health were apparent as indicated by the height difference at age 20 between students and conscripts and the general population in birth cohorts born between 1920–1940 (Figure 10.1c).[11] The gap in height started to narrow in the 1940 birth cohort. Because of the rising higher education enrolment rate, 'students' after World War II increasingly included individuals who would have been in the 'general population' in earlier decades. However, the narrowing trends were observed in both men and women while in women the higher education enrolment rates remained much lower than men in the early post-World War II period; therefore, it does appear that there was a real narrowing in the height gap according to socioeconomic background. The height inequality trend in the mid-century suggests that health inequalities were set to narrow.

10.3.1 Health Inequalities in Modern-day Japan

Previously, the material living environment, particularly sanitation, housing, and water supply, accounted for many of the health risks at population level. But in developed countries, these factors are more or less satisfied. Why then does health differ by the social position of individuals? Health is not solely a consequence of absolute material wellbeing. Even when the minimum needs for survival are satisfied, a lower social position often relates to relative disadvantage, in clustering of adverse factors in life, including suboptimal housing and living environment, lower education, unemployment, unsatisfactory and stressful work, health-damaging behaviours, low self-esteem, lack of future aspiration, and delayed healthcare-seeking behaviour.

The list is long. Although most of the Japanese population live with income above the poverty line, relative deprivation, such as having a lower income in comparison to others, may affect health through stress-related mechanisms.[30]

Observed trends in Japanese health inequalities differ, depending on socioeconomic indicators and health outcomes.[31] Trends in absolute and relative measures of health inequality lead to different conclusions because the former is calculated by subtraction while the latter is a ratio based on division of rates or proportions of ill health across social strata. For example, as average mortality declines, the relative difference (ratio) tends to increase even if absolute inequality (the gap) is constant. Bearing in mind these complexities in understanding historical trends, between the 1950s and 1990s, absolute as well as relative health inequalities declined in relation to regional socioeconomic characteristics and income, and some studies found low or no inequalities around the 1990s.[8,32-34] However, from the 1980s to 2001, the degree of health improvement was not uniform by occupational group. Clerical, sales, and service workers experienced slower improvement than advantaged groups such as managers and professionals; as a result, relative inequalities increased in relation to mortality[35] and self-rated health.[32]

Since the late 1990s, socioeconomic inequalities have widened, and from 2005 the pace of mortality improvement from leading causes of death has slowed.[36] Regional and occupational variation in health increased,[34,36,37] and there were polarized mortality trends, with administrative and to a lesser extent professional workers experiencing an increase in mortality (Figure 10.2).[34,37-39] We must be cautious about interpreting some aspects of the mortality trends. Administrative workers make up a small group, particularly so for women. The number of deaths below age 65 is small, and death rates may be unstable. However, it appears that the pattern of occupational inequalities in mortality has changed to a 'reverse' or U-shaped pattern where both the most and least advantaged groups have higher risk than the middle group. This pattern is different from that observed in Western countries.[37,38] Further, based on self-rated health, the social gradient in health has remained stable or may have narrowed in relation to income, especially in men,[40,41] with possible increasing inequalities in men and women in the decade before 2013 (Figure 10.3). The magnitude of health inequalities in the 1990s and 2000s were similar or a little smaller than Western countries in men and both sexes combined,[42,43] but inconsistent in women.[42] The trend in inequalities in poor self-rated health mirrors that for good health (Chapter 1.2.2, Figure 1.1).

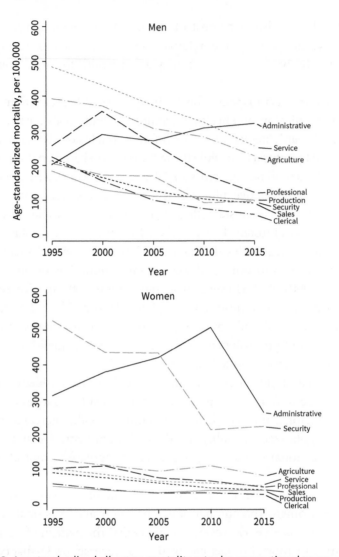

Figure 10.2 Age standardized all-cause mortality rates by occupational group, men and women aged 20–64, Japan 1995–2015

Occupational groups were classified according to the Japanese Standard Occupational Classification 2009 version. Administrative: administrative and managerial workers. Professional: professional and engineering workers. Clerical: clerical workers. Sales: sales workers. Service: service workers. Security: security workers (including police). Agriculture: agriculture, forestry, and fishery workers. Production: manufacturing, transport, machine, construction, mining, carrying, cleaning, and warehouse workers. Age-standardized mortality based on direct standardization using the entire 20–64 year population 1995–2015 as the standard.

Source: Portal site of official statistics of Japan. e-Stat. https://www.e-stat.go.jp/. Accessed 13 Sep 2019.

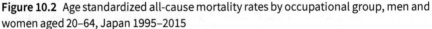

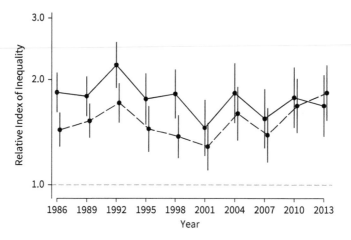

Figure 10.3 Relative inequalities in self-rated poor health, men and women aged 20–59, Japan 1986–2013

Solid line: men, dashed line: women. Relative Index of Inequality was calculated by taking the ratio of proportions reporting poor health between top and bottom of the income distribution, taking account of data in between, and weighting to Japanese population.

Source: Honjo and Hiyoshi, unpublished analysis of Comprehensive Survey of Living Conditions. Methods in Hiyoshi et al, J Epidemiol Community Health. 2013;67:960-965

10.3.2 Health Inequalities in a Super-ageing Low-growth Economy

Generally, in the later part of the twentieth century, the socioeconomic gradient in health in Japan narrowed, and the trend continued into the early 2000s. This trend may be thought remarkable because during these years Japan's economy lost its momentum and tended to stagnate. It might be considered that a lengthy economic slowdown places a strain on population health, in a 'social determinants' perspective, for example when welfare spending is constrained. This situation was exacerbated by rapid population ageing. During economic recessions, European countries experienced widening health inequalities.[44] Does this mean that Japan is still an exemplary country that narrowed health inequalities despite the challenging situations? The answer would be 'no'. The narrowing health inequality trends were due to limited improvement or even worsening health in high socioeconomic groups—not because health improved among lower socioeconomic groups. The most recent estimates of the trend in health inequalities in the 2010s, based on (subjective) self-rated health, suggest some widening (Figure 10.3).

The reasons for such trends are subject to discussion. Speculatively, they relate to economic, structural, and cultural aspects of Japan's situation. In particular, working conditions have become more difficult for those in executive and senior managerial positions, and lifetime regular employment is less accessible. During the economic downturns in the 1990s and 2000s, companies gradually adopted 'modernizing' cost-efficient practices by downsizing, restructuring, and cutting wages (Chapter 18). Older and higher grade workers were not always excluded from these changes. Age at promotion increased, the proportion of management workers declined, and the real value of salaries was reduced.[45]

While worsening working conditions in economic recessions are common across various social positions, earlier studies have reported certain vulnerabilities in those with high socioeconomic positions.[46,47] In Japan, strong emphasis is placed on the work ethic and high performance even with reduced resources. Therefore, it is not only unemployment and redundancy, but also remaining in work that is associated with increased stress. Especially in the patriarchal family model of the older generation, men unable to fulfill expectations as the breadwinner for the household may experience chronic and severe stress (Chapter 3). Lastly, favourable health-related behaviours, such as smoking, are generally linked with higher socioeconomic position in Western countries,[48] and such patterns of behaviour explain many of the health inequalities.[49] However, in Japan, the associations between behaviour and socioeconomic position are not consistent with the Western pattern, and this characteristic is likely to explain part of the phenomenon of narrower health inequalities.[50–52]

10.4 Limitations in Existing Evidence and Future Possibilities

Although there are now many Japanese studies of trends in health and health inequalities, limitations in the available data continue. For example, evidence on mortality differences by occupation requires information on the occupation of the deceased person and the size of the occupational group at the time of death. High quality information on this and other aspects of socioeconomic position is not yet available for the Japanese population. It is particularly difficult to analyse health among women in non-standard employment (Chapter 7). However, research using 'big data' such as electronic hospital records recently became possible. Linkage of these data with other official data sets including socioeconomic characteristics raises concerns about confidentiality and consent, that are now being discussed. There remains a lack of evidence on the health of several demographic groups, including children and older adults. The effects on health of recent changes in retirement and pension ages, and working after retirement, are poorly understood.

10.5 Countering Health Inequalities

In many developed countries there are policies specifically directed to counter social inequalities in health. Measures include provision of free or affordable health and social care, unemployment benefits, subsidized housing, free education, and support for social participation. Countries with such schemes are often referred to as welfare states. Although controversial, Japan was classified into the group of countries with conservative welfare regimes. In such countries, there is an emphasis on solidarity in order to reduce health risks in work and retirement.[53] The family is central to this system, with an expectation of support for individuals who need it. A male-breadwinner model of family structure is prevalent, with wife or another family member providing care for children, elderly, and dependents. The state intervenes only when family resources are exhausted. Hazards for workers and their family members, such as unemployment, sickness, and retirement, are taken care of by the social insurance system. Rights and privileges are tied to employment, and those who do not work are excluded from the insurance-based social security system.

The Japanese welfare system was established to counter disadvantage and poverty but may also reinforce the social structure and reproduce inequalities. For example, the family unit as the primary welfare provider, based on a male breadwinner and female home-maker, is around 100 years old. Gender division of labour is one aspect of the traditional family unit that has long been questioned and there has been some erosion of this model in younger generations, but it still holds a strong influence on daily life in Japan. Although the welfare system supports some of the unmet needs of families and individuals, disadvantage often passes to the next generation, and upward mobility is limited.[53] Therefore, although the welfare system is important, breaking the cycle of disadvantage probably depends on reforming many policies and systems in addition to the welfare system.

Many countries have implemented measures countering health inequalities, but few of these countries have succeeded in narrowing health inequalities. Since 2012, health inequalities have been recognized in health policies, and reduction of health inequalities became one of the goals in the second term of the National Health Promotion Movement in the twenty-first century. At this moment, the dominant preventive approach focuses on regional characteristics and changing the lifestyle of high-risk individuals, often defined by behaviours such as smoking. The inclusion of health inequalities as a policy target is a remarkable step, and such individual-level factors are important to consider as part of a chain of causal mechanisms. But without addressing wider societal causes of health inequalities, the policy is likely to not be very effective and may become victim-blaming. For example, the price of tobacco is low in Japan (Chapter 14). While Japan can capitalize on knowledge and measures for reducing health inequalities, developed mainly in Western countries, given its unique characteristics, there is a need to consider interventions based on the specific Japanese situation and its changing social values.

10.6 Conclusion

This chapter provided an overview of social and health development, and summarized evidence on time trends in socioeconomic health inequalities. Societal factors are important determinants of health and health inequalities. In Japan, a special combination of social structures, culture, and social policies resulted in remarkable progress in health, combined with relatively small health inequalities in the post-war period. Socioeconomic inequalities emerged during the more recent period of economic stagnation. Narrowing health inequalities at the start of this period appear to be due to the worsening health of some higher socioeconomic groups. Some evidence from recent representative surveys suggests health inequalities are growing. Monitoring health inequality trends is increasingly necessary, as is detailed investigation of causes and mechanisms. This information will support further development of policies to respond to Japan's unique health inequality trends. As the epidemiologist Geoffrey Rose wrote three decades ago, 'The primary determinants of disease are mainly economic and social, and therefore its remedies must also be economic and social. Medicine and politics cannot and should not be kept apart.'[54]

References

1. Bassino JP, Ma D. Japanese unskilled wages in international perspective 1741–1913. *Research in Economic History* 2005;23:229–48.

2. Johansson SR, et al. Disease and death in Japan, 1900–1960. *Population Stud.* 1987;41:207–35.

3. Ministry of Health, Labour and Welfare. The 22nd Life Tables 2015.

4. Office for National Statistics. How has life expectancy changed over time? 2015.

5. Human Mortality Database. University of California, Berkeley (US), and Max Planck Institute for Demographic Research (Germany).

6. Rubinger R. Illiteracy in Meiji Japan. *Monumenta Nipponica* 2000;55:163–97.

7. Roser M, et al. Literacy 2019. Available at: https://ourworldindata.org/literacy [last accessed 5 March 2020].

8. Mosk C, et al. Income and mortality: Japan. *Population Devel Rev* 1986;12:415–40.

9. Bassino JP. Inequality in Japan (1892–1941). *Econ Hum Biol* 2006;4:62–88.

10. Bolt J, et al. Maddison Project Database, version 2018: Rebasing 'Maddison': new income comparisons and the shape of long-run economic development 2018.

11. Kouchi M. Secular change and socioeconomic difference in height in Japan. *Anthropological Science* 1996;104:325–40.

12. Omran AR. The epidemiologic transition. *Milbank Memorial Fund Quarterly.* 1971;49:509–38.

13. Yokota K, et al. Evaluation of a community-based health education program for salt reduction through media campaigns. *Nihon Koshu Eisei Zasshi* 2006;53:543–53.

14. Lynch J, et al. Socioeconomic position. In: LF Berkman, et al., (eds.). *Social Epidemiology.* New York: Oxford University Press 2000.

15. Makino F. Income and wealth inequality in Japan. *Keizai Shirin.* 2017;85:105–39.

16. Minami R. Income distribution of Japan. *Japan Labor Review* 2008;5:5–20.

17. Murakami Y. New middle mass politics. *J Japanese Stud* 1982;8:29–72.

18. Statistics Bureau of Japan. Labour Force Survey: Historical data. Available at: https://www.stat.go.jp/english/data/roudou/lngindex.html [last accessed 5 March 2020].

19. Hirayama Y. Home ownership in Japan. *J Housing Built Environment* 2010;25:175–91.

20. Ishida H. Class structure and status hierarchies in Japan. *European Sociological Rev* 1989;5:65–80.

21. Hashimoto K. Increased class-stratification and reduced class mobility. *Japan Society Political Economy* 2008;44:29–40.

22. Ishida H, et al. Social class in Japan. In: Ishida H, et al., (eds.). *Social Class in Contemporary Japan.* New York: Routledge 2010:1–29.

23. Tachibanaki T. *Japan's Economic Inequality (Nihon no Keizai Kakusa).* Tokyo: Iwanami Shoten 1998.

24. Sato T. *Japan as an Unequal Society (Fubyodo Shakai Nippon).* Tokyo: Chuo Koron Shinsha 2000.

25. OECD. Income inequality and labour income share in G20 countries: trends, impacts and causes 2015.

26. OECD. Society at a glance 2011: OECD social indicators 2011.

27. Ministry of Health, Labour and Welfare. Overview of the comprehensive survey of living conditions 2016. Published in 2017.

28. OECD Family Database. Child poverty. Available at: https://www.oecd.org/els/CO_2_2_Child_Poverty.pdf [last accessed 24 March 2020].

29. Tachibanaki T. *Unequal Society (Kakusa Shakai)*. Tokyo: Iwanami Shoten 2006.

30. Kondo N, et al. Relative deprivation and perceived health among Japanese. *Soc Sci Med* 2008;67:982–7.

31. Fukuda Y, et al. Cause-specific mortality across municipal socioeconomic position in Japan, 1973–1977 and 1993–1998. *Int J Epidemiol* 2005;34:100–9.

32. Kondo N, et al. Economic recession and health inequalities in Japan: 1986–2001. *J Epidemiol Community Health* 2008;62:869–75.

33. Fukuda Y, et al. Health inequalities trends 1955–2000. *Biosci Trends* 2007;1:38–42.

34. Suzuki E, et al. Social and geographic inequalities in adult mortality in Japan, 1970–2005. *BMJ Open* 2012;2:e000425.

35. Hasegawa T. Japan: historical and current dimensions of health and health equity. In: T Evans, et al., (eds.). *Challenging Inequities in Health*: Oxford: Oxford Scholarship Online 2001.

36. Nomura S, et al. Population health and regional variations of disease burden in Japan, 1990–2015. *Lancet* 2017;390:1521–38.

37. Wada K, et al. Trends in cause specific mortality across occupations in Japanese men, 1980–2005. *BMJ* 2012;344:e1191.

38. Tanaka H, et al. Mortality inequalities by occupational class among men in Japan, South Korea and eight European countries, 1990–2015. *J Epidemiol Community Health* 2019;73:750–8.

39. Portal site of official statistics of Japan. e-Stat. Available at: https://www.e-stat.go.jp/ [last accessed 5 March 2020].

40. Kachi Y, et al. Income-related health inequalities in Japan, 1986–2007. *Soc Sci Med* 2013;81:94–101.

41. Hiyoshi A, et al. Inequalities in self-rated health in Japan 1986–2007. *J Epidemiol Community Health* 2013;67:960–5.

42. Martikainen P, et al. Socioeconomic differences in physical functioning and perceived health: Britain, Finland and Japan. *Soc Sci Med* 2004;59:1287–95.

43. Nakaya T, et al. Geographical inequalities of mortality by income in two developed island countries: a cross-national comparison of Britain and Japan. *Soc Sci Med* 2005;60:2865–75.

44. Heggebø K, et al. Socioeconomic inequalities in health during the Great Recession: a review. *Scand J Public Health* 2018; Epub ahead of print.

45. Oi M. Quantitative changes in managerial positions: their number, promotion speed and relative wage. *Japan J Labour Stud* 2005;545:4–17.

46. Vahtera J, et al. Effect of organisational downsizing on health of employees. *Lancet* 1997;350:1124–8.

47. Montgomery S, et al. Does financial disadvantage at older ages eliminate the potential for better health? *J Epidemiol Community Health* 2007;61:891–5.

48. Mackenbach J. Health Inequalities: Europe in Profile 2006.

49. Stringhini S, et al. Socioeconomic position with health behaviors and mortality. *JAMA* 2010;303:1159–66.

50. Martikainen P, et al. Socioeconomic differences in behavioural and biological risk factors: a Japanese and an English cohort. *Int J Epidemiol* 2001;30:833–8.

51. Fukuda Y, et al. High quality nutrient intake is associated with higher household expenditures by Japanese adults. *Biosci Trends* 2012;6:176–82.

52. Fukuda Y, et al. Household expenditure and marital status with cardiovascular risk factors in Japanese adults. *J Epidemiol* 2013;23:21–7.

53. Esping-Andersen G. *The Three Worlds of Welfare Capitalism*. Cambridge: Polity Press 1990.

54. Rose G. *Rose's Strategy of Preventive Medicine*. New York: Oxford University Press 1992.

11

Chronic Diseases and Risk Factor Trends in Japan

Cardiovascular Inequalities

Hiroyasu Iso, Kotatsu Maruyama, and Kazumasa Yamagishi

11.1 Introduction

Japan has achieved the highest longevity in the world,[1,2] which is attributable to the steepest decline in stroke mortality along with the lowest and modest decline in mortality from ischaemic heart disease since the 1960s. This striking trend was first emphasized in comparison with trends in England and Wales,[1] and was later investigated extensively.[2] These cardiovascular diseases are recognized as major lifestyle-related diseases, caused mostly by unhealthy behaviours such as smoking, heavy drinking, high sodium intake, unbalanced diet, physical inactivity, and other related risk factors such as obesity, hypertension, diabetes and dyslipidaemia (blood lipid abnormality).[3–5]

The 1964 Tokyo Olympics and the 1970 Osaka World Exposition resulted in substantial socioeconomic developments that helped in changing cardiovascular health in Japan dramatically.[6–8] The 2020 Tokyo Olympics, currently rescheduled for summer 2021, and the WORLD EXPO 2025 (in Osaka) provide opportunities to consider new strategies for the promotion of health in the face of population ageing both in Japan as well as other countries of the world.

This chapter highlights the success in the prevention and control of cardiovascular diseases and future issues related to rapid ageing in Japan, by providing an overview as well as a critique of the (1) profiles of cardiovascular diseases, risk factors and behaviours in the 1960s, taking into account the national, regional and occupational differences, (2) change in these profiles since the 1960s, (3) improvements in the Japanese diet following economic development, (4) roles of preventive activities through public health services and medical care, and (5) present and future issues related to health inequality for cardiovascular diseases.

Hiroyasu Iso, Kotatsu Maruyama, and Kazumasa Yamagishi, *Chronic Diseases and Risk Factor Trends in Japan* In: *Health in Japan*. Edited by: Eric Brunner, Noriko Cable, and Hiroyasu Iso, Oxford University Press (2021). © Oxford University Press. DOI: 10.1093/oso/9780198848134.003.0011.

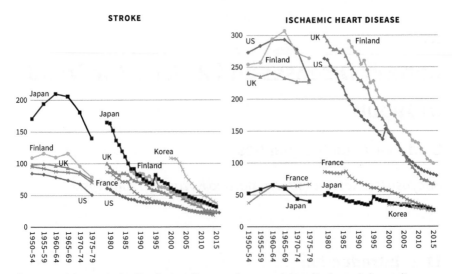

Figure 11.1 Age-standardized mortality rates from stroke and ischaemic heart disease, Japan and selected countries, 1950–2015

Data 1950–1979 from WHO World Health Statistics Annual 1993. Geneva: WHO. Age-standardized death rates based on 1990 United Nations standard populations. Data 1979–2015 from WHO Mortality Database. Age-standardized death rates based on the average of 2000–2025 United Nations standard populations. Available at: http://www.who.int/healthinfo/mortality_data/en/ [last accessed 21 July 2020].

11.2 Profiles of Cardiovascular Diseases, Risk Factors and Behaviours in the 1960s

11.2.1 Incidence of Cardiovascular Diseases and Mortality

Ten to 20 years after World War II, Japan had the highest mortality from stroke and the lowest mortality from ischaemic heart disease in the world. Mortality from stroke was two to three times higher, while mortality from ischaemic heart disease was only a quarter to one-fifth of that in the US, England, and Finland (Figure 11.1).[9]

Even within Japan, the incidence of stroke varied largely based on geography and occupation. It was approximately three times higher among rural men aged 40–69 years in Akita (northeast Japan) than among urban men aged 40–69 years in Osaka (western half of Japan),[3,8] and two-fold higher among blue-collared male workers aged 40–59 years than among white-collared male workers aged 40–59 years of Osaka.[3] However, no significant variations in the incidence of ischaemic heart disease were noted based on region and occupation.

11.2.2 Two Types of Vascular Pathology and Related Factors

Such large differences in the profiles of cardiovascular diseases by country, regional areas and occupation can be explained by the lower proportion of large vessel pathology (atherosclerosis) and the higher proportion of small vessel pathology (arteriolosclerosis) in Japan than in the US, England, and Finland. The prevalence of arteriolosclerosis is probably higher among rural residents than among the urban residents of Japan.

Atherosclerosis is characterized by lipid accumulation and inflammatory cell proliferation leading to the formation of 'plaque' and eventually blood clot, which causes ischaemic heart disease and ischaemic (large vessel) stroke.[10] High total cholesterol levels (from a diet rich in saturated fat such as meat), diabetes and smoking, and to a lesser extent, hypertension accelerate this type of pathology.

On the other hand, arteriolosclerosis is characterized by the death of smooth muscle cells, which constitute a major component of the vascular wall. This leads to weakening of the vascular wall and its subsequent rupture or cell proliferation due to an excessive healing process which cause intracerebral haemorrhage or ischaemic (small vessel) stroke. Hypertension, and to a lesser extent, diabetes and smoking accelerate arteriolosclerosis. Very low total cholesterol levels[11] (low intake of saturated fat)[12,13] and low intake of animal protein[12,14] were suggested being linked to this type of pathology and intracerebral haemorrhage.

11.2.3 Risk Factors and Behaviours

In the 1960s, the national mean levels of systolic blood pressure, the number one risk factor for stroke, were higher in those Japanese aged ≥20 years (142 mmHg in men and 141 mmHg in women)[15,16] than US whites aged 25–74 years (133 mmHg in men and 129 mmHg in women)[17,18] (Figure 11.2a).

Within Japan, large regional variations in diet provide a good explanation for the urban-rural differences in disease risk in the 1960s. The prevalence of hypertension (systolic blood pressure ≥140 mmHg, diastolic blood pressure ≥90 and/or medication) in rural men and women aged 40–69 years was 64% and 51%, respectively, while in urban men and women it was 38% and 37%, respectively.[8] This inequality in the incidence of hypertension was explained

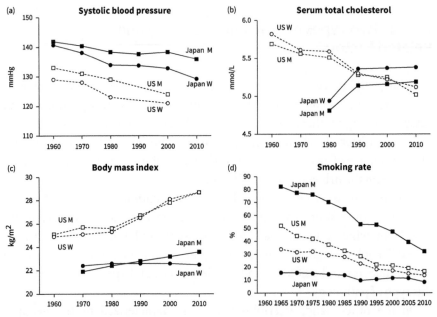

Figure 11.2 Vascular risk factors in Japan and the US, men and women, 1960–2010. Risk factor data from a series of national samples. M: men; W: women.

Sources: References 15–18 for (a) systolic blood pressure, references 15, 16, 22, 23 for (b) serum total cholesterol, references 15, 26, 27 for (c) body mass index, and references 28 for (d) smoking rate.

primarily by the higher salt intake (20 g/day) in rural men aged 40–69 years[6] than in urban men (13 g/day).[19] The low dietary intake of milk and dairy products (calcium), animal protein (meat), as well as high alcohol consumption (in men) were the other factors related to hypertension in the Japanese.[19,20]

In the 1960s, the national levels of blood total cholesterol, a major risk factor for ischaemic heart disease in US men and women aged 20–74 years were 5.69 mmol/L and 5.82 mmol/L, respectively[22,23] (Figure 11.2b). The prevalence of serum total cholesterol (>6.47 mmol/L) was much lower in Japanese rural men (7%) than in US railroad male workers (39%) aged 40–59 years.[21] Within Japan, the mean levels of serum total cholesterol showed large regional and occupational variations; those in rural men and women aged 40–69 years were 3.98 and 4.13 mmol/L respectively,[8] while 4.76 and 4.94 mmol/L in urban men and women, respectively.[7] Additionally, the mean total cholesterol levels in blue- and white-collared male workers aged 40–59 years were 4.81 mmol/ L and 5.20 mmol/L respectively.[3] In Japan, in the 1960s, the regional and socioeconomic disparities in blood cholesterol levels supported the idea that ischaemic heart disease was a 'disease of affluence'. In contrast, today, the risk of heart attack is linked to lower rather than higher education and income.

The striking diversity in cholesterol levels came from the extremely low intake of saturated fat (animal fat) in Japan compared to the US. Moreover, regional and occupational variations existed within Japan. While the dietary intake of saturated fat, a major determinant of blood total cholesterol, was 3% of the total calories consumed by Japanese rural men, it was 18% of the total calories consumed by US railroad male workers aged 40–59 years.[21] The Japanese national mean saturated fat intake levels in rural and urban residents aged 20 years were 9 g/day and 13 g/day, respectively.[24] These values in blue- and white-collared male workers aged 40–59 years were 11 g/day and 13 g/day respectively,[25] compared to ≥30 g/day in Americans.[12] The low intake of saturated fat by the Japanese is due to their traditional diet which includes a small portion of meat and dairy products and a large portion of rice and cereals, miso soup, salt-preserved or soy-sourced fish and vegetables.[6,24]

The national mean levels of body mass index (BMI) were 25.1 kg/m² and 24.9 kg/m² in US men and women aged 20–74 years respectively in the 1960s[26] (Figure 11.2c).The prevalence of high body weight was much lower in Japanese rural men (2%) than in US railroad male workers (32%) aged 40–59 years.[21] There were, however, no significant differences based on geography and occupation within Japan (BMI for rural and urban residents and male workers: 22–23 g/m²).[7,8] As for the prevalence of diabetes in the 1960s, there was no national-level data for Japan, the US, or England, as well as data for Japan based on region and occupation. Moreover, quantitative data on physical activity was also lacking, but jobs involving hard labour such as farming and manufacturing were very common in the 1960s before the introduction of widespread mechanization. Hard manual labour can trigger a sharp increase in blood pressure levels and raise the risk of stroke among hypertensive persons.

At a national level, the proportion of smokers aged ≥15 years was 82% in Japanese men and 16% in Japanese women while the corresponding proportions in US men and women were 52% and 34% respectively in 1965[28] (Figure 11.2d). Smoking was highly common among Japanese rural men (71–77%) compared to US railroad male workers (56%) aged 40–59 years in the 1960s.[21]

Japanese health profiles in the 1960s reveal the highest mortality from stroke and the lowest mortality from ischaemic heart disease worldwide, probably due to the high proportion of small vascular pathology and the low proportion of large vascular pathology. These Japanese profiles were attributable to the high prevalence of hypertension, smoking (in men), and the low prevalence of high blood cholesterol, obesity, as well as the traditional Japanese diet containing high salt, low animal protein and fat.

11.3 Trends for Cardiovascular Diseases, Risk Factors and Behaviours since the 1960s

11.3.1 Mortality and Incidence of Cardiovascular Diseases

As shown in Figure 11.1, Japan has had a substantial decline in mortality from stroke (down to one-eighth), and a moderate decline in ischaemic heart disease (down to half) between 1960 and 2015. In 2015, the mortality rate from stroke in Japan was comparable to that in the UK, US, and Finland, while mortality from ischaemic heart disease was only half or one-third of that in these other nations.

As for trends in the incidence of stroke and ischaemic heart disease, they varied by geography, occupation, and sex within Japan. Between the 1960s and 2000s, age-adjusted annual incidence of stroke declined from 9.7 to 2.3 per 1,000 (76%) and from 4.2 to 1.1 per 1,000 (76%) in rural men and women aged 40–69 years respectively, and from 2.7 to 1.2 per 1,000 (56%) and from 1.3 to 0.80 per 1,000 (38%) in urban men and women aged 40–69 years respectively.[8] In the 2000s, the incidence of stroke was still two-fold higher in rural than in urban men and women. While between the 1960s and 1990s, the age-adjusted annual incidence of ischaemic heart disease increased by 3.5 times from 0.4 to 1.4 per 1,000 in urban male workers aged 40–59 years,[7] between the 1960s and 2000s, it doubled from 0.6 to 1.2 per 1,000 in urban men aged 40–69 years.[8] However, between the 1960s and 2000s, no changes were seen in the trend for incident ischaemic heart disease among rural men and women and urban women.[8]

11.3.2 Risk Factors and Behaviours

The national mean levels of systolic blood pressure in Japanese men and women aged ≥30 years declined from 142 mmHg and 141 mmHg in the 1960s to 138 mmHg and 133 mmHg in the 2000s, respectively and continued to decline even after the 2000s[15] (Figure 11.2a). Similar blood pressure declines, albeit with lower mean levels than the Japanese, were observed in US men and women between the 1960s and 2000s.[17,18]

Within Japan, the mean levels of blood pressures declined substantially between the 1960s and 2010s, with a larger decline in rural residents,[8] and a similar decline in both blue- and white-collared male workers.[7] The prevalence of very high blood pressure levels decreased in rural residents between the 1960s and 1970s primarily due to screening and treatment for hypertension.[6] A large decrease in mean blood pressure levels was also seen in rural residents between the 1970s and 1980s probably due to lifestyle improvements.[29]

Between the 1960s and 1980s, salt intake declined from 20 g/day to 14 g/day in rural men aged 40–59 years and from 13 g/day to 12 g/day in urban men.[6,19] According to the Japan National Nutrition Survey, the mean salt intake decreased from 12.7 g/day in 2003 to 10.8 g/day in 2017 for men, and from 10.9 g/day to 9.1 g/day for women aged ≥20 years.[15]

The national mean levels of blood cholesterol in Japanese men and women aged ≥30 years increased from 4.81 mol/L and 4.94 mmol/L in the 1970s to 5.14 mmol/L and 5.36 mmol/L in the 2010s respectively,[15,16] and plateaued thereafter, reaching levels comparable to those in US men and women where the opposite trends were observed (a drop from 5.51–5.59 mmol/L to 5.02–5.12 mmol/L)[22,23] (Figure 11.2b).

Within Japan, mean total cholesterol levels for rural men and women aged 40–69 years increased from 3.98 mmol/L and 4.14 mmol/L in the 1960s to 5.12 mmol/L and 5.46 mmol/L in the 1990s, respectively. Similarly, in urban men and women, it increased from 4.76 mmol/L and 4.94 mmol/L to 5.46 mmol/L and 5.74 mmol/L, respectively.[8] From the 1960s to 2010s, the blood cholesterol levels in blue- and white-collared male workers aged 40–59 years increased from 4.81 mmol/L and 5.20 mmol/L to 5.28 mmol/L and 5.30 mmol/L, respectively.[7]

Changes in saturated fat intake correlated with changes in blood cholesterol levels,[24] and the Japan National Nutrition Survey showed similar results. The mean saturated fat intake increased from 9 g/day in the 1960s to 14 g/day in the 1980s in rural residents aged ≥20 years and from 13 g/day to 16 g/day in urban residents.[24] After the 1990s, the national level of saturated fat intake has not changed in Japanese men and women.[15]

Between the 1970s to 2010s, the national mean levels of BMI in Japanese men and women ≥20 years remained within the healthy range (22–23 kg/m^2) with a slight increase in men (still < 24 kg/m^2) and no change in women[15,30] (Figure 11.2c). However, during this period, the average BMI in US men and women aged 20–74 years increased from 25 kg/m^2 to 30 kg/m^2.[26,27,31] This large difference in mean BMI between the two countries in the 2010s corresponded to the substantial difference in the proportion of overweight (BMI ≥25 kg/m^2) individuals in Japan (20–30%)[15] versus the US (70–80%).[31] However, within Japan, changes in the prevalence of obesity (BMI ≥25 kg/m^2) did not vary significantly based on geography and occupation.

The prevalence of diabetes in rural men and women aged 40–79 years increased from 15% and 9% in the 1980s to 21% and 11% in the 2000s, respectively.[32] However, in rural men and women aged 40–69 years, very little change was observed; from 23% and 11% in the 1980s to 23% and 12% in the 2000s, respectively.[32] During the same period, the prevalence of diabetes went from 17% and 10% to 22% and 9% in urban men and women, respectively.[8] According to the Japan National Nutrition Survey, the prevalence of diabetes went from 10% and 7% in 2006 to 14% and 7% in 2015 for men and women ≥20 years, respectively.[15] The prevalence of diabetes in Japan is still lower than that in Western countries.[33]

At a national level, the proportion of current smokers in Japanese men and women aged ≥15 years dropped from 82% and 16% in 1965 to 32% and 8% in 2010[28] (and further declined to 29% and 7% in 2017[15]), respectively, while the corresponding proportions in US men and women went from 52% and 34% to 17% and 14%[28] (Figure 11.2d) respectively. Within Japan, the proportion of current smokers has declined in men, and has remained low in women regardless of geography between the 1970s and the 2000s; going from 68% and 3% in the 1970s to 53% and 3% in the 2000s for rural men and women aged 40–69 years, respectively, and from 67% and 10% to 49% and 10% for urban men and women[8] respectively. Mean alcohol consumption also slightly declined for both rural and urban men aged 40–69 years between the 1970s and 2000s.[8] According to the Japan National Nutrition Survey, the proportion of current habitual drinkers declined from 52% in 1990 to 33% in 2017 for men, and slightly increased from 6% to 8% for women aged ≥20 years.[15]

A substantial decline in stroke mortality, going from the highest to the lowest levels of mortality rate in the world and a moderate decline in ischaemic heart disease mortality remaining among the countries with the lowest rates since the 1960s can be attributed to a large decline in blood pressure, a moderate decline in smoking (for men) and an increase in blood cholesterol levels, but no or smaller increase in obesity and diabetes. A reduction in salt intake, combined with a moderate increase in the intake of animal protein and fat (saturated fat) also accounts for the changes in cardiovascular diseases and their risk factors.

11.4 Has Globalization Changed the Japanese Diet?

11.4.1 Economic Development and Diet

The rapid economic growth between the 1960s and the 1970s led to a remarkable improvement in access to fresh foods such as fish, meat, vegetables, and fruits due to the development of food preservation, transportation and markets. The improved economy stimulated the purchase of home refrigerators and fresh foods, which helped to reduce the reliance on foods preserved using salt, miso and soy source.[6] In the meantime, mechanization developed rapidly in many industries, including farming, leading to a significant decrease in work involving extremely hard manual labour. These circumstances helped in reducing salt intake and having more balanced diets, which contributed to lower blood pressure levels and reduced incidence of stroke and ischaemic heart disease.[6,34]

11.4.2 The Japanese Diet in the 1960s (Past) and in the 2010s (Present)

The traditional Japanese diet common in the 1960s was characterized mainly by rice and cereals with soybean soup, salt-preserved pickles, and salty dried fish (Figure 11.3). This traditional diet is still consumed, particularly by rural middle-aged and older residents.[15] The nutritional flaws of the traditional Japanese diet include high salt, low calcium and very low animal protein and

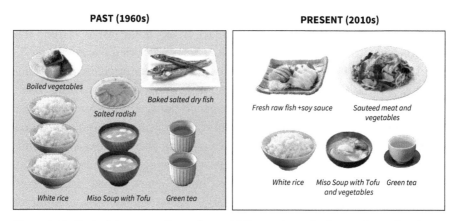

Figure 11.3 Typical Japanese dinner for a middle-aged man in the past (1960s) and present (2010s)

Past: white rice (150 g × 3 = 750 Cal), miso soup (150 g × 2 = 140 Cal + 4 g salt), salted radish (6 g × 15 = 30 Cal + 3 g salt), baked salted dry fish (15 g × 3 = 100 Cal + 2 g salt), boiled vegetables (50 Cal + 3 g salt). Total: 1070 Cal + 12 g salt.

Present: white rice (150 g × 1 = 250 Cal), miso soup with tofu and vegetables (150 g × 1 = 120 Cal + 1.5 g salt), fresh raw fish with soy sauce (60 g = 80 Cal + 1.5g salt), sautéed meat and vegetables (350 Cal + 2.5 g salt). Total: 800 Cal + 5.5 g salt.

Sources: Japan National Nutrition Survey, Energy and Salt Intake Estimated from the Standard Tables of Food Composition in Japan, 2015 (seventh revised edition).

fat. The modern Japanese diet, recognized as a healthy diet, is composed of fresh fish, meat, soy and vegetables, and is available during all four seasons.

The modern Japanese diet has low saturated fat (increased from the 1970s but still low; the distribution hardly overlaps with that in the American diet)[12,24] and a good overall nutritional balance.[35,36] This low intake of saturated fat keeps the chances of developing ischaemic heart disease low due to low levels of blood cholesterol (more specifically, low-density lipoprotein cholesterol, namely atherosclerosis-induced 'bad' type cholesterol).[34]

High fish intake may also keep the incidence of ischaemic heart disease low due to attenuation of blood clot formation.[37] According to the most extensive systematic review of randomized controlled trials conducted to date,[38] the supplementation of long-chain omega-3 fatty acids rich in fish suggested a reduction in risk of ischaemic heart disease events, but had little or no effect on mortality from cardiovascular disease.

11.4.3 Characteristics of the Modern Japanese Diet

The Japanese diet differs from the Mediterranean diet, another world-wide recognized healthy diet in terms of the seasoning used. While the former uses salt, soy sauce, and soy-bean paste, the latter uses vegetable oil (olive oil), pepper, and herbs. The modern Japanese diet still has higher salt and lower calcium content compared to the Mediterranean diet. In Japan, the fast food trend was introduced by franchise companies such as Kentucky Fried Chicken in 1970, MacDonald's in 1971, Yoshinoya Gyudon (bowl of rice topped with soy-and-sugar-sauced boiled beef) in 1973, Pizza-la in 1987, and many other companies which have appealed to younger generations. At the same time since 1970, franchise chains of family-friendly restaurants and convenience stores have appeared and provided not only Western but also Japanese style menus and 'bento' lunch with balanced nutrients, continuing the Japanese tradition. The proportion of ready-to-eat foods, including bento, increased from 4.4% in 1975 to 8.3% in 1991 and continued to increase thereafter, accounting for 11.8% of the total food sales in 2005. However, the prevalence of eating out increased from 10.2% to 15.6% and then began to decline thereafter.[39] These figures suggest that fast foods have not dominated the food industry in Japan.

According to the Japan National Nutrition Survey, the mean consumption of fish decreased from 94 g/day in 2001 to 64 g/day in 2017, and that of rice decreased from 356 g/day to 308 g/day. At the same time, the mean consumption of meat increased from 76 g/day to 99 g/day.[15]

The age-specific mean fish intake in 2017 was 50 g, 51 g, 53 g, 69 g, 80 g and 86 g for individuals in their twenties, thirties, forties, fifties, sixties, and seventies, respectively. For the same age groups, the corresponding mean rice intake was 332 g, 335 g, 317 g, 309 g, 282 g, and 279 g, respectively, while the meat intake was 129 g, 115 g, 115 g, 105 g, 92 g, and 75 g, respectively. The younger Japanese eat less rice, less fish and more meat as their main energy sources compared to the older Japanese.

The traditional Japanese diet has changed to a modern and healthier version along with the economic development since the 1960s. Despite the introduction of the fast-food industry in 1970, the Japanese, in general, have resisted fast foods, and have preferred to stay with a more or less traditional rice-based diet. However, a further decline in rice and fish intake and a further increase in meat intake may cause future increases in obesity, diabetes, and ischaemic heart disease.

11.5 Roles of Prevention Activities through Public Health Services and Medical Care

A frontier prevention programme for stroke in communities was launched in the early 1960s after the initiation of the 1961 universal health coverage.[6] This programme has employed screening and treatment for tuberculosis since the 1950s. It consisted of systematic blood pressure screening for the detection of hypertension by annual health check-ups for the middle-aged and elderly, referral of high-risk individuals to local physicians, health instructions for hypertension by physicians, access to public health nurses and nutritionists on an individual and group basis, adjunct activities by health volunteers, and community-wide media campaigns for health education.[40,41] One of the successful programmes achieved a substantial decline in blood pressure levels and approximately 50% or more reduction in the incidence of stroke[41] with cost-saving effects of public health services and medical care, compared to a reference community.[42]

Based on the above evidence, the Japanese government established the system in 1982 under the Health and Medical Service Act for the Aged, which made every municipality responsible for offering screening, preventive activities, and supportive medical care. This responsibility shifted to health insurers under the Act on Assurance of Medical Care for Elderly People in 2008 when the screening was focused on prevention and control of metabolic syndrome (abdominal obesity plus two or more metabolic risk factors based on the Japanese criteria) in order to prevent lifestyle-related diseases such as cardiovascular disease and chronic kidney disease.[43] In Japan, hypertension but not metabolic syndrome is still the major cause of cardiovascular diseases given the high salt intake, as well as the low prevalence of overweight and diabetes.[44]

11.6 Present and Future Issues in Health Inequality for Cardiovascular Diseases

Japan has been successful in reducing its mortality rates associated with stroke and ischaemic heart disease through substantial improvements in health behaviours (reduced salt intake and balanced intake of major nutrients) and cardiovascular risk factors. However, there are still regional and occupation-based inequalities in cardiovascular diseases and risk factors due to economic and psychosocial variations.

Since the 1990s, the estimated number of patients with diseases such as chronic heart failure, kidney disease, and dementia has increased substantially. According to the Patient Survey in Japan in mid-October from 1996 to 2017, the numbers of patients per day rose from 38,600 to 59,700 for chronic heart failure, 97,700 to 188,600 for kidney disease, and 54,000 to 135,500 for dementia. It is not clear how much of these increases are explained by ageing of the population.[45] Further, there is an increasing incidence of ischaemic heart disease probably caused by the reduced intake of fish, physical inactivity, and increased blood cholesterol levels (albeit small increase in BMI) among middle-aged men, as seen in urban male workers between the 1960s and 1990s,[7] and urban men between the 1960s and 2000s.[8]

To cope with these issues, Japan needs to develop a new model for the prevention and control of cardiovascular diseases and related chronic diseases considering its super-ageing population and reduced traditional social network due to an increase in nuclear families and enhanced individualism. Public health services and medical care efforts are focussed towards the early prevention of cardiovascular and related chronic diseases as well as their progress. The linkage, integration, and use of a database for public health services and medical care from pre-birth to old age (which is now segregated among different administrative sections) is urgently required. Our experiences in this area could provide valuable lessons to other countries, especially countries of Asia and the mid-East, which are also facing rapid population ageing.

11.7 Conclusions

Japan has been successful in substantially reducing the incidence of stroke from high levels and in moderately reducing the incidence of ischaemic heart disease from an already low level, a unique trend in the control of cardiovascular diseases. This trend has contributed to Japan's top ranking in terms of longevity. This great achievement coincides with reduced urban-rural inequalities in cardiovascular diseases, risk factors and behaviours. Important factors include rapid and profound socioeconomic developments and policies that support population health and the health care system, and the Japanese cultural characteristic of considerable resistance to the Westernization of their diet. However, advanced ageing, increasing economic inequality, and psychosocial factors such as increased mental stress and work-life imbalance are new challenges for the future prevention and control of cardiovascular and related diseases.

Acknowledgements

The authors thank Professor Emeritus Yoshio Komachi, a pioneer cardiovascular epidemiologist in Japan, and his colleagues, as well as other distinguished professors and researchers working on the epidemiology of cardiovascular diseases. The authors also thank Drs. Hironori Imano, Isao Muraki, Mina Hayama-Terada, Yasuhiko Kubota, Tomomi Kihara, Takeo Okada, Masahiko Kiyama, and Akihiko Kitamura for their contribution in the critical revision of this chapter.

References

1. Marmot MG, Smith GD. Why are the Japanese living longer? *BMJ* 1989;299:1547–51.
2. Ikeda N, Saito E, Kondo N, et al. What has made the population of Japan healthy? *Lancet* 2011;378:1094–105.
3. Komachi Y, Iida M, Shimamoto T, Chikayama Y, Takahashi H. Geographic and occupational comparisons of risk factors in cardiovascular diseases in Japan. *Jpn Circ J* 1971;35:189–207.
4. Yamagishi K, Muraki I, Kubota Y, et al. The Circulatory Risk in Communities Study (CIRCS): a long-term epidemiological study for lifestyle-related disease among Japanese men and women living in communities. *J Epidemiol* 2019;29:83–91.

5. Ninomiya T. Japanese legacy cohort studies: The Hisayama Study. *J Epidemiol* 2018;28:444–51.

6. Shimamoto T, Komachi Y, Inada H, et al. Trends for coronary heart disease and stroke and their risk factors in Japan. *Circulation* 1989;79:503–15.

7. Kitamura A, Iso H, Iida M, et al. Trends in the incidence of coronary heart disease and stroke and the prevalence of cardiovascular risk factors among Japanese men from 1963 to 1994. *Am J Med* 2002;112:104–9.

8. Kitamura A, Sato S, Kiyama M, et al. Trends in the incidence of coronary heart disease and stroke and their risk factors in Japan, 1964 to 2003: the Akita-Osaka study. *J Am Coll Cardiol* 2008;52:71–9.

9. World Health Organization. World Health Statistics Annual 1993. Geneva: World Health Organization, 1994. *WHO Mortality Database*. Available at: http://www.who.int/healthinfo/mortality_data/en/ [last accessed July 21, 2020].

10. Konishi M, Iso H, Komachi Y, et al. Associations of serum total cholesterol, different types of stroke, and stenosis distribution of cerebral arteries. The Akita Pathology Study. *Stroke* 1993;24:954–64.

11. Iso H, Jacobs DR, Jr., Wentworth D, Neaton JD, Cohen JD. Serum cholesterol levels and six-year mortality from stroke in 350,977 men screened for the multiple risk factor intervention trial. *N Engl J Med* 1989;320:904–10.

12. Iso H, Sato S, Kitamura A, Naito Y, Shimamoto T, Komachi Y. Fat and protein intakes and risk of intraparenchymal hemorrhage among middle-aged Japanese. *Am J Epidemiol* 2003;157:32–9.

13. Yamagishi K, Iso H, Kokubo Y, et al. Dietary intake of saturated fatty acids and incident stroke and coronary heart disease in Japanese communities: the JPHC Study. *Eur Heart J* 2013;34:1225–32.

14. Ozawa M, Yoshida D, Hata J, et al. Dietary protein intake and stroke risk in a general Japanese population: The Hisayama Study. *Stroke* 2017;48:1478–86.

15. Health Service Division, Ministry of Health, Labour and Welfare. National Health and Nutrition Survey (in Japanese). Available at: http://www.nibiohn.go.jp/eiken/kenkounippon21/eiyouchousa/keinen_henka_shintai.html [last accessed July 21, 2020].

16. Ministry of Health, Labour and Welfare. National Survey on Circulatory Disorders (in Japanese). Available at: https://www.mhlw.go.jp/toukei/list/junkanki_chousa.html [last accessed July 21, 2020].

17. Drizd T, Dannenberg AL, Engel A. Blood pressure levels in persons 18–74 years of age in 1976 to 1980, and trends in blood pressure from 1960 to 1980 in the United States. *Vital Health Stat 11* 1986;234:1–68.

18. Wright JD, Hughes JP, Ostchega Y, Yoon SS, Nwankwo T. Mean systolic and diastolic blood pressure in adults aged 18 and over in the United States, 2001–2008. *Natl Health Stat Report* 2011;35:1–24.

19. Komachi Y (Ed.). *Changes in Nutrition and Cardiovascular Disease in Japan* (in Japanese). Tokyo: Hoken Dojin Press 1987.

20. Umesawa M, Kitamura A, Kiyama M, et al. Association between dietary behavior and risk of hypertension among Japanese male workers. *Hypertens Res* 2013;36:374–80.

21. Keys A. Coronary heart disease in seven countries. *Circulation* 1970 (4 Suppl). doi:10.1016/s0899-9007(96)00410-8

22. Carroll MD, Lacher DA, Sorlie PD, et al. Trends in serum lipids and lipoproteins of adults, 1960-2002. *JAMA* 2005;294:1773–81.

23. Carroll MD, Kit BK, Lacher DA, Shero ST, Mussolino ME. Trends in lipids and lipoproteins in US adults, 1988–2010. *JAMA* 2012;308:1545–54.

24. Okayama A, Ueshima H, Marmot MG, Elliott P, Yamakawa M, Kita Y. Different trends in serum cholesterol levels among rural and urban populations aged 40–59 in Japan from 1960 to 1990. *J Clin Epidemiol* 1995;48:329–37.

25. Ueshima H, Iida M, Shimamoto T, et al. Dietary intake and serum total cholesterol level: their relationship to different lifestyles in several Japanese populations. *Circulation* 1982;66:519–26.

26. Ogden CL, Fryar CD, Carroll MD, Flegal KM. Mean body, weight, height and body mass index, United States 1960–2002. *Adv Data* 2004;347:1–17.

27. Fryar CD, Kruszon-Moran D, Gu Q, Ogden CL. Mean body weight, height, waist circumference, and body mass index among adults: United States, 1999–2000 through 2015–2016. *Natl Health Stat Report* 2018;122:1–16.

28. OECD Health Statistics: Non-medical determinants of health. Daily smokers (indicator). doi:10.1787/1ff488c2-en

29. Shimamoto T, Iso H, Sankai T, et al. Can blood pressure in the elderly be reduced? Findings from a long-term population survey in Japan. *Am J Geriatr Caridiol* 1994;3:42–50.

30. Yoshiike N, Seino F, Tajima S, et al. Twenty-year changes in the prevalence of overweight in Japanese adults: The National Nutrition Survey 1976–1995. *Obes Rev* 2002;3:183–90.

31. Flegal KM, Carroll MD, Kit BK, Ogden CL. Prevalence of obesity and trends in the distribution of body mass index among US adults, 1999–2010. *JAMA* 2012;307:491–7.

32. Muikai N, Doi Y, Ninomiya T, et al. Trends in the prevalence of type 2 diabetes and prediabetes in community-dwelling Japanese subjects: The Hisayama Study. *J Diabetes Invest* 2014;5:162–9.

33. Danaei G, Finucane MM, Lu Y, et al. National, regional, and global trends in fasting plasma glucose and diabetes prevalence since 1980: systematic analysis of health examination surveys and epidemiological studies with 370 country-years and 2.7 million participants. *Lancet* 2011;378(9785):31–40.

34. Iso H. Changes in coronary heart disease risk among Japanese. *Circulation* 2008;118:2725–9.
35. Nagata C, Wada K, Tamura T, et al. Dietary soy and natto intake and cardiovascular disease mortality in Japanese adults: the Takayama study. *Am J Clin Nutr* 2017;105:426–31.
36. Kurotani K, Akter S, Kashino I, et al. Quality of diet and mortality among Japanese men and women: Japan Public Health Center based prospective study. *BMJ* 2016;22:352:i1209.
37. Iso H, Kobayashi M, Ishihara J, et al. Intake of fish and n3 fatty acids and risk of coronary heart disease among Japanese: the Japan Public Health Center-Based (JPHC) Study Cohort I. *Circulation* 2006;113:195–202.
38. Abdelhamid AS, Martin N, Bridges C, et al. Polyunsaturated fatty acids for the primary and secondary prevention of cardiovascular disease. *Cochrane Database Syst Rev* 2018;7:CD012345.
39. Statsitcs Bureau of Japan. The Family Income and Expenditure Survey (in Japanese). Available at: https://www.stat.go.jp/data/kakei/index.html [last accessed July 21, 2020].
40. WHO News. Community-based efforts to reduce blood pressure and stroke in Japan. Available at: https://www.who.int/features/2013/japan_blood_pressure/en/ [last accessed July 21, 2020].
41. Iso H, Shimamoto T, Naito Y, et al. Effects of a long-term hypertension control program on stroke incidence and prevalence in a rural community in northeastern Japan. *Stroke* 1998;29:1510–18.
42. Yamagishi K, Sato S, Kitamura A, et al. Cost-effectiveness and budget impact analyses of a long-term detection and control program for stroke prevention. *J Hypertens* 2012;30:1874–9.
43. Kohro T, Furui Y, Mitsutake N, Fujii R, Morita H, Oku S, Ohe K, Nagai R. The Japanese national health screening and intervention program aimed at preventing worsening of the metabolic syndrome. *Int Heart J* 2008;49:193–203.
44. Noda H, Iso H, Saito I, Konishi M, Inoue M, Tsugane S; JPHC Study Group. The impact of the metabolic syndrome and its components on the incidence of ischemic heart disease and stroke: the Japan public health center-based study. *Hypertens Res* 2009;32:289–98.
45. Health Statistics Office, Ministry of Health, Welfare and Labour. Patient Survey (in Japanese). Available at: https://www.mhlw.go.jp/toukei/list/10-20.html [last accessed July 21, 2020].

12

Cancer Inequalities in Japan

Yuri Ito and Bernard Rachet

12.1 Context

12.1.1 Cancer: Not a Single Cause

Cancers are defined as diseases in which abnormal cells divide without control and invade nearby tissues. Cancer cells may spread to other parts of the body through the blood and lymphatic system. Cancer is a malignant and invasive non-communicable disease, which includes several types such as carcinoma, sarcoma, leukaemia, lymphoma, and central nervous system cancers.

The Japanese word for cancer is *Gan*, and was regarded with great fear because, for a long time, we were ignorant as to the causes of cancer and lacked curative treatment. The term *Gan* consists partly of the Chinese character for 'rock' (*iwa* or *gan* in Japanese), because cancer was detected at the late stage, and people thought of the tumour as a 'rock' in seventeenth-century Japan. In the 1800s, Seishu Hanaoka of Wakayama was the first surgeon to successfully remove a 'rock', when he performed a partial mastectomy under general anaesthesia. After furthering our understanding of some of the mechanisms of cancer incidence, risk factors for different cancers, and development of surgical and medical cancer treatment, we have started to control cancer. However, as with many other diseases, socioeconomic inequalities in cancer occurrence, detection, and treatment remain an important challenge for cancer control.

12.1.2 Measures of Cancer Burden

Cancer burden is measured by three main indicators: rates of mortality, incidence, and survival. The mortality rate is the number of cancer deaths

Yuri Ito and Bernard Rachet, *Cancer Inequalities in Japan* In: *Health in Japan*. Edited by: Eric Brunner, Noriko Cable, and Hiroyasu Iso, Oxford University Press (2021). © Oxford University Press. DOI: 10.1093/oso/9780198848134.003.0012.

in the population, based on vital statistics derived from death certification and the National Census. Cancer mortality is an important indicator of the impact of the disease on society. In Japan, reduction in cancer mortality was the main target in the National Cancer Control Plan. Cancer incidence and survival estimates are based on data collected by population-based cancer registries, which collect information on virtually all incident cancer cases diagnosed within a defined area. Incidence is the number of newly diagnosed cancer cases in the population in a defined time period. It is useful for the evaluation of primary prevention, e.g. as a consequence of reduced exposure to a risk factor for the cancer. Measured incidence is heavily influenced by early detection and the data quality of the cancer registry. Survival is the proportion of patients alive for a certain period after diagnosis/treatment. This indicator can be used for the evaluation of improvement in cancer diagnosis and treatment. All three indicators are important for meaningful evaluation of cancer control activities including primary prevention, screening, and cancer care.

Inequalities in cancer burden have several dimensions. Interpretation of the statistics is not easy when considering the combined influence of incidence and survival. Inequalities in incidence largely reflect differences in risk factors, though they can be directly impacted by the health system through early diagnosis and screening. Inequalities in cancer survival are also complex, with healthcare systems and inequalities in cancer care at their core. In this chapter, we will look at the trends in inequalities in these three measurements and try to interpret them, in a Japanese context.

In Japan, mortality data based on death certification are available from the 1950s onwards. Population data are based on National Census data which have been collected every five years since 1920. Population-based cancer registries were first started in a few prefectures in the 1950s, covering 13% of the national population in ten prefectures by 1960, and 28% by 2000. It was not until 2016, when the law of cancer registration was enacted in Japan, that all prefectures started to collect high quality data to measure cancer survival. Distribution and trends in cancer incidence showed wide variation among prefectures in Japan. Therefore, comparative data among prefectures is essential for cancer control based on regional variations.

Although only a limited number of prefectures are able to provide long-term population-based data, Japan contributes to international studies and atlases on mortality, incidence, and survival.[1-3]

12.1.3 Trends in Cancer Burden

After a steady increase, the all-cancer mortality rate started to decrease in the mid-1990s in men and the 1960s in women. There has been a dramatic increase in the all-cancer incidence rate in both sexes since the mid-2000s.[4] Putting these trends together, it is clear there has been a substantial improvement in cancer survival (prognosis) in recent decades. According to recent worldwide surveillance data, survival after stomach cancer diagnosis in Japan is the highest in the world. The screening programme may have contributed to this success. The other sites of solid cancer also showed high survival, as in Western countries, but haematological malignancy in adults showed lower survival.[3]

Trends in mortality rates of major cancer sites in Japan differ from Western countries but share some similarities with other East Asian countries (Figure 12.1). In Japan, lung cancer mortality increased until around 2000, and then showed a small decrease in both sexes, while trends in the UK, the US, and Australia showed a dramatic decrease, especially in men. This might be related to differences in tobacco control activities (Chapter 14).

Colorectal cancer mortality showed a striking increase in East Asian countries, while Western countries showed continuously decreasing trends. In Japan, colorectal cancer mortality was the lowest in the world in the 1960s, but then increased substantially, becoming one of the highest worldwide in the 1990s. This may be due to changes to a more Western diet and inefficient screening strategies in Japan.

Stomach cancer was once the leading cause of cancer death in Japan, but the mortality rate has decreased dramatically since the 1960s for both sexes. However, the mortality rate of stomach cancer in East Asian countries is still higher than in Western countries. Improvements in environmental hygiene, including cleaner water supply and widespread use of refrigerators in Japan, have led to a reduction in risk factors including *Helicobacter pylori* infection[5] and salt intake.[6] In addition, the screening programme led to an increase of early detection of stomach cancer. Improvements in treatment for stomach cancer also increased survival rates in Japan.

Breast cancer mortality is lower in Japan than in Western countries, but the gap has become smaller due to the dramatic decrease of mortality in Western countries in the past 30 years and gradual increase over the past 50 years in Japan. In Western countries, nationwide mammography screening and improved access to new treatments, such as adjuvant chemotherapy and tam-oxifen, has contributed to the notable decrease in breast cancer mortality. In Japan, increasing trends in mortality might correspond to increased preva-lence of risk factors, such as alcohol intake and reproductive factors including having no children and not breast feeding. Low participation rates in the screening programme may also contribute.

Cervical cancer mortality showed dramatically decreasing trends in many countries other than Japan. Stable trends and the highest mortality rate were observed in Japan. An unsuccessful screening programme is one of the reasons.

Prostate cancer mortality rates in Western countries were much higher than in Japan and Korea. Since the 1990s, the PSA test has been used for early de-tection, while both incidence and mortality rates jumped up in Western coun-tries. Some guidelines do not recommend PSA screening.[7] It may be that in recent years over-diagnosis due to false positive PSA tests has declined,[8] and mortality trends have followed (Figure 12.1).

12.1.4 Cancer Care, Cancer Policy, and Insurance Coverage

In Japan, universal healthcare coverage was introduced in 1961. Access to prevention, screening, and cancer care differ, compared to Canada, the UK, and Nordic countries. There are two types of health insurance in Japan, National Health Insurance and employment-based health insur-ance. National Health Insurance covers people who are unemployed or self-employed. In general, workers in large companies and civil servants benefit from comprehensive health insurance and regular opportunities for health checks and cancer screening. Small companies do not offer the same level of cover, and therefore provide fewer opportunities for screening (secondary prevention).

12.1.5 The Cancer Screening System in Japan

The first mass screening for stomach cancer started in the 1960s in Miyagi prefecture and was the first in the world. In 1983, the government started na-tionwide mass screening for stomach and cervical cancer followed by lung and breast cancer in 1987, and colorectal cancer in 1992. Although screening was introduced early, participation rates amongst the population remain low.

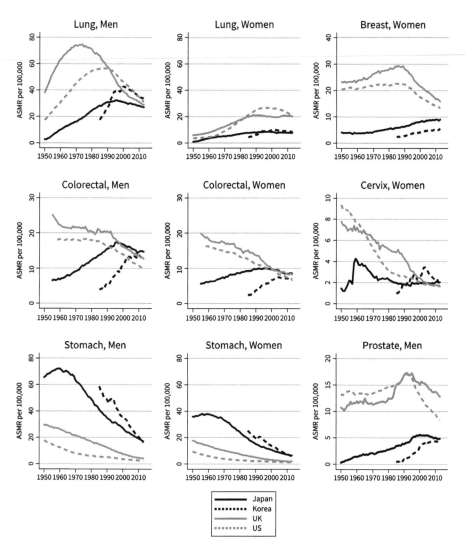

Figure 12.1 Age-standardized mortality rate for major cancer sites by sex in Japan and selected countries, 1950–2013

Age-standardized rates are based on the Segi's world population.

Source: World Health Organization Cancer Mortality Database. International Agency for Research on Cancer. http://www-dep.iarc.fr/WHOdb/WHOdb.htm

First, there are multiple settings where it is possible to attend cancer screening. Local government provides mass screening, but the target population is undefined. Large companies and government organizations are responsible for providing screening for their employees, but it is voluntary. Thus cancer screening participation is difficult to measure at a national level. One estimate suggests it may be very low, at around 40%.[9]

12.1.6 Diagnosis of Cancer

The prognosis of many cancers is improved by early diagnosis. Achieving this partly depends on accessibility and use of diagnostic tools and, for a few cancers, on screening programmes. Patients are usually referred to a specialized cancer care hospital following a first consultation in a primary care clinic or a cancer screening result. Access to cancer care in Japan is not restricted, which means that patients are free to choose any hospital, including a specialized cancer centre, based on their symptoms. The choice may affect the cancer prognosis, since poorer survival has been observed among patients treated in lower volume hospitals in Japan.[10] Another concern is the high proportion of people with a positive faecal occult blood test who do not seek diagnostic investigation for colorectal cancer. These factors linked to delayed diagnosis are however balanced by the large number of diagnostic medical devices, including CT and MRI scanners, per population in Japan. The availability of scanners may stimulate diagnostic activity, including opportunistic investigation. This explanation is consistent with the increase in early-stage tumour detection for some cancer sites.[11]

12.1.7 Cancer Care

The government set a target of equality in cancer care and introduced a National Cancer Control Plan in 2007. The plan supports prevention, early detection, equalization of cancer medical care, and research promotion. Designated cancer care hospitals providing a high standard level of care have been tasked to reduce inequity in cancer care. Gaps in cancer survival among prefectures were observed in the 1990s.[12] These gaps were reduced after the designated hospital scheme was established in 2007.[13] According to a recent report on treatment quality indicators from the National Cancer Centre, over 70% of specialist hospitals met the standard for cancer care.[14] Monitoring quality indicators for treatment and survival is essential to improve and assure cancer care and outcomes.

12.2 Trends in Inequalities in Mortality, Incidence, and Survival of Major Cancers

Socioeconomic inequalities in cancer incidence are directly related to inequalities in prevalence of cancer risks, mainly smoking, and inversely related to differences in screening uptakes. Reasons for socioeconomic inequalities in outcome after cancer diagnosis are likely to be different from those explaining inequalities in incidence. Both incidence and survival inequalities in cancer relate to inequalities in mortality.

12.2.1 Monitoring Inequalities in Cancer Using Population-based Data

Inequalities in cancer mortality at population level have been monitored with vital statistics and national census data using a geographical index of socioeconomic status.[15] This approach is necessary because individual socioeconomic information is not available in routinely collected population-based data. Inequalities in cancer incidence and survival have also been measured using the geographical index and population-based cancer registry data.

12.2.2 Inequalities in Cancer Mortality

We monitored socioeconomic inequalities in cancer mortality by cancer site using two measures. The absolute measure, or gap, is the difference in age-standardized mortality rates between the most deprived area and least deprived area. We also estimated relative inequalities in mortality as the ratio of rates in the most and least deprived area (Table 12.1, Figure 12.2). For comparison, absolute and relative inequalities in all-cause mortality are shown. Rates were age-standardized.

There was a large gap in all-cause mortality rates by geographical deprivation group in men but not in women. Absolute inequalities narrowed in men and widened in women from 1995–1999 to 2010–2014. All-cancer mortality showed a wide gap in men and a small gap in women, while gaps widened from 1995–1999 to 2010–2014 for both sexes. The proportion of the absolute difference in all-cause mortality accounted for by cancer mortality was calculated as absolute difference between the most and least deprived areas in all-cancer ASMR divided by the absolute difference between the most and least deprived areas in all-cause ASMR. The proportion was large and increased from 22% to 27% in men, and from 12% to 27% in women. The deprivation gap in cancer mortality was large compared to other main causes of death in Japan.[16]

Among major cancer sites, the largest absolute inequality in men was liver cancer (12.5 deaths per 100,000 person-years) in 1995–1999, but this

Table 12.1 Absolute and Relative Inequalities in All-cause and Cancer Mortality Using an Area Deprivation Index, Japan, 1995–1999 and 2010–2014

		ASMR[a]	Absolute inequality[b]		Relative inequality[c]	
			Estimate	95% CI	Estimate	95% CI
Men						
All causes	1995–1999	675	125	122	128	1.20	1.20	1.21
	2010–2014	527	117	115	119	1.25	1.25	1.26
All cancers	1995–1999	222	27.0	25.3	28.6	1.13	1.12	1.14
	2010–2014	176	31.6	30.4	32.7	1.20	1.19	1.20
Stomach	1995–1999	42.7	-1.3	-2.0	-0.6	0.97	0.95	0.99
	2010–2014	26.2	2.0	1.5	2.4	1.08	1.06	1.10
Colorectal	1995–1999	24.3	-0.7	-1.2	-0.2	0.97	0.95	0.99
	2010–2014	21.2	3.3	2.9	3.7	1.17	1.15	1.19
Liver	1995–1999	30.4	12.5	11.9	13.1	1.52	1.49	1.55
	2010–2014	17.1	7.9	7.6	8.3	1.60	1.57	1.64
Lung	1995–1999	47.2	8.8	8.1	9.6	1.21	1.19	1.23
	2010–2014	41.2	9.8	9.2	10.3	1.27	1.25	1.29
Leukaemia	1995–1999	5.2	1.8	1.5	2.0	1.41	1.34	1.48
	2010–2014	4.5	1.6	1.4	1.7	1.42	1.36	1.49

Women

		ASMR	Absolute inequality			Relative inequality		
All causes	1995–1999	355	23.6	21.9	25.3	1.07	1.06	1.07
	2010–2014	273	30.0	28.9	31.1	1.12	1.11	1.12
All cancers	1995–1999	107	2.8	1.9	3.8	1.03	1.02	1.04
	2010–2014	90.8	8.0	7.3	8.7	1.09	1.08	1.10
Stomach	1995–1999	17.0	-1.9	-2.3	-1.5	0.89	0.87	0.91
	2010–2014	9.6	-0.1	-0.3	0.1	0.99	0.97	1.01
Colorectal	1995–1999	14.0	-0.8	-1.1	-0.4	0.94	0.92	0.97
	2010–2014	12.2	0.6	0.4	0.9	1.05	1.03	1.07
Liver	1995–1999	9.2	2.7	2.4	2.9	1.34	1.30	1.38
	2010–2014	5.7	2.0	1.8	2.2	1.43	1.39	1.47
Lung	1995–1999	12.6	1.7	1.3	2.0	1.14	1.11	1.17
	2010–2014	11.5	2.3	2.0	2.5	1.22	1.19	1.25
Breast	1995–1999	10.2	-2.2	-2.6	-1.9	0.80	0.78	0.83
	2010–2014	11.8	-0.8	-1.2	-0.5	0.93	0.91	0.96
Cervical	1995–1999	2.6	0.5	0.3	0.6	1.19	1.12	1.27
	2010–2014	2.8	0.6	0.4	0.7	1.24	1.17	1.31
Leukaemia	1995–1999	3.1	1.2	1.1	1.4	1.51	1.42	1.60
	2010–2014	2.4	1.0	0.9	1.2	1.56	1.48	1.65

a. ASMR: age-standardized mortality rate per 100,000.

b. Absolute inequality: maximum difference due to inequalities in ASMR. Overall, the age-standardized all-cause mortality rate in men was 675/100,000 in 1995–1999. The difference in rates between areas with the highest and lowest deprivation index was 125/100,000.

c. Relative inequality: the ratio of ASMR between areas with the highest and lowest deprivation index was 1.20.

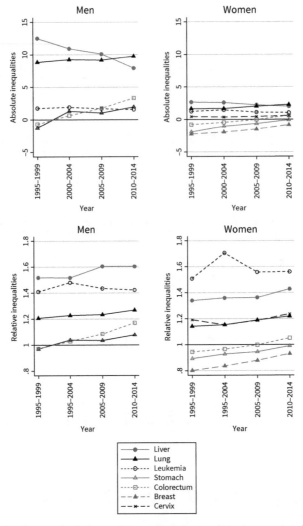

Figure 12.2 Absolute and relative socioeconomic inequalities in age-standardized mortality rates of selected cancer sites in Japan, 1995–2014

Absolute inequalities are the differences of age-standardized mortality rate per 100,000 between the most deprived and the least deprived area. Relative inequalities are the ratios of age-standardized mortality rate of the most deprived area to the least deprived area.

Source: Nakaya T and Ito Y. Synthesis. In: Nakaya T, Ito Y, eds. The Atlas of Health Inequalities in Japan, Springer 2019

decreased to 7.9 in 2010–2014. Relative inequality in liver cancer increased over this period. In 2010–2014, lung cancer mortality in men contributed 31% to the absolute deprivation gap in all-cancer mortality in men (absolute inequality in ASMR of lung cancer 9.8 divided by the absolute inequality in all-cancer ASMR 31.6 per 100,000). For women, absolute inequalities in all-cancer mortality were much smaller than in men, because some cancers showed negative differences. For example, women in the least deprived area had the highest breast cancer mortality rate. The absolute deprivation gap for cancer in women was small in 1995–1999, but it increased from 2.8 to 8.0 in 2010–2014. A striking change was observed in colorectal cancer in men and women. In 1995–1999, the absolute deprivation gap of colorectal cancer mortality was negative, but the absolute difference switched to a positive difference in 2010–2014 (Table 12.1).

12.2.3 Inequalities in Cancer Incidence

More affluent and better educated people are more likely to have regular cancer screening. As a result, cancer will often be diagnosed at an early stage. The stage at which the cancer is detected must be considered, in order to avoid distortion, or bias. For most types of cancer early detection greatly improves the chances of survival. Another more subtle bias may also operate. When a cancer is detected at an early stage, individuals will tend to survive for longer than those whose disease is diagnosed at a late stage, when symptoms appear. This 'lead time bias' means that over a period of years, survival may appear to increase because the proportion of cases detected early has risen due to improvement in a screening programme.

Lower socioeconomic status tends to be associated with later-stage cancer diagnosis.[17,18] Using the population-based cancer registry data in Osaka, similar results were observed for late-stage incidence rates of stomach, colorectal, lung, breast, and cervical cancer, although there are cancer screening programmes. Interestingly, the early-stage incidence rate showed an inverse contrast by deprivation quintile in men, but not in women. Higher incidence was observed in the less deprived than in the more deprived area for stomach, colon, and prostate cancer in men. Men but not women in the less deprived area tended to attend for screening and were diagnosed earlier than those in the more deprived area. This may be the consequence of work-related screening opportunities (Figure 12.3).

12.2.4 Inequalities in Cancer Survival

It was believed that universal health care protected the Japanese population from deprivation gaps in health outcomes after diagnosis. Following a report on deprivation gaps in cancer survival in England and Wales,[19] other

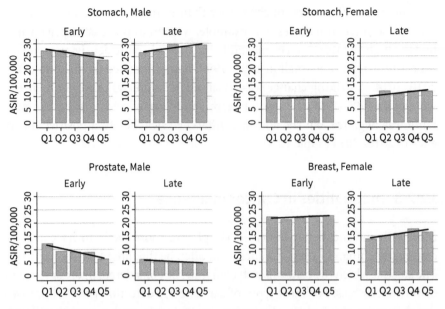

Figure 12.3 Stage-specific age-standardized incidence rate by area deprivation quintile for selected cancer sites in Osaka, Japan, 1999–2004

Early: localized stage. Late: regional or distant metastasis. Q1: least deprived area. Q5: most deprived area.

ASIR: age-standardized incidence rate per 100,000 person-years.

Source: Ito Y, Nakaya T, Kondo N, et al. Socio-Economic Differences In Stage-Specific Cancer Incidence In Osaka, Japan: 1993-2004. 37th International Association of Cancer Registries, Annual Scientific Conference 2015 2015:054 [O179].

countries reported deprivation gaps in cancer survival.[20] In Japan, wide deprivation gaps in cancer survival were reported in Osaka.[21] Cancers which had the highest five-year survival rates showed wider gaps in survival between the most and least deprived patients.

12.3 Inequalities in Risk Factors, Screening, and Treatment

12.3.1 Cancer Risk Factors in Japan

There are multiple risk factors for cancer. Hereditary factors modify susceptibility; however, many cancers are caused by environmental or behavioural factors, and some are preventable. The main known behavioural contributors to cancer in Japan are tobacco smoking, high alcohol consumption, and high salt intake. The population attributable fraction (PAF) quantifies the impact of a risk factor on disease occurrence in the population. PAF is a function of two measures: first, the excess risk of the disease attributable to the risk factor, second, the prevalence of risk factor in the population.

For the Japanese population in 2005, the most important behavioural risk factor for cancer death in men was smoking (34%), mainly related to lung, oesophageal, and oral cancer. The second most important risk factor was alcohol (9%), related to liver, oesophageal, oral, and pharyngeal cancer. Infection is the largest cause of female cancer death (19.4%); it is also large in men (23%) and is related to liver cancer (hepatitis B viruses (HBV) and hepatitis C viruses (HCV)), stomach cancer (*Helicobacter pylori*), and cervical cancer (human papilloma viruses (HPV)). Salt intake, overweight, and obesity (BMI > 25), low fruit intake, low vegetable intake, and physical inactivity are relatively minor factors[22] (Table 12.2).

In total, 57% of male cancer deaths and 30% of female cancer deaths were attributed to known and preventable causes. Among all known cancer risks, smoking is the largest attributable risk for cancer death in Japan, therefore, tobacco control should be the most important cancer control activity in Japan, but progress is quite slow (Chapter 14). As a result, lung cancer incidence and mortality, which has already declined in most Western countries, is a major problem in Japan, particularly for men.[11] Among cancers for which there is a preventive strategy, inequalities in the prevalence of risk factors is related to inequalities in cancer incidence and mortality. The deprivation gap in lung cancer mortality is strongly related to the deprivation gap in the prevalence of smoking (Chapter 14).

12.3.2 Inequalities in Liver Cancer Related to Hepatitis C Virus Prevalence and Alcohol Drinking

Trends in liver cancer incidence and mortality are unusual in Japan. Both incidence and mortality increased during the 1990s and then decreased dramatically. These trends are related to prevalence of HCV, which is the main cause of liver cancer in Japan. People born in the early 1930s have high risk of HCV infection due to transmission through blood transfusions and parenteral medical procedures.[23,24] The cohort born in 1925–1935 experienced peak incidence and mortality. Younger cohorts were much less at risk, due to the decrease in HCV prevalence, although the incidence rate is still higher than in Western countries. After World War II, HCV infection spread mainly in the western part of Japan. Deprived groups were at risk of transmitting the viruses through the economic necessity of selling their blood. In 2013, hazardous

Table 12.2 Impact of Preventable Risk Factors of Cancer Death in Japan (%)

Risk factor	Target cancers	Men	Women
Tobacco smoking	Oral and pharynx, oesophagus, stomach, colorectum, liver, pancreas, larynx, lung, cervix uteri, ovary, bladder, kidney, myeloid leukaemia	34.4	6.2
Passive smoking	Lung	0.4	1.6
Infection		23.2	19.4
Helicobacter pylori	Noncardia stomach, gastric MALT lymphoma		
Hepatitis B/C viruses	Liver		
Human papilloma virus	Oral cavity, oropharynx, anus, penis, vulva, vagina, cervix uteri		
Human T-cell leukaemia type I	Adult T-cell lymphoma/leukaemia		
Epstein–Barr virus	Nasopharynx, Burkitt lymphoma, Hodgkin lymphoma		
Alchol drinking	Oral and pharynx, oesophagus, colorectum, liver, female breast	8.6	2.5
Salt intake	Stomach	1.5	1.2
Body mass index	Colon, pancreas, postmenopausal breast, endometrial, kidney	0.5	1.1
Fruit intake	Oesophagus, stomach, lung	0.7	0.8
Vegetable intake	Oesophagus, stomach	0.7	0.4
Physical inactivity	Colon, breast, endometrial	0.2	0.4
Exogenous hormone use	Female breast	-	0.2
All above risk factors		**56.9**	**29.9**

Source: Inoue M, Sawada N, Matsuda T, et al. Attributable causes of cancer in Japan in 2005: --systematic assessment to estimate current burden of cancer attributable to known preventable risk factors in Japan. Annals of Oncology 2012;23(5):1362–9. doi: 10.1093/annonc/mdr437

drinking was more common among less educated men and women, but heavy episodic drinking was associated with higher socioeconomic status in men, and paid work in women.[25]

The population attributable risk for liver cancer death in Japan is estimated as high for HCV infection (> 70%) and lower for drinking (about 10%).[22] It appears that alcohol consumption accounts for little difference in liver cancer risk according to socioeconomic status, although interaction between alcohol consumption and HCV infection may be relevant.[26]

12.3.3 Inequalities in Cervical Cancer and Prevalence of Human Papilloma Virus

Universal vaccination against HPV is widely recommended and implemented throughout the world to prevent the incidence of cervical cancer. In Japan, HPV vaccination started in 2010 for 13–16 year-old girls, then continued for 12–16 year-old girls and by April 2013, about 70% of the targeted population were vaccinated. After reports of pain after the vaccination and other problems were spread through the media, the health ministry stopped the HPV vaccination programme.[27] To date (September 2019), the government has not re-started vaccinations, despite the World Health Organization's statement, in relation to the Japanese situation, that 'Policy decisions based on weak evidence, leading to lack of use of safe and effective vaccines, can result in real harm.'[28] Socioeconomic inequalities in cervical cancer incidence before the HPV vaccination era were reported.[29,30] Some evidence of a reduction in the deprivation gap in cervical cancer incidence after implementation of the universal vaccination programme was also reported.[31,32] Large socioeconomic inequalities in cervical cancer incidence were observed in Osaka.[33] Scaling up HPV vaccination could help to reduce the gap in the future in both Japan and other countries.[34]

12.3.4 Reverse Social Gradient in Breast Cancer Mortality

Higher breast cancer mortality has been observed in the least deprived areas in Japan (Table 12.1, Figure 12.2). This 'reverse gradient' is commonly reported in other countries.[35,36] The greater risk of death from breast cancer among more educated and higher socioeconomic status women has been related to risk factors for breast cancer including reproductive factors, but the exact reasons for this remain uncertain. Overall, participation in mammography screening in Japan is quite low. Less deprived women, especially in larger workplaces, were more likely to attend screening.[37] Correspondingly, a deprivation gap for breast cancer survival was observed in Osaka.[21]

12.3.5 Inequalities in Cancer Related to Screening

In Japan, cancer screening is a work-related issue. Most large companies provide cancer screening for their employees, and screening is less accessible to workers in small companies and the self-employed. This situation leads to inequalities in cancer screening attendance. 46% of men in the highest income quintile participated in stomach cancer screening, but only 24% in the lowest quintile. Employment status is also important as 51% of men working in large companies participated in stomach cancer screening, compared to only 29% of men who were unemployed, self-employed, or employed in a small company.[37,38] For women, an intervention study that paid out-of-pocket costs for cervical and breast cancer screening revealed inequalities in cancer screening attendance before the intervention and changes in inequalities afterwards.[37]

12.3.6 Occupation and Cancer Mortality

Several occupational exposures have been related to cancer incidence in Japan and other countries.[39] Exposure to these risk factors is managed by the Industrial Safety Act in Japan. In addition, occupation is also a key social determinant factor in cancer incidence and mortality. Unemployed people had the highest mortality for lung, gastric, and colorectal cancer, and service workers, administrative and managerial workers had high cancer mortality rates compared with manufacturing workers.[40]

12.3.7 Diagnosis and Treatment

Access to optimal diagnosis and treatment for cancer is a key factor that contributes to inequalities in cancer outcomes. The evidence remains scarce in Japan, although socioeconomic inequalities in cancer survival have been reported.[21] In other countries, more deprived patients may be more likely to receive suboptimal treatment.[41,42] Although stage at diagnosis plays an important role in these socioeconomic inequalities, other factors such as comorbidities are likely play a part,[43-46], and further studies are needed. Linkage between cancer registry data and clinical databases could provide new insights into the nature of this type of health inequality.

12.4 Policy Implications

As observed in the trends in inequalities in cancer burden, some were attributed mainly to inequalities in prevalence of risk factors, as is the case with smoking and lung cancer. Others were related to delay in diagnosis due to inadequate cancer screening, while inequalities in cancer care appear also to contribute. The range of factors involved suggests health policies need to address the cancer-related aspects of health inequality.

Some high-income countries including the UK, Canada, the US, Taiwan, and Korea, have already focused on the socioeconomic inequalities in cancer. They are monitoring several indicators using population-based official statistics. In Japan, the third (latest) version of the National Cancer Control Plan did not include the keyword 'inequalities (*Kakusa*)'. We cannot act to reduce inequalities in cancer without monitoring and setting targets for these indicators. In the third Osaka Prefecture Cancer Control Plan, a target was set to 'reduce the inequalities in cancer mortality and incidence', based on monitoring regional inequalities in cancer mortality and incidence. Since the second Healthy Japan 21 plan included the target 'reduction in health inequalities', it is more important to monitor and evaluate health inequalities based on population-based statistics. Based on substantial evidence of risk factors, screening, and treatment of cancer, we are making progress to reveal the mechanisms of cancer inequalities that will support evidence-based measures to reduce it.

12.5 Conclusion

Cancer incidence and mortality are generally declining in Japan. Cancer survival has increased and is now among the highest in the world. However, behind this overall improvement, socioeconomic inequalities in all three indicators are observed. The mechanisms underlying these inequalities are complex and vary according to the cancer indicator. Generally, inequalities in incidence depend largely on the prevention of risk factors and on efficient screening programmes. Policy in these areas has been traditionally weak in Japan. Inequalities in cancer survival are more likely to be due to characteristics of the healthcare system than to individual factors, even in countries with universal health coverage such as Japan. Since 2007, Japan has implemented a process of accreditation for hospitals delivering cancer care in order to improve the general level of care and its standardization. It may increase the equity of cancer care and narrow the inequalities in cancer survival. However, there is a need for more evidence-based policies in order to reduce the inequalities in cancer burden and strengthen research capacity in this area.

References

1. WHO. Mortality database. Available at: https://www.who.int/healthinfo/statistics/mortality_rawdata/en/ [last accessed 6 March 2020].
2. Forman D, Bray F, Brewster DH, et al. (eds.). *Cancer Incidence in Five Continents, Vol. X* (electronic version). Lyon: IARC 2014.
3. Allemani C, Matsuda T, Di Carlo V, et al. Global surveillance of trends in cancer survival 2000–14 (CONCORD-3): analysis of individual records for 37,513,025 patients diagnosed with one of 18 cancers from 322 population-based registries in 71 countries. *Lancet* 2018;391(10125):1023–75. doi: 10.1016/s0140-6736(17)33326-3
4. Katanoda K, Hori M, Matsuda T, et al. An updated report on the trends in cancer incidence and mortality in Japan, 1958–2013. *Jpn J Clin Oncol* 2015;45(4):390–401. doi: 10.1093/jjco/hyv002
5. Watanabe M, Ito H, Hosono S, et al. Declining trends in prevalence of *Helicobacter pylori* infection by birth-year in a Japanese population. *Cancer Sci* 2015;106(12):1738–43. doi: 10.1111/cas.12821
6. Inoue M, Tsugane S. Epidemiology of gastric cancer in Japan. *Postgrad Med J* 2005;81(957):419–24.
7. Moyer VA, US Preventive Services Task Force. Screening for prostate cancer: recommendation statement. *Ann Intern Med* 2012;157(2):1–44. doi: 10.7326/0003-4819-157-2-201207170-00464
8. Barocas DA, Mallin K, Graves AJ, et al. Effect of the USPSTF Grade D recommendation against screening for prostate cancer on incident prostate cancer diagnoses in the United States. *J Urol* 2015;194(6):1587–93. doi: 10.1016/j.juro.2015.06.075
9. OECD. OECD Health Statistics 2018. Available at: http://stats.oecd.org/index.aspx?DataSetCode=HEALTH_STAT [last accessed 6 March 2020].
10. Ioka A, Tsukuma H, Ajiki W, et al. Hospital procedure volume and survival of cancer patients in Osaka, Japan: a population-based study with latest cases. *Jpn J Clin Oncol* 2007;37(7):544–53.
11. Kinoshita FL, Ito Y, Nakayama T. Trends in lung cancer incidence rates by histological type in 1975–2008: a population-based study in Osaka, Japan. *J Epidemiol* 2016;26(11):579–86. doi: 10.2188/jea.JE20150257
12. Ito Y, Ioka A, Tsukuma H, et al. Regional differences in population-based cancer survival between six prefectures in Japan: application of relative survival models with funnel plots. *Cancer Sci* 2009;100(7):1306–11.
13. Recent trends in regional differences in cancer survival in Japan: population-based cancer registry data in 1993–2008: plenary session 1. The 39th annual

meeting of the International Association of Cancer Registries 2017, Utrecht, Netherlands.

14. Division of Health Services Research, Center for Cancer Control and Information Services NCC. Annual report on study group for the quality indicators of cancer treatment in 2014. Project for establishing a quality measurement system for cancer care in Japan 2018. Available at: https://www.ncc.go.jp/jp/cis/divisions/health_s/health_s/010/index.html [last accessed 6 March 2020].

15. Nakaya T, Honjo K, Hanibuchi T, et al. Associations of all-cause mortality with census-based neighbourhood deprivation and population density in Japan: a multilevel survival analysis. *PloS one* 2014;9(6):e97802. doi: 10.1371/journal.pone.0097802

16. Nakaya T, Ito Y. Synthesis. In: T Nakaya, Y Ito (eds.). *The Atlas of Health Inequalities in Japan*. New York: Springer 2019.

17. Kweon SS, Kim MG, Kang MR, et al. Difference of stage at cancer diagnosis by socioeconomic status for four target cancers of the National Cancer Screening Program in Korea: results from the Gwangju and Jeonnam cancer registries. *J Epidemiol* 2017;27(7):299–304. doi: 10.1016/j.je.2016.07.004

18. Clegg LX, Reichman ME, Miller BA, et al. Impact of socioeconomic status on cancer incidence and stage at diagnosis: selected findings from the surveillance, epidemiology, and end results: national longitudinal mortality study. *Cancer Causes Control* 2009;20(4):417–35. doi: 10.1007/s10552-008-9256-0

19. Coleman M, Babb P, Damiecki P, et al. Cancer survival trends in England and Wales 1971–1995: deprivation and NHS region. London: The Stationery Office 1999.

20. Woods LM, Rachet B, Coleman MP. Origins of socio-economic inequalities in cancer survival: a review. *Ann Oncol* 2006;17(1):5–19.

21. Ito Y, Nakaya T, Nakayama T, et al. Socioeconomic inequalities in cancer survival: a population-based study of adult patients diagnosed in Osaka, Japan, during the period 1993–2004. *Acta Oncol* 2014;53(10):1423–33. doi: 10.3109/0284186x.2014.912350

22. Inoue M, Sawada N, Matsuda T, et al. Attributable causes of cancer in Japan in 2005: systematic assessment to estimate current burden of cancer attributable to known preventable risk factors in Japan. *Ann Oncol* 2012;23(5):1362–9. doi: 10.1093/annonc/mdr437

23. Tanaka H, Imai Y, Hiramatsu N, et al. Declining incidence of hepatocellular carcinoma in Osaka, Japan, from 1990 to 2003. *Ann Intern Med* 2008;148(11):820–6.

24. Ito Y, Ioka A, Nakayama T, et al. Comparison of the trends in cancer incidence and mortality in Osaka, Japan, using an age-period-cohort model. *Asian Pac J Cancer Prev* 2011;12(4):879–88.

25. Kinjo A, Kuwabara Y, Minobe R, et al. Different socioeconomic backgrounds between hazardous drinking and heavy episodic drinking: prevalence by sociodemographic factors in a Japanese general sample. *Drug Alcohol Depend* 2018;193:55–62. doi: 10.1016/j.drugalcdep.2018.08.015

26. Yun EH, Lim MK, Oh JK, et al. Combined effect of socioeconomic status, viral hepatitis, and lifestyles on hepatocelluar carcinoma risk in Korea. *Br J Cancer* 2010;103(5):741–6. doi: 10.1038/sj.bjc.6605803

27. Ueda Y, Yagi A, Ikeda S, et al. Beyond resumption of the Japanese Government's recommendation of the HPV vaccine. *Lancet Oncol* 2018;19(12):1563–64. doi: 10.1016/s1470-2045(18)30573-4

28. Global Advisory Committee on Vaccine safety. Statement on safety of HPV vaccines 2015 (updated 17 December 2015). Available at: http://www.who.int/vaccine_safety/committee/GACVS_HPV_statement_17Dec2015.pdf [last accessed 6 March 2020].

29. Simard EP, Fedewa S, Ma J, et al. Widening socioeconomic disparities in cervical cancer mortality among women in 26 states, 1993–2007. *Cancer* 2012;118(20):5110–16. doi: 10.1002/cncr.27606

30. Pukkala E, Malila N, Hakama M. Socioeconomic differences in incidence of cervical cancer in Finland by cell type. *Acta Oncol* 2010;49(2):180–4. doi: 10.3109/02841860903386390

31. Cameron RL, Kavanagh K, Cameron Watt D, et al. The impact of bivalent HPV vaccine on cervical intraepithelial neoplasia by deprivation in Scotland: reducing the gap. *J Epidemiol Community Health* 2017;71(10):954–60. doi: 10.1136/jech-2017-209113

32. Malagon T, Drolet M, Boily MC, et al. Changing inequalities in cervical cancer: modeling the impact of vaccine uptake, vaccine herd effects, and cervical cancer screening in the post-vaccination era. *Cancer Epidemiol Biomarkers Prev* 2015;24(1):276–85. doi: 10.1158/1055-9965.epi-14-1052

33. Ito Y, Nakaya T, Kondo N, et al. Socio-economic differences in stage-specific cancer incidence in Osaka, Japan: 1993–2004. 37th International Association of Cancer Registries annual scientific conference 2015:054 [O179].

34. Simms KT, Steinberg J, Caruana M, et al. Impact of scaled up human papilloma virus vaccination and cervical screening and the potential for global elimination of cervical cancer in 181 countries, 2020–99: a modelling study. *Lancet Oncol* 2019;20(3):394–407. doi: https://doi.org/10.1016/S1470-2045(18)30836-2

35. Lundqvist A, Andersson E, Ahlberg I, et al. Socioeconomic inequalities in breast cancer incidence and mortality in Europe: a systematic review and meta-analysis. *Eur J Public Health* 2016;26(5):804–13. doi: 10.1093/eurpub/ckw070

36. Strand BH, Kunst A, Huisman M, et al. The reversed social gradient: higher breast cancer mortality in the higher educated compared to lower educated.

A comparison of 11 European populations during the 1990s. *Eur J Cancer* 2007;43(7):1200–7. doi: 10.1016/j.ejca.2007.01.021

37. Tabuchi T, Hoshino T, Nakayama T, et al. Does removal of out-of-pocket costs for cervical and breast cancer screening work? A quasi-experimental study to evaluate the impact on attendance, attendance inequality and average cost per uptake of a Japanese government intervention. *Int J Cancer* 2013;133(4):972–83. doi: 10.1002/ijc.28095

38. Fukuda Y, Nakamura K, Takano T, et al. Socioeconomic status and cancer screening in Japanese males: large inequality in middle-aged and urban residents. *Environ Health Prev Med* 2007;12(2):90–6. doi: 10.1007/bf02898155

39. Loomis D, Guha N, Hall AL, et al. Identifying occupational carcinogens: an update from the IARC Monographs. *Occup Environ Med* 2018;75(8):593–603. doi: 10.1136/oemed-2017-104944

40. Eguchi H, Wada K, Prieto-Merino D, et al. Lung, gastric and colorectal cancer mortality by occupation and industry among working-aged men in Japan. *Scientific Reports* 2017;7:43204. doi: 10.1038/srep43204

41. Morris E, Quirke P, Thomas JD, et al. Unacceptable variation in abdominoperineal excision rates for rectal cancer: time to intervene? *Gut* 2008;57(12):1690–7.

42. Lejeune C, Sassi F, Ellis L, et al. Socio-economic disparities in access to treatment and their impact on colorectal cancer survival. *Int J Epidemiol* 2010;39(3):710–17. doi: 10.1093/ije/dyq048

43. Ellis L, Canchola AJ, Spiegel D, et al. Racial and ethnic disparities in cancer survival: the contribution of tumor, sociodemographic, institutional, and neighborhood characteristics. *J Clin Oncol* 2018;36(1):25–33. doi: 10.1200/jco.2017.74.2049

44. Li R, Daniel R, Rachet B. How much do tumor stage and treatment explain socio-economic inequalities in breast cancer survival? Applying causal mediation analysis to population-based data. *Eur J Epidemiol* 2016;31(6):603–11. doi: 10.1007/s10654-016-0155-5

45. Fowler H, Belot A, Njagi EN, et al. Persistent inequalities in 90-day colon cancer mortality: an English cohort study. *Br J Cancer* 2017;117(9):1396–404. doi: 10.1038/bjc.2017.295

46. Belot A, Fowler H, Njagi EN, et al. Association between age, deprivation and specific comorbid conditions and the receipt of major surgery in patients with non-small cell lung cancer in England: a population-based study. *Thorax* 2019;74(1):51–9. doi: 10.1136/thoraxjnl-2017-211395

13

Physical Activity, Sport, and Health in Japan

Shigeru Inoue, Hiroyuki Kikuchi, and Shiho Amagasa

13.1 Introduction

Various health benefits of physical activity have been well documented.[1] Physical activity has been attracting a lot of interest in ageing Japan, in terms of maintaining older adults' independence and physical performance, which enables social participation and leads to successful ageing. Thus, the promotion of physical activity is currently a critical public health issue in Japan. Historically, the 1964 Tokyo Olympics caused a growing trend towards physical activity to promote public health. Now would be good time to look back at the history of physical activity and related policies in Japan and to discuss future challenges with a view to the 2020 Tokyo Olympic and Paralympic Games. This chapter presents (1) a brief history of physical activity policies, (2) an overview of physical activity among Japanese, (3) socio-environmental determinants of physical activity, (4) health and physical education in Japan, (5) Olympic Games and physical activity, and (6) future challenges for physical activity in a super-aged society.

13.2 A Brief History of Physical Activity Policies

Physical activity policies in Japan could be summarized in four phases since the end of World War II.

13.2.1 Reconstruction of Japan, 1945–1951: Years of Malnutrition

Malnutrition was the greatest challenge right after World War II. During this period, Japan faced serious threats of poverty and poor medical care,

Shigeru Inoue, Hiroyuki Kikuchi, and Shiho Amagasa, *Physical Activity, Sport, and Health in Japan* In: *Health in Japan*. Edited by: Eric Brunner, Noriko Cable, and Hiroyasu Iso, Oxford University Press (2021). © Oxford University Press. DOI: 10.1093/oso/9780198848134.003.0013

which caused an epidemic of infection diseases. Tuberculosis had been the leading cause of deaths until 1950. Policies focused on improving nutritional status. Nutritionists were nationally certified, and a school lunch programme was started to improve child development and health status. During this phase, the promotion of physical activity was not a major public health concern.

13.2.2 The 1964 Tokyo Olympic Movement, 1951–1980s: Growing Interest in Exercise as 'Positive Health'

In 1951, stroke became the leading cause of death along with the rapid decrease of tuberculosis due to improvements in nutrition, hygiene, and medication. Health checkup systems (i.e. secondary prevention) for the prevention of non-communicable diseases (NCDs) had been developed (Chapter 11). Exercise guidance was expected to be conducted as a part of nutrition guidance by nutritionists around that time. However, the 1964 Tokyo Olympics provided great attention to the role of exercise on public health.[2] Right after the Olympic Games, the Cabinet endorsed the 'Positive Health' concept by stating 'Our health is not given by others, but is achieved by ourselves'. Achieving higher physical fitness levels through sports or exercise is essential to obtain this positive health.[3] This period was the time that exercise appeared in the health agenda.

13.2.3 Exercise for Health Promotion, 1980s–2000s: Increased Concern with Primary Prevention through Exercise

In the 1980s, Japan started to put additional efforts into primary prevention as well as secondary prevention of NCDs. In 1988, the Japanese government launched 'Active 80 Health Plan', aiming to achieve a healthy lifespan of 80 years. This plan focused on three behaviours; nutrition, exercise, and rest, which meant that exercise was placed as one of priorities for public health. In 1988, 'Health Fitness Programmer' started to professionally provide an effective exercise programme, and 'Recommended Exercise for Health Promotion' was established in 1989. At this stage, interest was mainly in exercise prescription, less in physical activity (see Box 13.1).

13.2.4 Physical Activity into Public Health, 2000s: Moving Towards the Entire Population

In the 1990s, policy makers recognized the importance of a physically active way of life, beyond the value of leisure-time exercise. The Health Japan 21 policy launched in 2000 set national goals for physical activity, including (1) to increase the average number of steps taken by 1,000 steps/day, and (2) to increase the proportion of regular exercisers by 10 points of percentage. In line with Health Japan 21, Japanese physical activity guidelines were issued in 2006. These guidelines recommended that adults engage in 23 metabolic equivalents (METs)-hour/week of moderate-to-vigorous physical activity (MVPA), which represents twice the amount recommended by WHO guidelines, and parallel to approximately 60 minutes/day of walking.

In 2008, all health insurers were mandated to provide Specific Health Checkups focusing on the prevention and control of metabolic syndrome. The programme targets people aged 40–74 (approximately 56 M people). Intensive professional support to reevaluate their lifestyles is individually given to those with abdominal obesity and certain risk factors of metabolic syndrome (approximately 1 M people annually). Recent studies using a national database showed that the Specific Health Checkups are effective in improving the profiles of metabolic syndrome.[4,5]

Not only individual approaches but also population approaches (to change the whole population) are sought. Following global trends towards an ecological approach, the Japanese government added a new national goal to increase the number of prefectures that address improvement of activity-friendly environments in Health Japan 21 (second term) starting in 2013. That same year, Japanese physical activity guidelines were updated. The recommended volume of MVPA did not change from the previous guidelines. The guidelines included 'Plus 10', a key message for adding ten minutes per day of physical activity to their life-style.[6] Policy to promote physical activity and sport participation became more closely coordinated in preparation for the 2020 Tokyo Olympic and Paralympic Games. The Japan Sports Agency, established in 2015, aims to realize through sport a society where people are healthy in body and mind.[7] The agency has the task of encouraging greater collaboration between education, health, and other sectors, and to promote popular and elite sport across the country, including sport for people with disabilities.

13.3 Physical Activity in Japan

The National Health and Nutrition Survey (NHNS) has been conducted annually since 1945, using a stratified random sample from the whole Japanese population of about 18,000 people.[11] It includes physical measurement, blood pressure, blood sampling, interviews and questionnaires for lifestyle behaviours, nutrient intake, and pedometry. The NHNS used a three-day food weighing method until 1994; currently a one-day food weighing and proportional method is used. With regard to physical activity, self-reported exercise habit and pedometry has been assessed since 1986 and 1989 respectively.

According to the 2017 survey, 35.9% of men and 28.6% of women were regular exercisers, defined as $\geq$ 30 minutes/day, $\geq$ 2 days/week, over a year. Mean step-count estimated with pedometry for one day was 6,846 steps/day in men and 5,867 steps/day in women. The one-day survey may lead to measurement bias, but the time trend is likely to be adequately captured, because bias is similar each year. In all age groups, men are more likely to exercise regularly and to take more steps than women. As expected, the step count tends to decrease with age. There is a slight dip in step count in women's child-rearing years. However, older adults are more likely to exercise regularly than middle-aged adults. Looking at the trend longitudinally, peak step counts in adults ($\geq$ 15 years) since 1995, when the current monitoring system was established, were 8,202 steps/day among men (1997) and 7,392 steps/day among women (1998). Considering the ageing population, age-adjusted step counts have decreased by about 700 steps/day in the past two decades. In recent years, there has been little further decline.

International comparison based on self-report suggests that the Japanese are physically inactive as a nation.[13-16] The Japanese also appear to spend time in sedentary behaviours such as sitting.[13] Prevalence of insufficient physical activity was 38% (men 36%, women 40%) in Japan according to WHO guidelines (Box 13.1), higher than the global prevalence (28%).[16] In other countries, the prevalence of inactivity was 38% in the UK, 43% in the US, 47% in Brazil, 32% in Australia, 14% in China, 33% in India, 18% in Russia, 32% in Iran, and 25% in Nigeria. Japanese adults had the longest sitting time (median: 420 minutes/day) among 20 countries. Information bias from self-reported physical activity is likely to differ from one culture to another, and therefore cross-national comparison is difficult.[17,18] Different sampling strategies between countries may also be problematic.

Smartphone technology makes it possible to measure physical activity objectively.[19] A massive study (N > 700,000) in 111 countries generated 68 M days

---

Box 13.1 Key Terms and Definitions: Physical Activity [8-10]

Physical activity	Any bodily movement produced by skeletal muscles that leads to energy expenditure. Classified as light, moderate, or vigorous intensity, according to level of energy expenditure. The main physical activity settings are leisure, travel, work, and home.
Intensity of physical activity	The Metabolic Equivalent of Task (MET) is a unit of activity intensity. 1 MET is the energy expenditure while sitting at rest, approximately 1 kcal/kg body weight/hour. The intensity of an activity is defined as the ratio of energy expenditure relative to resting: • light (1.6–2.9 MET): standing, household chores, slow walking • moderate (3.0–5.9 MET): walking, cycling • vigorous ($\geq$ 6.0 MET): running, swimming.
Exercise	A subset of physical activity that is planned, structured, repetitive, and with a specific purpose.
Physical activity recommendations	World Health Organization recommends 150 minutes/week of moderate-intensity physical activity or 75 minutes/week of vigorous-intensity activity, or an equivalent combination of both.
Sedentary behaviour	Any waking behaviour characterized by energy expenditure $\leq$ 1.5 METs, while in a sitting, reclining, or lying posture.

of data derived from built-in smartphone accelerometers.[20] The Japanese were ranked fourth highest (6,010 steps/day), following Hong Kong, China, and the Ukraine, among 46 countries with more than 1,000 participants. Mean steps/day were 5,444 in the UK and 4,774 in the US. This study found relatively small inequality in step counts in Japan and, across countries, smaller activity inequality was associated with higher mean daily-step count (Figure 13.1). In addition,

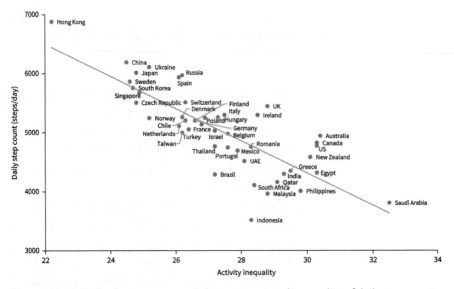

Figure 13.1 Relation between mean daily step count and inequality of daily step counts in selected countries

Daily step counts measured on smartphones. Activity inequality by country is summarized with the GINI coefficient of the ranked step count values: the higher the number, the greater the variation.

Source: Althoff T et al. Nature 2017;547:336–39.

activity inequality was a stronger correlate of national obesity prevalence than mean step count. Furthermore, neighbourhoods with an environment favourable to walking, i.e. with higher 'walkability', appeared to promote lower inequality and a smaller gender gap in physical activity. Speculatively, the high walkability of Japanese cities contributes to relatively high physical activity levels.

In summary, Japanese physical activity levels have decreased slightly in the past two decades, however, the mean level remains higher than in other countries. Considering the health benefits of physical activity, this may have contributed in part to high Japanese longevity.

13.4 Socio-environmental Determinants of Physical Activity

Despite physical activity equality among Japanese, area-difference is obvious and suggests socio-environmental determinants of physical activity. There is a clear positive association between the size of towns and cities and mean step counts. Adults were found to walk about 740 steps (12%) more per day in a large city than in a town, adjusting for age.[21] Environmental factors could explain some part of this area-difference. As seen in Western studies, the neighbourhood physical activity environment, such as walkability (the function of density, land use mix, and street connectivity), sidewalk, aesthetic, public transport, crime, traffic safety, and exercise facilities are associated with physical activity in Japan.[22] Large cities generally have these walkable features. In addition to city size, natural environmental factors such as extremely high/low temperatures and precipitation including snow may determine a population's activity level. For example, in Hokkaido and Okinawa, located in the north and south regions of Japan and with low and high temperatures respectively, people walk less. Car-dependent societies are formed in low density rural areas where residences are far from destinations such as shopping areas, schools, and workplaces, and in areas where people can live without difficulties using cars even in severe summer/winter weather.

Car dependence is a barrier to walking and other modes of active travel, particularly in towns and smaller cities (Figure 13.2).[23] More and more people have started to use a car rather than walking and public transport. An example of this occurs in Kanazawa (38.8% in 1974 versus 67.2% in 2007), which is an old city, famous for the Kenrokuen Garden, which has a population of about 450,000 and is located in a snowy area on the coast of the Japan Sea. When looking at cross-sectional area differences, the cities with smaller populations were more likely to be car-dependent when compared to metropolitan cities including Tokyo, Osaka, and Nagoya.

Out-of-town shopping centres and online shopping is a threat to the survival of retailing in many countries, and also results in fewer opportunities to walk for residents. In Japan, approval of three acts relating to city planning in 2000 triggered the development of large commercial complexes placed out-of-town one after another. This accelerated the loss of shopping streets in downtown areas and made life difficult for socially disadvantaged people without access to cars (e.g. older adults). This change deprived people of opportunities for daily walking, and even worse, it became more difficult for vulnerable people without adequate mobility to buy fresh foods, especially in rural areas. No matter how advanced information technologies and home delivery services are, fewer opportunities for walking and social interaction will remain. The term 'Shuttered Street', representing a local shopping street where there are many closed stores, illustrates this change in community structure. While the Japanese government went on to reconsider these city planning acts in 2006, in order to address these issues, the restructuring of communities remains one of the greatest challenges. In 2014, the government established the grand design of land use towards 2050 to structure a sustainable super-aged society. 'Compact and Network' is a key strategy which leads to walkable communities as well as social interaction opportunities. A compact city

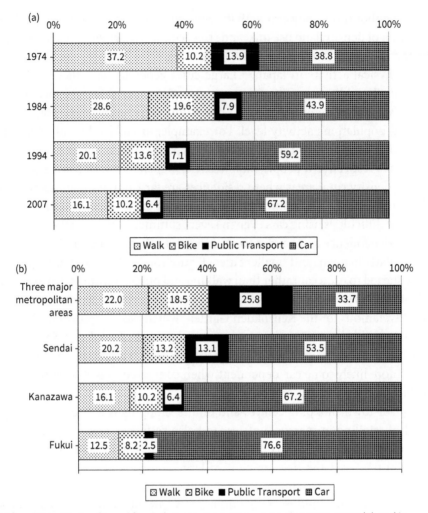

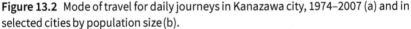

Figure 13.2 Mode of travel for daily journeys in Kanazawa city, 1974–2007 (a) and in selected cities by population size (b).

B shows cross-sectional comparisons of the mode of travel by population size: Fukui 253,997; Kanazawa 455,497; Sendai 1,025,098; three major metropolitan areas: Tokyo 8,396,594; Osaka 2,628,811; Nagoya 2,215,062.

Source: Person Trip survey. Ministry of Land, Infrastructure, Transport and Tourism, 2009. Accessed 31 July 2019.

is characterized by a relatively high residential density with mixed land use where city functions are located in a small area.

There are some unique findings on socio-environmental determinants of physical activity among the Japanese. In contrast to previous research that demonstrated walking as a favourable feature of dense places, excessive population density observed among youth living in Tokyo may lead to lower physical activity.[24] The underlying mechanism could be that an overly densely populated area is (1) very close to destinations, (2) prevents children from playing outside because of safety concerns regarding traffic and crime, and (3) provides small playing space at schools and in communities. Lower physical activity in extremely densely populated areas may be relevant to other super-crowded cities in the world. Older Japanese adults living in low walkable and rural areas accumulated more sporadic MVPA and light-intensity physical activity (e.g. household chores, standing), behaviours which are currently overlooked by WHO guidelines but which do have health benefits,[25] and less sedentary behaviour than those living in high walkable and urban areas.[26] Characteristics which promote sporadic MVPA and light activities, such as some forms of social contact, detached larger houses with yards and private gardens, and other traditional Japanese cultures, may coexist with rural and low walkable areas.

As mentioned in section 13.3, it is estimated that the Japanese are in general physically active, with low levels of inequality. However, recent changes in community structure have resulted in a slight decline of physical activity among the Japanese. Developing activity-friendly communities through a socio-environmental approach is important for the health of the Japanese population through reversal of this decline.

13.5 Health and Physical Education in Japan

The Japanese school education system has made a significant contribution to childhood physical activity and health in later life. The prevalence of childhood obesity has increased slightly (Chapter 4) but maintains a lower prevalence of obesity compared to other developed countries according to the OECD 2011 report.[27] Despite the difference in the definition of obesity, the prevalence of overweight among the Japanese is 16.2% for boys and 14.4% for girls (cf. OECD mean; 22.9% for boys and 21.4% for girls; in the US 35.0% and 35.9%; in the UK 22.7% and 26.6% respectively). School life is equally providing all children with various opportunities for physical activity; physical education classes, extracurricular exercise activities, and other school routines such as active commuting, break/recess, and cleaning. These opportunities for physical activity play an important role in children's health, building their ability to have fun through exercise and sport throughout life, with minimum inequality of physical activity. In addition, schools function at the centre of communities. Social interactions occur among children, their parents, and community residents through school activities and school events run in collaboration with the community (e.g. athletics festivals). For example, an athletics meeting, *Undokai*, held on weekends annually, is historically a community event. There is a culture that the entire neighbourhood is responsible for child rearing.

Ministry curriculum guidelines require that children take about 100 classes per year of physical education and engage in a variety of exercise (e.g. gymnastics, track and field, swimming, ball games, and dancing). In Japan, physical education has been designed to ensure children have a certain amount of exercise time and experience a variety of activities regardless of whether they like it or not, whereas there are still several countries where physical education is not required subject or each school decides the content of classes independently. It is unique that Japanese physical education is not only 'physical education' but 'health education'.

Although extracurricular activity is self-disciplined, 65.2% of junior high school students and 41.9% of high school students belong to extracurricular sports teams. School-based sport participation may contribute to health during adulthood.[28] Participation in sporting activities out of school is susceptible to annual household income, whereas at school this is not the case (Figure 13.3).[29] That is, physical education and

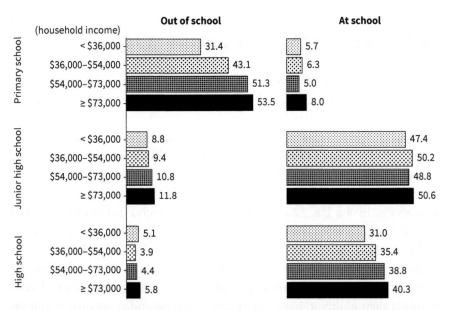

Figure 13.3 Sports participation rate according to annual household income by setting and type of school, 2017

Annual household incomes converted at 110 JPY/US$. Questionnaire survey among 12,360 parents with children aged 7–18 years. Most common types of sport among junior high school students in 2018 were soccer, baseball, and basketball for boys, and tennis, volleyball, and basketball for girls.

Source: 3rd Survey on Activities Outside Schools 2017. Benesse Education Research and Development Institute. 2017. Accessed 31 July 2019.

extracurricular sports activities can contribute to attenuating the association of parent's income gap and child's physical activity inequality. It is a general rule that the commuting distance to school is within 4 km in elementary school and within 6 km in junior high school, which equates with one hour of walking/cycling time. Almost all students (elementary school 93%, junior high 88%) commute to school by walking or cycling. They spend approximately 50 minutes actively commuting a day. Active commuting to school has helped combat childhood obesity by providing regular physical activity.[30]

In summary, Japanese education provides children with opportunities for exercise and physical activity in-class, and out-of-class, contributing to low inequality in physical activity in youth and later life.

13.6 Olympic Games and Physical Activity

Japan has already hosted three Olympic Games, Tokyo 1964, Sapporo Winter Games 1972, and Nagano Winter Games 1998, and is due to host another, Tokyo 2020. Looking back, each one left legacies such as infrastructure and promotion of sports. In particular, the first Tokyo Olympics was a turning point in terms of physical activity policy and left an immense legacy.

13.6.1 The Legacy of Tokyo 1964

The 1964 Tokyo Olympics left not only tangible legacies of infrastructures such as transportation systems and sports facilities, but also various intangible legacies such as sports culture. From the viewpoint of health, it stimulated the momentum of health-enhancing exercise. Exercise policies had been mainly covered within education sectors to improve physical strength, which was a relic of the past for developing strong soldiers before Tokyo 1964. However, this momentum made health sectors regard exercise as their issue and as integral to a health-related lifestyle. Health policies relating to physical activity appeared around this time (see section 13.2). From the viewpoint of sports, legal acts relating to sports promotion were developed. The Sport Promotion Act, the first sports-related law in Japan, was promulgated in 1961 prior to the Olympic Games. It included the requirement for sports promotion planning at national and local government level, including setting up the Sports Promotion Council at local government level, sports instructor systems for community residents, National Sports Competitions, Sports Days, and so on. For example, the National Sports Competition is an inter-prefectural competition annually hosted by one of 47 prefectures in rotation. As a result, each prefecture has sports associations to enhance its competition power and facilities to host national games, which promote sports all over Japan.

13.6.2 The Challenges of Tokyo 2020

Tokyo is hosting the Olympic and Paralympic Games with the vision 'Sport has the power to change the world and our future'. Based on this vision, the Action and Legacy Plan consists of five domains; (1) Sport and Health, (2) Urban Planning and Sustainability, (3) Culture and Education, (4) Economy and Technology, and (5) Recovery, Nationwide Benefits, and Global Communication. Various sectors such as sports, education, culture, health, transportation, city planning, and industry are encouraged to work on each domain. A unique concept of 'Sport and Health' is to recognize three aspects of sports, which are 'doing', 'watching', and 'supporting' sports to increase the number of the population who are familiar with sports culture.

A variety of approaches have started the move forward with this plan. Local governments are developing sports promotion planning based on the Basic Act on Sport. The Tokyo government is targeting 70% of sports participation by 2020 from 56% in 2016. For 'doing' sports, the plan includes (1) information delivery, (2) sports events as a motivator, (3) development and management of sports facilities, (4) physical activity in schools, and (5) supporting athletes' sports. They have tried to make the best use of existing facilities through effective management of this resource, rather than developing new facilities, in response to criticism against cost. The Japan Sports Agency put up a slogan, 'Sports in Life' to create a society where people enjoy sports as a part of their life and live healthier. To promote the slogan, they defined sports as not only competitions, but also physical activity including daily walking. For example, they started the 'Fun + Walk' project in 2017 in order to combine walking with various daily matters of concern such as commuting, shopping, eating out, travelling, and playing music. Commuting while wearing a suit, sneakers, and backpack is spreading among business people. A programme has also been started to certify companies which address sports promotion among employees as a 'Sports Yell Company'.

While much of this progress is commendable, there are some negative concerns. One is a lack of stronger and more comprehensive physical activity promotion within a theoretical framework. Another is the insufficiently scientific assessment of achievements. Survey methods have not always been well-designed, and the redefinition of sports to include walking and stair climbing was carried out during the monitoring period. To date, there have been few studies which scientifically examine the effects of mega-sports events. In reality, there has been no clear scientific evidence to date to support the link between the Olympics and promotion of physical activity. Bauman et al.[31] reported no effect from the Sydney Olympics and suggested that mega-sporting events, by themselves, may be unlikely to have a sustained influence on a population's physical activity levels in host cities and nations. They also suggested that multi-year integrated and well-funded programmes accompanying the Olympics are needed. As the Olympics holds huge potential to promote health, more academic discussion is required in the future.

13.7 Future Challenges for Physical Activity in a Super-aged Society

Japan is now facing the world's highest rate of ageing. The number of care receivers on the Long-term Care Insurance System exceeded more than six million (almost one in five of those $\geq$ 65 years) in 2015.[32] Physical activity has the potential to prevent a decline in cognitive[33] and physical functions.[34]

The Japanese Sports Agency reports that today's older adults' physical performance is estimated to be as high as those who are ten years younger once had in 1998.[35] More than half (51%) of individuals aged $\geq$ 60 do not recognize themselves as old and 57% of them regarded those aged $\geq$ 70 or $\geq$ 75 as older adults.[36] It was proposed to redefine older adults as those aged 75 years and above.[37] In 2018, the Japanese government issued the 'ageless society' plan by emphasizing that those aged 65 or older would not be conventionally regarded as older adults, but would be encouraged to stay healthy and work.

The second Health Japan 21 plan set out goals for older adults such as increasing their daily number of steps (7,000 steps/day for elderly men and 6,000 steps/day for elderly women), increasing the proportion of those who regularly exercise (58% for elderly men and 48% for elderly women), and increasing the proportion of those who participate in community activities (80% for elderly men and women) by 2022. The promotion of physical activity is expected to play one of the key roles for a successful super-ageing society.

References

1. Lee IM, Shiroma EJ, Lobelo F, Puska P, Blair SN, Katzmarzyk PT. Effect of physical inactivity on major non-communicable diseases worldwide: an analysis of burden of disease and life expectancy. *Lancet* 2012;380:219–29.
2. Japan Olympic Committee. History. Japan Olympic Committee. Available at: https://www.joc.or.jp/english/historyjapan/ [last accessed 6 March 2020].
3. Japan Health Promotion & Fitness Foundation. National policy for health and physical fitness. Available at: http://www.health-net.or.jp/undou/about/taisaku.html [last accessed 6 March 2020].
4. Tsushita KS, Hosler A, Miura K, et al. Rationale and descriptive analysis of specific health guidance: the nationwide lifestyle intervention program targeting metabolic syndrome in Japan. *J Atheroscler Thromb* 2018;25:308–22.
5. Nakao YM, Miyamoto Y, Ueshima K, et al. Effectiveness of nationwide screening and lifestyle intervention for abdominal obesity and cardiometabolic risks in Japan: the metabolic syndrome and comprehensive lifestyle intervention study on nationwide database in Japan (MetS ACTION-J study). *PLoS One* 2018;13:e0190862.
6. Miyachi M, Tripette J, Kawakami R, Murakami H. +10 min of physical activity per day: Japan is looking for efficient but feasible recommendations for its population. *J Nutr Sci Vitaminol* 2015;61:S7–S9.
7. Japan Sports Agency. Background of establishing the Japan Sports Agency 2015. Available at: http://www.mext.go.jp/sports/en/index.htm [last accessed 6 March 2020].
8. Caspersen CJ, Powell KE, Christenson GM. Physical activity, exercise, and physical fitness: definitions and distinctions for health-related research. *Public Health Rep* 1985;100:126–31.
9. Tremblay MS, Aubert S, Barnes JD, et al. Sedentary behavior research network (SBRN)—terminology consensus project process and outcome. *Int J Behav Nutr Phys Act* 2017;14:75.
10. Pate RR, O'Neill JR, Lobelo F. The evolving definition of 'sedentary'. *Exerc Sport Sci Rev* 2008;36:173–8.
11. Ministry of Health, Labour and Welfare. The national health and nutrition survey. Available at: https://www.mhlw.go.jp/bunya/kenkou/kenkou_eiyou_chousa.html [last accessed 6 March 2020].
12. Takamiya T, Inoue S. Trends in step-determined physical activity among Japanese adults from 1995 to 2016. *Med Sci Sports Exerc* 2019;51:1852–9.

13. Bauman A, Ainsworth BE, Sallis JF, et al. The descriptive epidemiology of sitting. A 20-country comparison using the International Physical Activity Questionnaire (IPAQ). *Am J Prev Med* 2011;41:228–35.

14. Bauman A, Bull F, Chey T, et al. The international prevalence study on physical activity: results from 20 countries. *Int J Behav Nutr Phys Act* 2009;6:21.

15. Hallal PC, Andersen LB, Bull FC, Guthold R, Haskell W, Ekelund U. Global physical activity levels: surveillance progress, pitfalls, and prospects. *Lancet* 2012;380:247–57.

16. Guthold R, Stevens GA, Riley LM, Bull FC. Worldwide trends in insufficient physical activity from 2001 to 2016: a pooled analysis of 358 population-based surveys with 1.9 million participants. *Lancet Glob Health* 2018;6:e1077–e86.

17. Sallis JF, Saelens BE. Assessment of physical activity by self-report: status, limitations, and future directions. *Res Q Exerc Sport* 2000;71:S1–14.

18. Lee PH, Macfarlane DJ, Lam TH, Stewart SM. Validity of the International Physical Activity Questionnaire Short Form (IPAQ-SF): a systematic review. *Int J Behav Nutr Phys Act* 2011;8:115.

19. Amagasa S, Kamada M, Sasai H, et al. How well iPhones measure steps in free-living conditions: cross-sectional validation study. *JMIR Mhealth Uhealth* 2019;7:e10418.

20. Althoff T, Sosic R, Hicks JL, King AC, Delp SL, Leskovec J. Large-scale physical activity data reveal worldwide activity inequality. *Nature* 2017;547:336–9.

21. Ihara M, Takamiya T, Ohya Y, et al. A cross-sectional study of the association between city scale and daily steps in Japan: data from the National Health and Nutrition Survey Japan (NHNS-J) 2006–2010. *Nihon Koshu Eisei Zasshi* 2016;63:549–59.

22. Inoue S, Ohya Y, Odagiri Y, et al. Association between perceived neighborhood environment and walking among adults in 4 cities in Japan. *J Epidemiol* 2010;20:277–86.

23. Ministry of Land, Infrastructure, Transport and Tourism. Person trip survey 2009. Available at: http://www.pref.ishikawa.jp/toshi/person2009/kanazawa%20ptH21.9.11/kekka4.html [last accessed 6 March 2020].

24. Sato H, Inoue S, Fukushima N, et al. Lower youth steps/day values observed at both high and low population density areas: a cross-sectional study in metropolitan Tokyo. *BMC Public Health* 2018;18:1132.

25. Amagasa S, Machida M, Fukushima N, et al. Is objectively measured light-intensity physical activity associated with health outcomes after adjustment for moderate-to-vigorous physical activity in adults? A systematic review. *Int J Behav Nutr Phys Act* 2018;15:65.

26. Amagasa S, Inoue S, Fukushima N, et al. Associations of neighborhood walkability with intensity- and bout-specific physical activity and sedentary behavior of older adults in Japan. *Geriatr Gerontol Int* 2019;19:861–7.

27. OECD. *Health at a Glance 2011: OECD Indicators*. Paris: OECD Publishing 2011.

28. Gero K, Iso H, Kitamura A, Yamagishi K, Yatsuya H, Tamakoshi A. Cardiovascular disease mortality in relation to physical activity during adolescence and adulthood in Japan: does school-based sport club participation matter? *Prev Med* 2018;113:102–8.

29. Benesse Education Research and Development Institute. The 3rd Survey on the Activities Outside Schools 2017. Available at: https://berd.benesse.jp/shotouchutou/research/detail1.php?id=5210 [last accessed 6 March 2020].

30. Mori N, Armada F, Willcox DC. Walking to school in Japan and childhood obesity prevention: new lessons from an old policy. *Am J Public Health* 2012;102:2068–73.

31. Bauman A, Bellew B, Craig CL. Did the 2000 Sydney Olympics increase physical activity among adult Australians? *Br J Sports Med* 2015;49:243–7.

32. Ministry of Health, Labour and Welfare. Long-term care, health and welfare services for the elderly 2017. Available at: https://www.mhlw.go.jp/english/policy/care-welfare/care-welfare-elderly/index.html [last accessed 6 March 2020].

33. Blondell SJ, Hammersley-Mather R, Veerman JL. Does physical activity prevent cognitive decline and dementia?: a systematic review and meta-analysis of longitudinal studies. *BMC Public Health* 2014;14:510.

34. Ip EH, Church T, Marshall SA, et al. Physical activity increases gains in and prevents loss of physical function: results from the lifestyle interventions and independence for elders pilot study. *J Gerontol A Biol Sci Med Sci* 2013;68:426–32.

35. The Japan Sports Agency. Results of physical fitness test 2017. Available at: http://www.mext.go.jp/sports/b_menu/toukei/chousa04/tairyoku/kekka/k_detail/1409822.htm [last accessed 6 March 2020].

36. Cabinet Office of Japan. Investigation into the health status of older adults 2014. Available at: https://www8.cao.go.jp/kourei/ishiki/h26/sougou/gaiyo/index.html [last accessed 6 March 2020].

37. Ouchi Y, Rakugi H, Arai H, et al. Redefining the elderly as aged 75 years and older: proposal from the Joint Committee of Japan Gerontological Society and the Japan Geriatrics Society. *Geriatr Gerontol Int* 2017;17:1045–7.

14

Tobacco Control Policy and Tobacco Product Use Disparity in Japan

Takahiro Tabuchi

14.1 Introduction

Tobacco smoking continues to be a major contributor to mortality, morbidity, and social inequalities in health.[1–4] Reducing socioeconomic inequalities in health has become a priority for public health worldwide. The World Health Organization (WHO)'s Commission on Social Determinants of Health has recommended monitoring and evaluating socioeconomic inequalities in health and health related behaviours.[5] Japan's new health promotion strategy, Health Japan 21 (second term)[6] is in line with this recommendation. Reducing smoking rates and socioeconomic inequality in smoking will lead to major health gain in Japan. Impact on health inequality depends on response to intervention across the socioeconomic strata.[5,7]

The WHO Framework Convention on Tobacco Control is an evidence-based global public health treaty which suggests solutions to tobacco-related problems for countries and governments.[8,9] Several tobacco control measures, such as tobacco taxation, smoke-free legislation, and anti-tobacco media campaigns, have been shown to contribute to an improvement in people's health.[8] Although these measures have been investigated for effectiveness in reducing socioeconomic inequality in smoking,[10–12] results have been inconsistent.

This chapter examines the historical situation and current status of the smoking epidemic in Japan. It pays special attention to smoking disparities in Japan, and the associated factors behind them, particularly the tobacco control measures adopted, and the interference of the tobacco industry in Japanese policy making. Heated tobacco products (HTPs) have become a new public health issue in Japan and worldwide, adding to the importance of continuing research and monitoring to support policy development.

Takahiro Tabuchi, *Tobacco Control Policy and Tobacco Product Use Disparity in Japan* In: *Health in Japan.* Edited by: Eric Brunner, Noriko Cable, and Hiroyasu Iso, Oxford University Press (2021). © Oxford University Press. DOI: 10.1093/oso/9780198848134.003.0014.

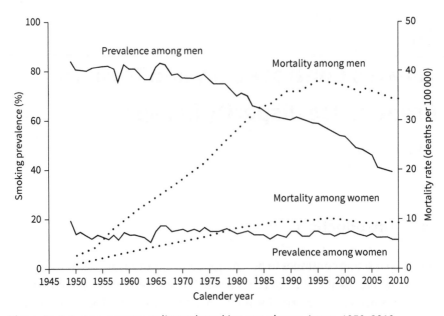

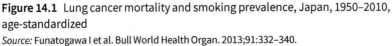

Figure 14.1 Lung cancer mortality and smoking prevalence, Japan, 1950–2010, age-standardized

Source: Funatogawa I et al. Bull World Health Organ. 2013;91:332–340.

14.2 Smoking Prevalence and Socioeconomic Inequalities in Japan

Regarding characteristics of Japanese smokers, the historical pattern of smoking prevalence in Japanese populations is linked to lung cancer mortality in Japan (see Figure 14.1).[13] The prevalence of smoking among men aged ≥ 20 years ranged from 74% to 85% over the three decades from 1949 but since then has gradually decreased, falling to 37% in 2010.

Early initiation to tobacco use is uncommon among recent birth cohorts of males, who showed relatively low prevalence of smoking. In women, the prevalence of smoking was generally low and early initiation of tobacco use was uncommon in absolute terms. The prevalence proportion for smoking among women ranged between 10% and 20% over the six decades from 1949 and showed no clear trend, up or down, over this period with relatively high percentages of smoking prevalence. For both men and women, age-standardized lung cancer mortality rates increased between 1950 and 1996 and then slightly decreased between 1996 and 2010[13] (see Figure 14.1).

Socioeconomic inequality in smoking has been monitored throughout the world, including Japan. Socio-demographic factors such as education, income, occupation, gender, ethnicity, and age have been used as analytical dimensions to estimate inequalities in smoking.[3,10,11] For example, educational attainment is a representative socioeconomic factor.[14] The US surgeon general's report showed educational gradients in smoking using four education levels among adults aged 18 years or more:[3] it was reported that 31.5% (36.2% for men and 26.5% for women) of adults who received education of less than high school standard were current smokers, compared with 10.4% (11.1% for men and 9.7% for women) of college graduates. Similar patterns were reported in European countries.[15] In Japan, among men aged 25–64 (Figure 14.2a), junior

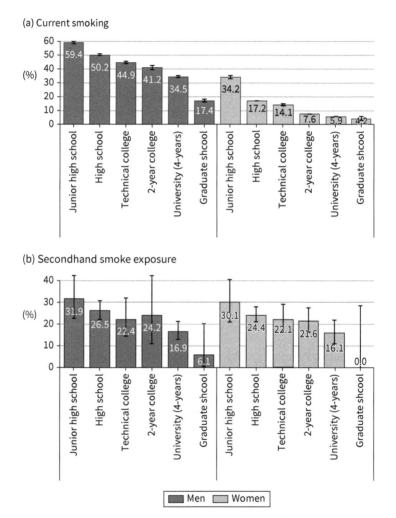

Figure 14.2 Socioeconomic inequality in smoking in Japan, 2010. (a) Education and current smoking (%); (b) education and secondhand smoke exposure (%).

(a) current smoking prevalence (%) among men and women aged 25–64 years (with direct age standardization); (b) frequent secondhand smoke exposure (%) at home or work among men and women aged 25–64 years. Linked data from 2010 Comprehensive Survey of Living Conditions (CSLC) and 2010 National Health and Nutritional Survey (NHNS). NHNS based on smaller sample than CSLC, thus (b) error bars (95% confidence interval) wider than (a).

Source: Tabuchi T, Iso H, Brunner E. J Epidemiol 2018;28:170–175.

high school graduates had the highest current smoking prevalence (59.4%), and graduate school graduates had the lowest (17.4%); high school graduates had the second highest (50.2%); among women, junior high school graduates had the highest (34.2%), and graduate school graduates had the lowest (4.2%).[16]

Socioeconomic inequality in frequent second-hand smoking exposure ('almost every day') at home and/or workplace was striking among non-smokers aged 20–69, based on data from two nationally representative cross-sectional studies which were conducted by the Japanese Ministry of Health, Labour and Welfare in 2010 (see Figure 14.2b).[17] Among both sexes, a high percentage of second-hand smoke exposure was observed in the low education group (30–32% in junior high-school graduates and 24–27% in high-school graduates), and a low percentage of exposure was observed in the high education group (0–6% in graduate school graduates and 16–17% in university graduates). This requires us to monitor socioeconomic inequality in second-hand smoking as well as active smoking.

14.3 Tobacco Control Measures and Interference by the Tobacco Industry in Japan

The World Health Organization's Framework Convention on Tobacco Control (FCTC) came into effect in 2005, and Japan was one of the parties included. However, regulation of tobacco in Japan has lagged behind other participant countries (Table 14.1).[18] Warnings of the risk of smoking displayed on cigarette packaging comprise only text; neither photographs of disease nor plain packaging are implemented. Tobacco smoking is allowed indoors; Japan Tobacco Inc., the Ministry of Finance being their largest shareholder, has persistently resisted regulation, and an amendment to the Health Promotion Act, which has created a new policy for restricting second-hand smoking which comes into force in 2020, has allowed many exceptions to the policy. For example, restaurants with a floor area of ≤100 m², which applies to more than half of all restaurants, are exempt from the regulation. Protection of tobacco control policies from tobacco companies' commercial and other vested interests has been and continues to be a big problem in Japan from a public health point of view (Table 14.1).

Second-hand smoke (i.e. environmental tobacco smoke) was recognized as 'carcinogenic in humans (Group 1)' in 2004 by the International Agency for Research on Cancer.[19] Causal relationships of exposure to indoor second-hand smoke with lung cancer, ischaemic heart disease, stroke, paediatric

Table 14.1 Evaluation of Tobacco Control Measures in Japan, the UK, Australia, and Thailand 2017

	Japan	UK	Australia	Thailand
M: Monitor tobacco use and prevention policies	1 (Best)	1 (Best)	1 (Best)	1 (Best)
P: Protect people from tobacco smoke	4 (Worst)	1 (Best)	1 (Best)	1 (Best)
O: Offer help to quit tobacco use	2	1 (Best)	1 (Best)	2
W[1]: Warn about dangers of tobacco (warning label)	3	1 (Best)	1 (Best)	1 (Best)
W[2]: Warn about dangers of tobacco (anti-tobacco media campaign)	4 (Worst)	1 (Best)	1 (Best)	1 (Best)
E: Enforce bans on tobacco advertising, promotion, and sponsorship	4 (Worst)	2	2	2
R: Raise taxes on tobacco products	2	1 (Best)	2	2

*Four grades evaluation: 1(Best) to 4 (Worst); details are available in the MPOWER report 2017.

respiratory disease, sudden infant death syndrome, and other conditions have been scientifically established through comprehensive evaluations conducted by international agencies and governmental organizations.[3,20]

However, the tobacco industry has been promoting organized campaigns against legislation to prevent indoor second-hand smoke exposure.[21] As of March 2019, Japan Tobacco Inc. (JT)'s website shows that 'a statistical relation between exposure to environmental tobacco smoke and the increase in disease incidence among non-smokers has not been proven' by referencing the discredited Enstrom and Kabat study and a controversial IARC study from 1998.[21–23] In May 2016, when the Japanese Ministry of Health estimated the number of deaths in Japan from exposure to second-hand smoke as 15,000 per year, JT responded that they needed more research, to promote *bun-en* ('separate-smoking' spaces), and improve 'smokers' manners' to 'realize a harmonious society'.[24] Regarding a meta-analysis study by the National Cancer Centre Japan, demonstrating the health hazards arising from second-hand smoke exposure in Japan,[25] the above-mentioned claim by JT was clearly revealed to be a scientific error. The National Cancer Centre Japan made a counterargument by correcting their error and showed their interference to tobacco control through the media.[21]

Japan's tobacco control has been weak by international standards. However, Japan has finally decided to promote the smoke-free rule regarding public smoking in recent years, especially after the 2018 revised Health Promotion Act was adopted. As of March 2019, in addition to two prefectures (Kanagawa and Hyogo) and one city (Bibai in Hokkaido), Tokyo metropolis, Osaka, Yamagata, Yamaguchi, and Shizuoka prefectures, along with Chiba city, have adopted ordinances to prevent second-hand smoking.[26–28] Furthermore, some prefectures and cities, such as Okayama prefecture and Toyohashi city, have been proceeding with smoke-free ordinances in Japan.

14.4 Heated Tobacco Products in Japan: A New Era of Nicotine Products

Electronic cigarettes (e-cigarettes) are battery-operated devices that contain an inhalation-activated mechanism that heats a cartridge, producing an aerosol. Since their introduction to the market in 2004, e-cigarettes have become popular, especially among adolescents and young adults in North American and European countries.[29–31] In Japan, e-cigarettes with nicotine liquid have been prohibited by the Pharmaceutical Affairs Act since 2010, while non-nicotine e-cigarettes were available to the public, even to minors, because there was no regulation for non-nicotine e-cigarettes in Japan. Under these circumstances, e-cigarette use was not popular in Japan.

In December 2013, JT began online sales in Japan of a new heated tobacco product, 'Ploom', that vaporizes tobacco leaf. Furthermore, in 2014, Philip Morris International introduced a novel heated tobacco product, 'IQOS', that heats specific tobacco leaf stick, in Japan and Italy.[32,33] Japan became the only country selling two new brands of HTPs. Launched in 2015, the Japan 'Society and New Tobacco' Internet Survey (JASTIS)[34] was specifically designed to estimate the prevalence of use of novel heated tobacco and e-cigarettes in Japan.

Since e-cigarettes have been marketed to consumers as a means of evading smoke-free policies,[35,36] the use of e-cigarettes in places where conventional tobacco smoking is prohibited could potentially re-normalize tobacco smoking, sustain the dual use of e-cigarettes and tobacco, maintain nicotine addiction, and complicate enforcement of smoke-free policies.[37–39] In an online survey conducted in 2015, more than a quarter of Japanese e-cigarette users reported ever using them in smoke-free restaurants and workplaces, and about one in six said they used e-cigarettes frequently in such smoke-free public places.[40]

Mass media influences people's behaviour through direct and indirect product marketing.[41,42] The prevalence of heated tobacco products use dramatically increased in 2017; from 0.3% in 2015 to 3.6% in 2017 for IQOS.[32] A popular TV programme called *Ame-talk* triggered IQOS diffusion in

Japan.[32] The IQOS was picked up on this popular programme in April 2016, with many popular Japanese comedians also discussing their IQOS use, which seems to have led to increased interest in the product by viewers.

In addition to the prevalence of products, population interest in HTPs in Japan was explored using Google search query data.[32] The weekly Google search volume for words related to heated tobacco/e-cigarettes in Japan from 2013 to 2017 is shown in Figure 14.3.

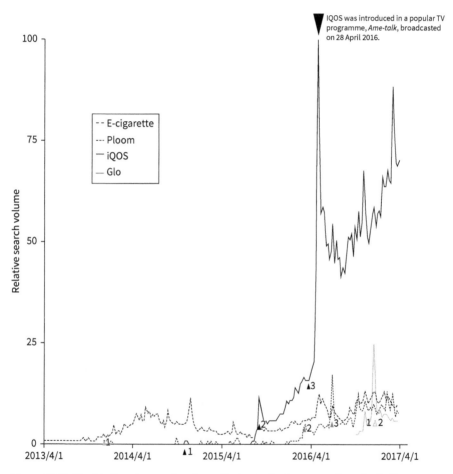

Figure 14.3 Weekly Google search volume for heated tobacco products including e-cigarettes, Japan, 2013–2017

Ploom sales began online in December 2013 and Ploom tech sales began in March 2016. Both soon stopped because of product shortages. Ploom tech sales restarted in June 2016. IQOS was sold only in Nagoya city from November 2014, with sales expanded to 12 prefectures in September 2015, and further expansion to 35 prefectures in April 2016. IQOS results omitted before November 2014. British American Tobacco announced November 2016 that Glo would be sold from 12 December 2016. Glo's results omitted before October 2016.

Source: Tabuchi T et al. Tobacco Control 2018;27(e1):e25–e33.

Over this period, the highest search volume spike for IQOS (i.e. search volume = 100) was observed in the week of 24–30 April 2016, when IQOS was introduced in the TV programme *Ame-talk*; after the spike, the IQOS search volume maintained high values. For e-cigarettes, small spikes were occasionally seen, particularly around 2014, but there was no conspicuous upward trend. Small spikes corresponding to release time periods were observed for Ploom (search volume = 17; 26 June to 2 July 2016) and glo (search volume = 25; 11–17 December 2016).

14.5 Policy Implications: Tobacco Control Measures and Smoking Inequality

Tobacco control interventions tend to have different effects on the rich and poor.[11] Raising the price of cigarettes through taxation is one of the most effective measures to reduce overall smoking rates, but it has been shown repeatedly that tobacco taxation may have the potential to benefit the poor, but yielded mixed results for socioeconomic differences, especially for other tobacco control measures such as smoke-free policies:[43] i.e. increased price due to tobacco taxation consistently shows great potential to reduce smoking inequalities by income.

However, this was not true for other socioeconomic factors such as education. Furthermore, other tobacco control measures such as smoke-free policies were assessed as unlikely to reduce socioeconomic inequalities in smoking without specific efforts to reach socioeconomically disadvantaged smokers.[11,43] If the smoke-free policy covers all workplaces, it will narrow socioeconomic inequalities in smoking. However, smoke-free legislation in bars and restaurants is less likely to be enforced in socioeconomically disadvantaged areas.[43]

On the other hand, smoking cessation interventions targeted at socially disadvantaged groups have been evaluated, and a systematic review[44] concluded that smoking cessation interventions (such as brief advice and behavioural support) for socially disadvantaged groups may be effective; however, overall the findings are inconsistent including the above-mentioned systematic reviews. Further research for both total population and vulnerable socially disadvantaged groups is necessary[45] to provide concrete evidence to the public. This research approach can contribute to not only reducing smoking prevalence but also to narrowing the socioeconomic inequalities in smoking.

In October 2010, the tobacco tax was increased in Japan and the tobacco industry simultaneously increased the price for its own benefit. The price of a pack (20 cigarettes) of the most popular brand in Japan, *Mild Seven* (the brand name was changed to *Mevius* in 2013), increased from 300 yen to 410 yen (37% increase).[46] The 2010 tobacco price increase and its effect on cessation has been reported in two studies.[47,48] Previous studies (mostly conducted in Western developed countries) generally found that tobacco price increases promoted smoking cessation more among the poor and the young than among the affluent and the old.[11,43,49] Importantly, these two Japanese studies may not be interpreted as they completely follow the results from previous studies.[47,48] This might be due to the low tobacco price in Japan, even after the price increase in 2010, according to the affordability index.[7]

Of all the developed countries surveyed for the index, Japan had the most affordable cigarette price in 2009, i.e. people only had to work for 11.5 minutes to earn the price of a pack of 20-cigarettes.[7] Even after the 2010 price increase (410 JPY, GB£2.97, US$3.78), this figure increased to around 16 minutes, whereas in other developed countries such as Australia (1,320 JPY, GB£9.55, US$12.14), Canada (US$10.51), the UK (US$10.99), and New Zealand (US$10.35) it was 30 minutes or more.[7] The impact of a price increase on purchases only lasted for four months after the tobacco price was raised by 95 cents in California.[50]

14.6 Conclusions: Implications for Future Research

14.6.1 Equity Perspective

The evidence is clear that tobacco price increase (taxation) reduces smoking inequality by income.[11,43] A tobacco price increase is the first priority policy. However, previous reviews and empirical studies have not fully evaluated a long-tailed time-course of the effect of tobacco control interventions, suggesting a research gap in the field of tobacco control measures and socioeconomic inequality in smoking.

The 'inverse equity hypothesis'[51] recognizes that inequality may evolve, depending on the period of implementation. Usually, population-based interventions are initially primarily accessed by the affluent and well-educated, so there is an initial increase in socioeconomic inequality (early period). These inequalities narrow when the deprived population can access the intervention after the affluent have gained maximum benefit (late period).

Following the inverse equity hypothesis, continuous and sustained interventions may reduce inequality in the later period of the policy. Similarly, based on the strategy of proportionate universalism,[52] inequality reduction may be achieved if the measures continue long-term expansion to the best practical level (i.e. covering and reaching all socioeconomic subgroups).

Re-evaluation of the impact of the interventions to reduce smoking inequality using a long time-course perspective which takes account of the inverse equity hypothesis, and of vulnerable or hard-to-reach populations, will be beneficial in future research on health promotion and equity effectiveness. Tackling socioeconomic inequality in smoking may be a key public health target in the reduction of overall inequality in health.[45]

14.6.2 New Tobacco Products Made All Tobacco Control Measures Difficult

Japan needs to consider the interactions between new tobacco products use and tobacco control policy status, i.e. whether Japan has implemented the measures recommended by the WHO MPOWER policy package, such as tobacco taxation and smoke-free policies. Regarding taxation, the price of cigarettes will strongly affect new tobacco product use, or a strict smoke-free policy in schools may encourage students to use new tobacco products, which can be easily concealed.[53] Assessment of the differential pricing of cigarettes and new tobacco products is also needed, together with data on how pricing affects new tobacco products use,[54] especially among younger people who would choose new tobacco products if they were much cheaper than cigarettes.

In order to monitor all nicotine-containing product use, in addition to combustible cigarettes and e-cigarettes, we should all watch HTPs such as IQOS, glo, and PloomTECH, developed by tobacco companies Philip Morris International, British American Tobacco, and Japan Tobacco respectively. IQOS are currently sold in more than 40 countries or regions worldwide, particularly in high income countries.[55] After becoming popular and widely used in Japan,[32] IQOS have also gained widespread acceptance in the Republic of Korea.[56] Given the marketing strategies of the big tobacco companies, the worldwide market share of HTPs as nicotine-containing products is likely to grow, which is concerning for public health.

The big tobacco companies have increasingly bought e-cigarette companies. For example, the tobacco company Altria (the parent company of Philip Morris International) took a 35% stock share in the e-cigarette company

JUUL, the makers of the most popular e-cigarette brand in the US.[57] As a result, all major nicotine-containing products, conventional cigarettes, other tobacco products such as snus, e-cigarettes, and HTPs, have become part of the big tobacco companies' range of products. This is concerning because the use of e-cigarettes and/or HTPs is strongly influenced by the marketing strategies of tobacco companies.[58,59] The time period since the first appearance of e-cigarettes and HTPs on the market has been relatively short and thus our knowledge of the dissemination of these new products and our appropriate responses in relation to their regulation is limited.[60]

Worldwide, our society has already entered a 'new era of new tobacco products' after the 'era of the conventional cigarette'.[60] Regarding the regulation of e-cigarettes and/or HTPs, a consensus has not yet been reached in Japan and beyond. Worldwide, we should continue to gather information and evidence on these products in order to evaluate the best approach, and carefully determine our attitudes towards each nicotine-containing product, especially from Japan.

To conduct monitoring of health behaviours and health inequalities in Japan, we need to focus not only on combustible cigarettes but also on heated tobacco products, which are increasingly widely used. In addition, careful consideration of the tobacco industry's interference in tobacco-related policy making is important.

References

1. Jha P, Peto R. Global effects of smoking, of quitting, and of taxing tobacco. *N Engl J Med* 2014;370(1):60–8.
2. Ikeda N, Inoue M, Iso H, et al. Adult mortality attributable to preventable risk factors for non-communicable diseases and injuries in Japan: a comparative risk assessment. *PLoS Med* 2012;9(1):e1001160.
3. US Department of Health and Human Services, Centers for Disease Control, Office on Smoking and Health. The health consequences of smoking—50 years of progress. A report of the Surgeon General. Rockville 2014.
4. GBD 2015 Risk Factors Collaborators. Global, regional, and national comparative risk assessment of 79 behavioural, environmental and occupational, and metabolic risks or clusters of risks, 1990–2015: a systematic analysis for the Global Burden of Disease Study 2015. *Lancet* 2016;388(10053):1659–724.
5. Commission on Social Determinants of Health. Closing the gap in a generation: health equity through action on the social determinants of health. Final report of the Commission on Social Determinants of Health. Geneva: WHO 2008.

6. Ministry of Health, Labour and Welfare. Health Japan 21 (second term) 2012. Available at: http://www.mhlw.go.jp/bunya/kenkou/kenkounippon21.html [last accessed 6 March 2020].

7. Eriksen M, Mackay J, Ross H. *The Tobacco Atlas*, 4th edn. Atlanta: American Cancer Society 2012.

8. WHO. MPOWER 2015. Available at: http://www.who.int/tobacco/mpower/en/ [last accessed 6 March 2020].

9. Eriksen M, Mackay J, Schluger N, Gomeshtapeh F, Drope J. *The Tobacco Atlas* (5th edn.): *Revised, Expanded, and Updated*. Atlanta: American Cancer Society 2015.

10. David A, Esson K, Perucic A, Fitzpatrick C. Tobacco use: equity and social determinants. In: Blas E, Kurup A (eds.). *Equity, Social Determinants and Public Health Programmes*. Geneva: WHO 2010:199–217.

11. Thomas S, Fayter D, Misso K, et al. Population tobacco control interventions and their effects on social inequalities in smoking: systematic review. *Tob Control* 2008;17(4):230–7.

12. Durkin S, Brennan E, Wakefield M. Mass media campaigns to promote smoking cessation among adults: an integrative review. *Tob Control* 2012;21(2):127–38.

13. Funatogawa I, Funatogawa T, Yano E. Trends in smoking and lung cancer mortality in Japan, by birth cohort, 1949–2010. *Bull World Health Organ* 2013;91(5):332–40.

14. Kagamimori S, Gaina A, Nasermoaddeli A. Socioeconomic status and health in the Japanese population. *Soc Sci Med* 2009;68(12):2152–60.

15. Huisman M, Kunst AE, Mackenbach JP. Educational inequalities in smoking among men and women aged 16 years and older in 11 European countries. *Tob Control* 2005;14(2):106–13.

16. Tabuchi T, Kondo N. Educational inequalities in smoking among Japanese adults aged 25–94 years: nationally representative sex- and age-specific statistics. *J Epidemiol* 2017;27(4):186–92.

17. Tabuchi T, Nakamura M. Disparity of secondhand smoke exposure at home and/ or workplace according to age, education and medical insurance in Japan. *JACR Monograph* 2014;20:39–48.

18. WHO. MPOWER 2017. Available at: http://www.who.int/tobacco/mpower/en/ [last accessed 6 March 2020].

19. International Agency for Research on Cancer. *IARC Monographs on the Evaluation of Carcinogenic Risks to Humans*. Vol. 83: *Tobacco Smoke and Involuntary Smoking*. Lyon 2004.

20. Review Committee on the Health Effects of Tobacco Smoking. Tobacco smoking and health: a report (in Japanese) 2016. Available at: http://www.mhlw.go.jp/stf/shingi2/0000135586.html [last accessed 6 March 2020].

21. Iso H, Matsuo K, Katanoda K, Fujiwara T. New policy of the Journal of Epidemiology regarding the relationship with the tobacco industry. *J Epidemiol* 2018;28(1):1–2.

22. Enstrom JE, Kabat GC. Environmental tobacco smoke and tobacco re-lated mortality in a prospective study of Californians, 1960–1998. *BMJ* 2003;326(7398):1057.

23. Ong EK, Glantz SA. Tobacco industry efforts subverting International Agency for Research on Cancer's second-hand smoke study. *Lancet* 2000;355(9211):1253–9.

24. Japan Tobacco Inc. JT's opinion and comments on tobacco control (in Japanese). Available at: https://www.jti.co.jp/tobacco/responsibilities/opinion/index.html [last accessed 6 March 2020].

25. Hori M, Tanaka H, Wakai K, Sasazuki S, Katanoda K. Secondhand smoke ex-posure and risk of lung cancer in Japan: a systematic review and meta-analysis of epidemiologic studies. *Jpn J Clin Oncol* 2016;46(10):942–51.

26. Murata Y. *Environmental Research in Passive Smoking* (in Japanese). Kyoto: Sekaishisosha 2012.

27. Yamada K, Mori N, Kashiwabara M, et al. Industry speed bumps on local tobacco control in Japan? The case of Hyogo. *J Epidemiol* 2015;25(7):496–504.

28. Kashiwabara M, Armada F, Yoshimi I. Kanagawa, Japan's tobacco control legisla-tion: a breakthrough? *APJCP* 2011;12(8):1909–16.

29. Drope J, Cahn Z, Kennedy R, et al. Key issues surrounding the health impacts of electronic nicotine delivery systems (ENDS) and other sources of nicotine. *CA Cancer J Clin* 2017;67(6):449–71.

30. Glasser AM, Collins L, Pearson JL, et al. Overview of electronic nicotine delivery systems: a systematic review. *Am J Prev Med* 2017;52(2):e33–e66.

31. Grana R, Benowitz N, Glantz SA. E-cigarettes: a scientific review. *Circulation* 2014;129(19):1972–86.

32. Tabuchi T, Gallus S, Shinozaki T, Nakaya T, Kunugita N, Colwell B. Heat-not-burn tobacco product use in Japan: its prevalence, predictors and perceived symptoms from exposure to secondhand heat-not-burn tobacco aerosol. *Tob Control* 2018;27(e1):e25–e33.

33. Liu X, Lugo A, Spizzichino L, Tabuchi T, Pacifici R, Gallus S. Heat-not-burn tobacco products: concerns from the Italian experience. *Tob Control* 2019;28(1):113–14.

34. Tabuchi T, Shinozaki T, Kunugita N, Nakamura M, Tsuji I. Study profile: the Japan 'Society and New Tobacco' Internet Survey (JASTIS): a longitudinal internet co-hort study of heat-not-burn tobacco products, electronic cigarettes and conven-tional tobacco products in Japan. *J Epidemiol* 2019;29(11):444–50.

35. Grana RA, Ling PM. 'Smoking revolution': a content analysis of electronic cigar-ette retail websites. *Am J Prev Med* 2014;46(4):395–403.

36. Crowley RA, Health Public Policy Committee of the American College of Physicians. Electronic nicotine delivery systems: executive summary of a policy position paper from the American College of Physicians. *Ann Intern Med* 2015;162(8):583–4.

37. WHO. Electronic nicotine delivery systems 2014. Available at: http://apps.who. int/gb/fctc/PDF/cop6/FCTC_COP6_10-en.pdf [last accessed 6 March 2020].

38. Bhatnagar A, Whitsel LP, Ribisl KM, et al. Electronic cigarettes: a policy statement from the American Heart Association. *Circulation* 2014;130(16):1418–36.

39. Bam TS, Bellew W, Berezhnova I, et al. Position statement on electronic cigarettes or electronic nicotine delivery systems. *Int J Tuberc Lung Dis* 2014;18(1):5–7.

40. Kiyohara K, Tabuchi T. Electronic cigarette use in restaurants and workplaces where combustible tobacco smoking is not allowed: an Internet survey in Japan. *Tob Control* 2018;27(3):254–7.

41. Chapman S. *Public Health Advocacy and Tobacco Control: Making Smoking History*. Oxford: Blackwell Publishing 2007.

42. National Cancer Institute. *The Role of the Media in Promoting and Reducing Tobacco Use*. Tobacco Control Monograph No. 19. Bethesda: US Department of Health and Human Services, National Institutes of Health, National Cancer Institute 2008. NIH Pub. No. 07-6242.

43. Hill S, Amos A, Clifford D, Platt S. Impact of tobacco control interventions on socioeconomic inequalities in smoking: review of the evidence. *Tob Control* 2014;23(e2):e89–97.

44. Bryant J, Bonevski B, Paul C, McElduff P, Attia J. A systematic review and meta-analysis of the effectiveness of behavioural smoking cessation interventions in selected disadvantaged groups. *Addiction* 2011;106(9):1568–85.

45. Tabuchi T, Iso H, Brunner E. Tobacco control measures to reduce socioeconomic inequality in smoking: the necessity, time-course perspective, and future implications. *J Epidemiol* 2018;28(4):170–5.

46. Ito Y, Nakamura M. The effect of increasing tobacco tax on tobacco sales in Japan. *[Nihon koshu eisei zasshi] Japanese Journal of Public Health* 2013;60(9):613–18.

47. Tabuchi T, Nakamura M, Nakayama T, Miyashiro I, Mori J, Tsukuma H. Tobacco price increase and smoking cessation in Japan, a developed country with affordable tobacco: a national population-based observational study. *J Epidemiol* 2016;26(1):14–21.

48. Tabuchi T, Fujiwara T, Shinozaki T. Tobacco price increase and smoking behaviour changes in various subgroups: a nationwide longitudinal 7-year follow-up study among a middle-aged Japanese population. *Tob Control* 2017;26(1):69–77.

49. International Agency for Research on Cancer. *IARC Handbooks of Cancer Prevention Tobacco Control Volume 14: Effectiveness of Tax and Price Policies for Tobacco Control*. Lyon: France International Agency for Research on Cancer 2011.

50. Reed MB, Anderson CM, Vaughn JW, Burns DM. The effect of cigarette price increases on smoking cessation in California. *Prevention Science : The Official Journal of the Society for Prevention Research* 2008;9(1):47–54.

51. Victora CG, Joseph G, Silva ICM, et al. The inverse equity hypothesis: analyses of institutional deliveries in 286 national surveys. *Am J Public Health* 2018;108(4):464–71.

52. Fair Society. Healthy lives strategic review of health inequalities in England post-2010. Available at: www.ucl.ac.uk/marmotreview [last accessed 6 March 2020].

53. Barrington-Trimis JL, Leventhal AM. Adolescents' use of 'Pod Mod' e-cigarettes—urgent concerns. *N Engl J Med* 2018;379(12):1099–102.

54. Huang J, Tauras J, Chaloupka FJ. The impact of price and tobacco control policies on the demand for electronic nicotine delivery systems. *Tob Control* 2014;23(3):41–7.

55. Philip Morris: Heated tobacco products. Available at: https://www.pmi.com/smoke-free-products/iqos-our-tobacco-heating-system [last accessed 6 March 2020].

56. Kim J, Yu H, Lee S, Paek YJ. Awareness, experience and prevalence of heated tobacco product IQOS among young Korean adults. *Tob Control* 2018;27(1):s74–s7.

57. Huang J, Duan Z, Kwok J, et al. Vaping versus JUULing: how the extraordinary growth and marketing of JUUL transformed the US retail e-cigarette market. *Tob Control* 2019;28(2):146–51.

58. Nicksic NE, Snell LM, Rudy AK, Cobb CO, Barnes AJ. Tobacco marketing, e-cigarette susceptibility, and perceptions among adults. *Am J Health Behav* 2017;41(5):579–90.

59. Elias J, Dutra LM, St Helen G, Ling PM. Revolution or redux? Assessing IQOS through a precursor product. *Tob Control* 2018;27(1):s102–s110.

60. Tabuchi T. Commentary on Gravely et al. (2019). Beginning a new era of nicotine products: beyond the four national-level determinants of nicotine vaping products (NVPs) use. *Addiction* 2019;114:1074–5.

15

Mental Health and Wellbeing in Japan

Social, Cultural, and Political Determinants

Norito Kawakami and Akihito Shimazu

15.1 Introduction

This chapter intends to provide an overview of mental health status and mental health care in Japan over the last 50 years. The chapter consists of five sections and a summary. The first section reports on the number of patients under treatment for mental disorders and the prevalence of mental disorders based on community-based epidemiologic studies in Japan. The second section describes the history and current status of treatment of mental disorders in Japan. The third section focuses on suicide in Japan, which has been an important public health problem. In the fourth section, various emerging problems related to mental health among adolescents and young adults are considered. The fifth section focuses on the happiness and psychological wellbeing of people in Japan, associating these with the collective and hierarchical nature of Japanese culture. In each section, we try to report trends over the last 50 years, the social determinants, and the comparison with other countries, based on government statistics and epidemiological studies. The chapter concludes with some future perspectives on mental health in Japan.

15.2 Prevalence of Mental Disorders in Japan

15.2.1 Number of Patients Treated in Japan

There were 3.48 million people (2.7% of the total population of Japan) receiving treatment for mental disorders in 2017. Ninety-three per cent are treated as outpatients, and 7% are inpatients (N = 240,000). The most common

Norito Kawakami and Akihito Shimazu, *Mental Health and Wellbeing in Japan* In: *Health in Japan*. Edited by: Eric Brunner, Noriko Cable, and Hiroyasu Iso, Oxford University Press (2021). © Oxford University Press. DOI: 10.1093/oso/9780198848134.003.0015.

ICD-10 diagnostic group of mental disorders was mood disorder (36.7%), followed by neurotic, stress-related, and somatoform disorders (29.9%), and schizophrenia and related disorders (22.8%). Among inpatients with mental disorders, schizophrenia and related disorders are most common (60.9%). Diagnosed mood disorder increased from 441,000 in 1999 to 1,276,000 in 2017. Neurotic, stress-related, and somatoform diagnoses are also increasing. The number of patients with schizophrenia and related disorders has been relatively stable over the last 20 years.

15.2.2 Prevalence of Mental Disorders in Japan

Large-scale, cross-sectional, community-based surveys of mental disorders were conducted twice in Japan, first in 2002–2005 (N = 4,130)[1] and second in 2013–2015 (N = 2,450).[2] They provide prevalence estimates of common mental disorders (CMD), such as mood, anxiety, and substance use disorders, in the community. These surveys reported that 12-month prevalence (the proportion of people who experienced a disorder in the past 12 months) of any CMD did not increase (5.6% and 5.2%, respectively) in the ten years after the baseline survey.[1,2]

It has been reported that high socioeconomic status (SES) is associated with lower prevalence of depression across countries.[3] This was true in Japan when we used a symptom measure of depression.[4] The association between SES and prevalence of CMD based on clinical diagnostic criteria (DSM-IV) was not clear.[1,2,5]

The 12-month prevalence of CMD in Japan was lower than in Western high-income countries e.g. the US, Australia, and many European countries.[6] The pattern is consistent with findings in other Asian countries e.g. China, Korea, Singapore, and Taiwan. It is still unclear what explains the lower prevalence of CMD in Asian countries. Possible explanations include: (1) low prevalence due to sample selection bias e.g. depressed people missing from survey samples; (2) information bias e.g. depressed people do not report their diagnosis or symptoms, consciously and/or unconsciously; (3) small sample size, which by chance resulted in a low estimate; (4) confounding in reporting, i.e. Asian people have a cultural tendency to report fewer symptoms.[7] Some argue that the low prevalence of CMD in Asian countries may be real, with a protective effect of a collective culture on CMD.[8] This is an interesting research question for future studies of cross-cultural mental health.

15.3 Treatment of Mental Disorders in Japan

15.3.1 Treatment of Mental Disorders: From Hospital to the Community

The history of treatment for people with mental disorders, particularly those with severe mental illness (SMI) such as schizophrenia, started before the middle ages. At the beginning of the Meiji era, the *Seishin Byosha Kango Ho* Act (Confinement and Protection of the Mentally Ill Act) made the family responsible for the care of a member with SMI. This lead to a practice of confinement in a room in their home. This was forbidden after 1950 by the *Seishin Eisei Ho* (Mental Hygiene Act). However, this Act introduced a new confinement policy, a system of involuntary admission to hospital, either by official order or the intention of the family. Following this Act, the number of patients admitted involuntarily at the family's request increased. Treatment costs were covered by the social welfare system in most cases. The number of beds at mental hospitals increased dramatically, in response (see Figure 15.1). Most mental hospitals were privately owned.

Until recently, inpatient care was central to the treatment of SMI in Japan. There were about 1,000 mental hospitals with 331,700 beds in 2017. The

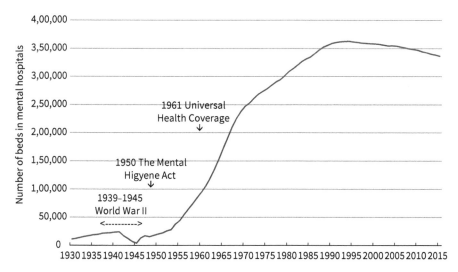

Figure 15.1 Number of beds in mental hospitals in Japan, 1930–2015

Okinawa not included 1946–1971. Bed numbers not adjusted for size and age-structure of the population.

Source: Statistics and Information Department, Minister's Secretariat, Ministry of Health, Labour and Welfare.

number of beds in mental hospitals per 1,000 of the population was 2.6, considerably higher than in other high-income countries (usually <1 per 1,000). The average length of stay in mental hospitals was 267.7 days; one in five inpatients in mental hospitals stayed for ten years or longer. The proportion of inpatients confined and restrained remains high.

Several mental health policies were introduced to encourage change from hospital-based to community-based care. The amendment of the Mental Hygiene Act in 1965, following an incident when US Ambassador Edwin O. Reischauer was injured by a young man with a history of mental disorder, introduced some community-based mental health care. Public health centres were given responsibility for psychiatric care and prefectural mental health centres were set up. The death of two inpatients caused by violence of nursing staff in 1983 called into question the respect of human rights in mental hospitals. These incidents led to *Seishin Hoken Ho* (Mental Health Act) in 1987, that introduced formal protection of the human rights of inpatients, and a system of rehabilitation for inpatients. *Seishin Hoken Fukushi Ho* (Mental Health and Welfare Act) of 1995 strengthened the outpatient psychiatric service and rehabilitation programmes after discharge from mental hospitals. More recently, in 2004, the health ministry launched a new initiative 'Vision for Reform of Mental Health and Welfare Service' to accelerate the discharge of psychiatric inpatients.

As such, the Japanese government has shifted its mental health policy from hospital-based care to community-based care. The number of outpatient mental clinics outnumbered the number of mental hospitals in 1993, and is steadily increasing. The number of beds in mental hospitals is slowly decreasing since its peak in 1994. Since 1993, mental disorders have been included in the welfare regimen for people with disability. At present, people with mental disability are covered by the integrated schema of welfare services for three types of disability (physical, mental, and learning) under the Act for Comprehensive Welfare for Persons with Disabilities (2012). The service supported about 860,000 people with mental disability to live in the community in 2015.

15.3.2 Diagnosis and Mode of Treatment of Mental Disorders

After the introduction of modern medicine from Germany in the beginning of the Meiji era, the so-called 'traditional diagnosis' system has been used by psychiatrists in Japan for many years. The traditional diagnosis system was based on Emil Kraepelin's work, and classifies mental disorders into endogenous and exogenous disorders by their causes, where endogenous mental disorders are further classified into schizophrenia and manic-depressive disorder. For government statistics, the International Classification of Diseases (ICD) system is used. After the introduction of the Diagnostic and Statistical Manual of Mental Disorders (DSM) by the American Psychiatric Association in 1980, DSM has been the most frequently used diagnostic system both for clinical practice and research.[9] The ICD is also used for clinical practice, but slightly less frequently than the DSM. About 10% of psychiatrists still use the traditional diagnosis system in their daily clinical practice.

In Japan, the mode of treatment of mental disorders is mainly pharmaceutical. Some reports indicate that the prescription of psychotropic drugs has increased in the last 5–10 years. Prescription of the new SSRI antidepressants increased rapidly after 1999.[10] Psychotherapy and case management are provided for inpatients. Outpatient services include group psychotherapy and occupational therapy, and currently about 110,000 outpatients use psychiatric day care programmes which offer such therapies. In addition, about 25,000 patients with mental disorders use home-visit nursing services. There is a need for the quality of non-pharmaceutical treatments to be improved.

15.3.3 Treatment Rate of Mental Disorders

The treatment rate (more precisely, the treatment proportion in any healthcare setting in the past 12 months) for CMD was lower in Japan compared to other high-income countries (37% for Japan[1] and more than 50% in other countries for severe cases).[11] This has often been attributed to the more negative attitude among Japanese people to mental disorders than in other countries.[12] Low perceived need was a major reason for not seeking treatment.[13] In addition, a low treatment rate in primary care (non-psychiatrist outpatient services) was particularly low compared to the US.[14]

However, a recent survey found that the treatment rate was higher (45% among severe cases),[2] possibly because of a nationwide community campaign to identify and treat depression in residents, increase liaison between psychiatrists and other doctors, and provide early consultation for people with depression in the workplace. These moves were facilitated by the Suicide Prevention Act (2008). No clear association was reported between SES (such as educational attainment and income) and treatment rate.[1,2] Some studies reported that people with high SES were less likely to seek treatment.[4] The authors[4] argued that barriers to accessing mental health services among people with low income may be relatively low due to universal health insurance, while high-income people may have barriers due to difficulty in taking time off from work and the social stigma of seeking mental healthcare. These points need further elucidations.

15.4 Suicide and its Social Determinants in Japan

Japan is known for its unique culture-bound suicide behaviour of *seppuku*.[15] It developed in Japan as a culturally sanctioned role-behaviour in highly formal and closed organizations and groups. *Seppuku* is becoming rare in contemporary Japan, while it is argued that suicide related to one's role-performance still continues.[15]

Age-standardized suicide rates in Japan were 14.3 per 100,000 of the population for both sexes, 20.5 for men, and 8.1 for women in 2016[16] (see also Figure 1.4). Japanese rates have improved since 2010, but are still higher globally (10.6 for both sexes, 13.5 for men, and 7.7 for women in 2016), and ranked 14th among countries with the data.

Suicide rates have fluctuated in the past 60 years. There were three peaks after World War II (Figure 15.2). In the first peak in the mid-1950s, suicide

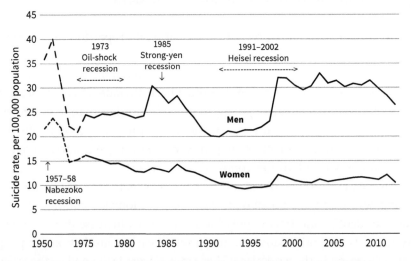

Figure 15.2 Age-adjusted suicide rate, men and women, Japan, 1950–2012

Rates are age-adjusted using world standard population 2015 (United Nations World Population Prospects, 2019). Dotted lines indicate that yearly data are not available. *Nabezoko* (pan-bottom) lingering recession of 1957–1958. Recessions in Japan are named.

Source: Statistics and Information Department, Minister's Secretariat, Ministry of Health, Labour and Welfare.

among younger men and women increased, mainly due to discord in the parent-child relationship e.g. parents against the marriage their child wanted. The recent peak in suicide rate was between 1998 and 2010, following the long *Heisei* recession. The rise in suicide rate was most prominent among middle-aged men. They were often the bread-winners of their family and were at high risk of suicide when economic problems, such as redundancy, affected them. The recent downward trend of suicide rates among men since 2010 is often attributed to improvements in the economy and unemployment rates. The recent decline in suicide rate is also linked with suicide prevention measures of municipalities under the Suicide Prevention Act (2008, revised 2016), reported to be effective among men.[17]

Low SES was strongly associated with suicide during the 'lost decades'. For instance, an ecological study found that a high deprivation at municipality level was associated with suicide rates.[18] The rate was extremely high among people who were unemployed. A nationwide 'psychological autopsy' study found that suicide was associated with complicated debt.[19] Community characteristics have also been linked to the suicide rate. An ecological study in Tokyo showed that the social trust score at ward level was negatively associated with the male suicide rate.[20,21] The role of social capital is less clear in rural areas.[21] Social capital in the community may prevent suicide of men in urban areas where social capital levels are usually lower. However, social capital may have a downside in rural areas. Japan has a strong tradition of community ties and social norms. High social capital may bring excessive community demands and discrimination against people in marginalized positions. There may also be a contagion effect, i.e. suicide in the community.[22]

15.5 Behavioural Disorders and Problems among Younger Generations in Japan

15.5.1 Developmental Disorder

Developmental disorder is a group of conditions related to brain development that may cause delays in learning, social interaction, and communication. Diagnoses include pervasive developmental disorder (PDD), autistic spectrum disorder (ASD), and attention-deficit hyperactivity disorder (ADHD). The Japanese ministry of education reported after a 2012 survey that there could be 6.5% of students in elementary and middle schools with developmental disorders or similar conditions. Developmental disorder is also considered a problem in the workplace, causing secondary mental and behavioural problems. Prevalence of developmental disorders among children aged 4–12 years old in Japan were reported at 0.13–0.37% for ASD and 1.81% for PDD,[23] comparable with Europe, America, and Asia.[24] Developmental disorders are believed to be increasing in Japan, however, evidence for such a trend over the past 30 years is lacking.[23] The apparent increase seems to be due to a widening definition of the disorder.[24] There is some advocacy that people labelled with 'developmental disorder' may be better described as having unique features of personality.

15.5.2 Child Abuse

According to the National Police Agency, 4,571 children and adolescents aged 18 or younger were protected by police in 2018, with 1,380 child abuse incidents including 36 deaths. Annually, more than 100,000 reports of child abuse were made by citizens to child consultation centres under the Child Welfare Act. Numbers have steadily increased in the past ten years. Experience of child abuse is associated with increased risk of CMD at later ages.[25] Child abuse is also associated with increased risk of suicidal ideation.[26] People exposed to physical abuse as a child tend to use physical discipline with their children,[27] thus abuse may transmit across generations. Prevalence studies reported a lower to similar prevalence of child sexual abuse in Japan compared to other countries,[28] while a comparison is difficult due to different measures used. The reason for the increasing number of child abuse reports in Japan is unclear, beside increased awareness.

15.5.3 School Non-attendance and Bullying

School non-attendance for 30 or more days per year, not attributable to health or economic reasons, was 1.5% among elementary and middle school students, and 1.5% among high school students in 2017, with a rising trend. School bullying is an issue in school mental health, with higher prevalence in elementary schools (4.9%) compared to middle- and high schools (2.4% and 0.2% respectively) in 2017, also with an increasing trend. One study reported both victims and perpetrators of school bullying were more prevalent in Japan than in the US and South Africa.[29] School bullying is associated with higher internalizing disorders, such as depression and anxiety among victimized students, and sometimes among bullying students.[30]

15.5.4 *Hikikomori*

Hikikomori refers to severe and prolonged social withdrawal. It was originally considered as a culture-bound phenomenon in Japan, but a similar phenomenon is found in many other countries.[30] A survey conducted in 2002–2006 in Japan reported that 1.2% of community residents aged 20–49 years old ever experienced *hikikomori* in their lifetime.[31] More than half of *hikikomori* were found to have mental disorders before or during the *hikikomori* episode.[31] *Hikikomori* is strongly associated with autism spectrum and ADHD.[32] However, it is unclear if all cases of *hikikomori* are explained by mental disorders. Interestingly, *hikikomori* cases are more common among children of highly educated parents.[33]

15.5.5 Problems Related to Internet Use among Adolescents

Seven out of ten people in Japan used a social network service such as LINE, Facebook, or Twitter according to the 2016 government survey, with higher proportions among people aged 10–39 years old (81–98%). Prevalence of Internet addiction (problematic Internet use) was reported as 6.2% in males and 9.8% in females among middle- and high school students.[34] These figures are comparable to those reported in other countries.[35] Texting (SNS messaging) was strongly associated with Internet addiction. Cases of suicide among adolescents were reported and sometimes associated with SNS cyberbullying by peers.

15.6 Wellbeing and Happiness in Japan

15.6.1 The Nature of Wellbeing and Happiness in Japan

The nature of wellbeing and happiness in Japan has been extensively examined in the field of cultural psychology. Numerous findings have accumulated based on comparison of Japanese and US participants.[36] In relation to self and social relationships, wellbeing is likely to be enhanced by attunement to one's surrounding cultural context.[37] In the East, wellbeing is relational, intersubjective, and collective in scope and it is described as social harmony tied to self-criticism, discipline, and adjusting to others. In the West, wellbeing is viewed as personal and individual in scope and, thus, associated with experiences of personal achievement and self-esteem. A unique concept in Japan is 'minimalist wellbeing'.[38] This concept of wellbeing underscores the transitory nature of happiness as well as the gratitude, calm, and peacefulness that can come from immersing oneself in nothingness.

A further dimension of wellbeing in the Eastern context is dialectical emotions, which involve a balanced experience of positive and negative emotions.[39] In contrast, the more common bipolar pattern is prominent in the West, wherein positive and negative affect are inversely related. These studies suggest that the nature of wellbeing and happiness in Japan is different from that in other Western countries.

15.6.2 Why Japanese People Report Low Life Satisfaction

Much attention has been devoted to the question of whether and how the experience of wellbeing differs across cultures.[36] Questionnaire surveys reveal differences in degrees of positivity among Japanese and Western respondents.

The Japanese scored lowest on general self-efficacy, the belief of being able to control challenges and demands by taking adaptive action,[40] among 25 countries.[41] In addition, among 16 countries, Japanese employees scored lowest on work engagement, a positive and fulfilling work-related state of mind (characterized as vigour, dedication, and absorption).[42,43] Evidence of cultural differences in survey responses comes from research[44] examining responses to positive and negative items from the Centre for Epidemiologic Studies Depression Scale (CES-D)[45] among American and Japanese workers. Responses to negatively worded items, e.g. lonely, crying, were comparable in the two groups, whereas the Japanese responses to positively worded items markedly differed from those of US workers.

One possible explanation for the low scores on instruments measuring wellbeing and happiness is the tendency to suppress expression of positive affect among Japanese people. Maintenance of social harmony is one of the most important values in Japanese society, and the Japanese have been taught since childhood to understate their own virtues and not to behave assertively.[44] As a result, the Japanese may make a relativistic judgement of affect and situation through comparison with others, leading to suppression of positive affect expression. The suppression of positive affect appears to represent a moral distinction and socially desirable behaviour in Japanese society.[43]

Hence, we should be cautious when interpreting low wellbeing and happiness scores among Japanese (Chapter 1.2.2).

15.6.3 Cultural Differences in Determinants of Wellbeing in Japan and the Western Context

The above studies illustrate cultural differences in the nature of wellbeing in Japan and the West, and correspondingly determinants of wellbeing are also likely to differ across cultures. Happiness is construed in terms of interpersonal connectedness with more embedding of the self in social relationships in the East Asian context, whereas happiness in the West is construed as a personal achievement with more autonomy and independence.[46] We can say that it is commitment to social roles, social obligations, and a readiness to respond to social expectations that are important determinants of wellbeing in Japan.[36]

15.7 Summary

Mental disorders are common in Japan as well as in other parts of the world. In Japan, one in 37 people currently receives treatment for any mental disorder, while one in 20 people have experienced any CMD in the past year. While the number of psychiatric patients has increased, particularly with mood disorder, this seems attributable to improving detection and treatment. The trend in prevalence of mental disorders during the last 10–15 years of economic slowdown and social changes is unclear.

Historically, mental hospitals played a central role in treatment, isolating people from the community in inpatient units. The number of beds in mental hospitals remains greater in Japan than in other high-income countries. Concerns to protect the human rights of patients and to provide more efficient treatment has gradually shifted policy from inpatient treatment to community-based care. The welfare regimen also plays an important role in supporting life in the community for people with mental disorders.

Suicide rates, particularly among men, have fluctuated in Japan, largely influenced by economic factors. SES seems to be a strong determinant of suicide in Japan. The suicide rate is still higher in Japan than in other countries, while it is improving after its peak in 2012. The improvement may partly be attributable to recent suicide prevention measures at national and municipality levels.

In Japan, people retain a characteristic perception and cognition of wellbeing in a family- and community-oriented collective culture, that is also a basis of a sense of meaningfulness in life (*Ikigai*). While reported prevalence of CMD is usually lower in Asian collectivist countries than Western countries, it is still not clear if collectivism is beneficial to mental health in Japan. At least there seem to be two faces to this aspect of the culture. For instance, collectivism and high social capital may be protective against suicide in urban areas, but not always in rural areas.

Japan faces diverse behavioural problems among younger generations, both at home and school, in a rapidly changing social, economic, and cultural environment. It is necessary for policy makers and professionals in the mental health field to work together across other sectors such as education to tackle these problems. It is also important to monitor impacts of new individualistic cultures and subcultures such as *Otaku* on the mental health and wellbeing of future Japanese generations.

Mental health services in Japan face many challenges. Current national priorities (Box 15.1) include a diverse set of topics including reform of mental health services, action to reduce stigma around mental disorders,

---

Box 15.1 Current National Priorities in Mental Health Care and Welfare in Japan

1. Reform of mental health services: from inpatient treatment to support for life in the community:
   a. Improvement in understanding of and lowering stigma for mental disorders among people in Japan.
   b. Reform of mental health care, e.g. to control the number of beds in mental hospitals.
   c. Effective mental healthcare and welfare services.
   d. Improving the involuntary admissions system.
2. Disorder-specific measures
   a. Depressive disorder;
   b. Post-traumatic stress disorder (PTSD);
   c. Dependence (alcohol, other drugs, gambling);
   d. Eating disorder;
   e. Developmental disorder.
3. Suicide prevention.
4. Integration of mental health in a local medical care plan.
5. Training manpower for mental health.

and reforming the system of involuntary hospital admission. In addition to system reform, there are several disorder-specific measures which are already underway, or being planned, such as services for substance use disorders (alcohol, other drugs, gambling). Capacity to support mental health in the community will depend on increased training of psychiatric social workers and certified public psychologists.

References

1. Ishikawa H, Kawakami N, Kessler RC. Collaborators WMHJS. Lifetime and 12-month prevalence, severity and unmet need for treatment of common mental disorders in Japan: results from the final dataset of World Mental Health Japan Survey. *Epidemiol Psychiatr Sci* 2016;25(3):217–29.

2. Ishikawa H, Tachimori H, Takeshima T, et al. Prevalence, treatment, and the correlates of common mental disorders in the mid 2010s in Japan: the results of the world mental health Japan second survey. *J Affect Dis* 2018;241:554–62.

3. Lorant V, Deliège D, Eaton W, Robert A, Philippot P, Ansseau M. Socioeconomic inequalities in depression: a meta-analysis. *Am J Epidemiol* 2003;157(2):98–112.

4. Fukuda Y, Hiyoshi A. Influences of income and employment on psychological distress and depression treatment in Japanese adults. *Environ Health Prev Med* 2012;17(1):10–17.

5. Honjo K, Kawakami N, Tsuchiya M, Sakurai K. Group W-JS. Association of subjective and objective socioeconomic status with subjective mental health and mental disorders among Japanese men and women. *Int J Behav Med* 2014;21(3):421–9.

6. Demyttenaere K, Bruffaerts R, Posada-Villa J, et al. Prevalence, severity, and unmet need for treatment of mental disorders in the World Health Organization World Mental Health Surveys. *JAMA*. 2004;291(21):2581–90.

7. Chang SM, Hahm BJ, Lee JY, et al. Cross-national difference in the prevalence of depression caused by the diagnostic threshold. *J Affect Disord* 2008;106(1–2):159–67.

8. Chiao JY, Blizinsky KD. Culture-gene coevolution of individualism-collectivism and the serotonin transporter gene. *Proc Biol Sci* 2010;277(1681):529–37.

9. Nakane Y, Nakane H. Classification systems for psychiatric diseases currently used in Japan. *Psychopathology* 2002;35(2–3):191–4.

10. Nakagawa A, Grunebaum MF, Ellis SP, et al. Association of suicide and antidepressant prescription rates in Japan, 1999–2003. *J Clin Psychiatry* 2007;68(6):908–16.

11. Wang PS, Aguilar-Gaxiola S, Alonso J, et al. Use of mental health services for anxiety, mood, and substance disorders in 17 countries in the WHO world mental health surveys. *Lancet* 2007;370(9590):841–50.

12. Griffiths KM, Nakane Y, Christensen H, Yoshioka K, Jorm AF, Nakane H. Stigma in response to mental disorders: a comparison of Australia and Japan. *BMC Psychiatry* 2006;6:21.

13. Kanehara A, Umeda M, Kawakami N. Group WMHJS. Barriers to mental health care in Japan: results from the World Mental Health Japan Survey. *Psychiatry Clin Neurosci* 2015;69(9):523–33.

14. Naganuma Y, Tachimori H, Kawakami N, et al. Twelve-month use of mental health services in four areas in Japan: findings from the World Mental Health Japan Survey 2002–2003. *Psychiatry Clin Neurosci* 2006;60(2):240–8.

15. Fusé T. Suicide and culture in Japan: a study of *seppuku* as an institutionalized form of suicide. *Social psychiatry* 1980;15(2):57–63.

16. WHO. Global Health Observatory Data Repository. Registry of Research Data Repositories. Available at: http://doi.org/10.17616/R3S32Q [last accessed 24 March 2020].

17. Ono Y, Sakai A, Otsuka K, et al. Effectiveness of a multimodal community intervention program to prevent suicide and suicide attempts: a quasi-experimental study. *PLoS One* 2013;8(10):e74902.

18. Fukuda Y, Nakamura K, Takano T. Cause-specific mortality differences across socioeconomic position of municipalities in Japan, 1973–1977 and 1993–1998: increased importance of injury and suicide in inequality for ages under 75. *Int J Epidemiol* 2005;34(1):100–9.

19. Kameyama A, Matsumoto T, Katsumata Y, et al. Psychosocial and psychiatric aspects of suicide completers with unmanageable debt: a psychological autopsy study. *Psychiatry Clin Neurosci* 2011;65(6):592–5.

20. Okamoto M, Kawakami N, Kido Y, Sakurai K. Social capital and suicide: an ecological study in Tokyo, Japan. *Environ Health Prev Med* 2013;18(4): 306–12.

21. Sanpei M, Kawakami N, Shimomitsu T, et al. Social capital in the community and suicide rate: an urban and non-urban difference. Paper presented at the 71st Annual Conference of the Japan Association of Public Health 2012, Yamaguchi, Japan.

22. Villalonga-Olives E, Kawachi I. The dark side of social capital: a systematic review of the negative health effects of social capital. *Soc Sci Med* 2017;194:105–27.

23. Honda H, Shimizu Y, Imai M, Nitto Y. Cumulative incidence of childhood autism: a total population study of better accuracy and precision. *Dev Med Child Neurol* 2005;47(1):10–18.

24. Elsabbagh M, Divan G, Koh Y-J, et al. Global prevalence of autism and other pervasive developmental disorders. *Autism Research: Official Journal of the International Society for Autism Research* 2012;5(3):160–79.

25. Fujiwara T, Kawakami N. Group WMHJS. Association of childhood adversities with the first onset of mental disorders in Japan: results from the World Mental Health Japan, 2002–2004. *J Psychiatr Res* 2011;45(4):481–7.

26. Obikane E, Shinozaki T, Takagi D, Kawakami N. Impact of childhood abuse on suicide-related behavior: analysis using marginal structural models. *J Affect Disord* 2018;234:224–30.

27. Umeda M, Kawakami N, Kessler RC, Miller E. 2002–2006 WMHJSG. Childhood adversities and adult use of potentially injurious physical discipline in Japan. *J Fam Violence* 2015;30(4):515–27.

28. Tanaka M, Suzuki YE, Aoyama I, Takaoka K, MacMillan HL. Child sexual abuse in Japan: a systematic review and future directions. *Child Abuse Negl* 2017;66:31–40.

29. Dussich JP, Maekoya C. Physical child harm and bullying-related behaviors: a comparative study in Japan, South Africa, and the United States. *Int J Offender Ther Comp Criminol* 2007;51(5):495–509.

30. Kozasa S, Oiji A, Kiyota A, Sawa T, Kim SY. Relationship between the experience of being a bully/victim and mental health in preadolescence and adolescence: a cross-sectional study. *Ann Gen Psychiatry* 2017;16:37.

31. Koyama A, Miyake Y, Kawakami N, et al. Lifetime prevalence, psychiatric comorbidity and demographic correlates of 'hikikomori' in a community population in Japan. *Psychiatry Res* 2010;176(1):69–74.

32. Umeda M, Shimoda H, Miyamoto K, et al. Comorbidity and sociodemographic characteristics of adult autism spectrum disorder and attention deficit hyperactivity disorder: epidemiological investigation in the World Mental Health Japan 2nd Survey. *Int J Dev Disabil* 2019. Available at: https://www.tandfonline.com/doi/full/10.1080/20473869.2019.1576409 [last accessed 24 March 2020].

33. Umeda M, Kawakami N. 2002–2006 WMHJSG. Association of childhood family environments with the risk of social withdrawal ('hikikomori') in the community population in Japan. *Psychiatry Clin Neurosci* 2012;66(2):121–9.

34. Mihara S, Osaki Y, Nakayama H, et al. Internet use and problematic Internet use among adolescents in Japan: a nationwide representative survey. *Addict Behav Rep* 2016;4:58–64.

35. Cheng C, Li AY. Internet addiction prevalence and quality of (real) life: a meta-analysis of 31 nations across seven world regions. *Cyberpsychol Behav Soc Netw* 2014;17(12):755–60.

36. Ryff CD, Love GD, Miyamoto Y, et al. Culture and the promotion of wellbeing in East and West: understanding varieties of attunement to the surrounding context. In: Fava GA, Ruini C (eds.), *Increasing Psychological Wellbeing in Clinical and Educational Settings: Interventions and Cultural Contexts*. Dordrecht: Springer Netherlands 2014:1–19.

37. Kitayama S, Markus HR. The pursuit of happiness and the realization of sympathy: cultural patterns of self, social relations, and wellbeing. In: Diener E, Suh EM (eds.). *Culture and Subjective Wellbeing.* Cambridge, MA: The MIT Press 2000:113–61.

38. Kan C, Karasawa M, Kitayama S. Minimalist in style: self, identity, and wellbeing in Japan. *Self and Identity* 2009;8(2–3):300–17.

39. Miyamoto Y, Ryff CD. Cultural differences in the dialectical and non-dialectical emotional styles and their implications for health. *Cognition & Emotion* 2011;25:22–39.

40. Bandura A. *Self-efficacy: The Exercise of Control.* New York, NY: W H Freeman/ Times Books/ Henry Holt & Co. 1997.

41. Scholz U, Dona BG, Sud S, Schwarzer R. Is general self-efficacy a universal construct? Psychometric findings from 25 countries. *Eur J Psychol Assess* 2002;18(3):242–51.

42. Schaufeli WB, Salanova M, González-romá V, Bakker AB. The measurement of engagement and burnout: a two sample confirmatory factor analytic approach. *J Happiness Stud* 2002;3(1):71–92.

43. Shimazu A, Miyanaka D, Schaufeli WB. Work engagement from a cultural perspective. In: Albrecht S 9ed.), *Handbook of Employee Engagement: Perspectives, Issues, Research and Practice.* Northampton: Edward-Elgar 2010:364–72.

44. Iwata N, Roberts CR, Kawakami N. Japan-U.S. comparison of responses to depression scale items among adult workers. *Psychiatry Res* 1995;58(3):237–45.

45. Radloff LS. The CES-D scale: a self-report depression scale for research in the general population. *Applied Psychological Measurement* 1977;1(3):385–401.

46. Uchida Y, Norasakkunit V, Kitayama S. Cultural constructions of happiness: theory and empirical evidence. *J Happiness Stud* 2004;5:223–39.

16

Japan's Engagement with Global Health

Evolution and Outlook in the Era of Sustainable Development Goals

Hiroki Nakatani

16.1 Introduction: Relevance of Global Health to the Japanese

The United Nations (UN) is still well respected in Japan, and many will remember their school days when teachers urged them to memorize the definition of health in the Constitution of the World Health Organization, 'a state of complete physical, mental, and social wellbeing and not merely the absence of disease or infirmity'. However, until recently, health in international settings was rarely discussed among citizens, the business community, and even political leaders. The common perception of international health projects and the dedicated workers in this field is as a noble cause serving the underprivileged, yet an outlier of our communities. Perception is now slowly changing, and this section aims to explain how and why.

In Japan, the terms 'international health' and 'global health' are used interchangeably, and the term *Kokusai Hoken* is used. Outside Japan, international health typically refers to health issues in developing countries and mitigation through foreign aid in the form of official development assistance (ODA). Global health, on the other hand, refers to all aspects of health in a global context.

First, let us see how international commitment is viewed by the Japanese public, which is rather surprising. Japan has been a strong advocate of health in G7 summits and is a founding member of many international health-related organizations such as the Global Fund to Fight AIDS, Tuberculosis, and Malaria (Global Fund). However, there is a discrepancy between government commitment and public opinion. An opinion poll on diplomacy is conducted annually. In the 2018 survey,[1] the ranking of reasons (from preset choices) for Japanese engagement in development assistance was in the

Hiroki Nakatani, *Japan's Engagement with Global Health* In: *Health in Japan*. Edited by: Eric Brunner, Noriko Cable, and Hiroyasu Iso, Oxford University Press (2021). © Oxford University Press. DOI: 10.1093/oso/9780198848134.003.0016.

following descending order: securing essential resources such as energy, building trust for Japan in the international community, a tool of Japanese diplomacy, economic revitalization of Japan, appreciation for the assistance given to Japan during hardship such as the Tohoku Earthquake in 2011, and finally moral responsibility toward the international community. Although this survey did not specifically address attitudes to global health commitments, ranking 'moral responsibility' the lowest suggests instrumental purposes are considered more important than ethical ones by the public.

Another survey,[2] conducted by the Ministry of Foreign Affairs, asked 1,000 citizens aged over 18 years to rank among sustainable development goals (SDGs) the priority areas for Japanese development aid. The order of ranking was: education (44.8%), marine plastic waste (40.5%), disasters (37.9%), climate change (34.5%), women's empowerment (22.7%), followed by health (16.5%). However, trend analysis of the survey series showed a decrease in the percentage of people who are against provision of development aid, currently about 20%. It appears Japanese citizens generally see ODA as a source of soft power and a useful tool to maintain national and economic interests in an increasingly tough diplomatic environment.[3]

A search of publications on major databases may give an indication of perceptions of global health among academics and health professionals. A search on *Igaku-Chuo-Zasshi (Ichushi)*, the major Japanese bibliographic database operated by Japan Medical Abstracts Society, shows a paucity of publications on global health and international health. The number of articles containing 'global health' in the title during 2014–2018 was 1,925 in PubMed and only 99 in *Ichushi*, while the same search for 'international health' yielded 186 and 75 articles respectively. This suggests that 'global health' is more commonly used abroad. On the other hand, a search on *Ichushi* for the earlier period of 2008–2013 found 24 articles for 'global health' and 87 for 'international health'. Comparing the frequency of use of these terms over time, 'global health' is gaining popularity in Japan as well. Among university students from Japan, Chinese Taipei, and Fiji, a survey revealed a narrow definition of international health.[4] While 89% of Japanese medical students and 96% of nursing students responded 'helping developing countries', their counterparts from other countries responded predominantly 'provision of service for non-natives' and 'exchange of knowledge internationally'.

Public health is one of the core subjects taught in all schools of health sciences in Japan, and usually some lectures on international health or global health are included. Often lecturers are invited from other institutions, usually one of 14 postgraduate schools or departments of public health which has a subspecialty of international health or global health. As mentioned before, 'global health' and 'international health' are used interchangeably in Japan. For example, a textbook edited by the Japan Association for International Health has a Japanese title of *Kokusai Hoken Iryou Gaku*[5] (English translation: *Study of International Health*) with an English subtitle *Textbook of Global Health*. In fact, a section in the textbook was dedicated to discussing the difference between international health and global health. The writer, Dr Daisuke Nonaka, reviewed five definitions of global health by Brown (2006),[6] the UK Government (2008),[7] Institute of Medicine (2009),[8] Koplan (2009),[9] and the European Commission (2010),[10] and identified several elements that have different weights in these definitions. They are (1) targeting all countries (not only developing countries); (2) multiple actors including state actors and non-state actors such as civil society organizations; (3) issues including global problems that cannot be solved by one nation, social determinates of health, and mitigation of inequity among/within nations; (4) approaches including multisectoral approaches, health promotion and disease prevention, population and individual approaches, and an evidence-based approach. If one compares the Japanese perception of international health with the above-mentioned elements of global health, it is evident that the Japanese focus remains largely on developing countries. Efforts to expand the concept of international health to a wider global context are urgently required, if the sustainability of Japanese commitment to global health is not to be challenged.

16.2 Japan's Engagement with Global Health: Past and Present

16.2.1 Japan's Official Development Assistance

Japan's ODA budget was US$14.2 billion in 2018, making Japan the fourth largest donor country internationally and the largest in Asia.[11] This represents 0.28% of Japan's gross national income, of which health ODA accounted for about 5% of the total. This allocation is below the Development Assistance Committee (DAC) average of 8%, which ranks Japan in eighteenth place in relative terms and fifth place in absolute amount.

The Japanese position is weaker when one looks at the total volume of global health financing that includes not only government but also emerging private philanthropies and other sources such as the Bill and Melinda Gates Foundation. According to the Institute of Health Metrics and Evaluation, the total volume in 2018 is an estimated US$38.9 billion,[12] only 3% of which

(US$1.2 billion) comes from Japan. Further analysis of these data reveals that the Japanese resources are channelled mainly through the Global Fund (31.7%) and development banks (15.2%), while the amount channelled through non-governmental organizations (NGOs) and foundations is relatively small (5.3%).

The Japanese approach is very different from other major donors such as the US and the UK, where the NGOs and foundations receive the second largest share of ODA after their own official aid agencies. Therefore, financially speaking, Japanese global health resources are substantial but relatively modest in scope of resource allocation, focusing predominately on three major infections; HIV/AIDS, tuberculosis, and malaria. However, through hosting G7 summits, the scope of global engagement is expanding. Resources for health systems and universal health coverage (UHC) are channelled through the development banks and an ear-marked contribution to the WHO. Funding partnerships has begun, such as the Global Health Innovative Technology Fund (GHIT), Global Alliance for Vaccines and Immunizations (GAVI), UNITAID, Stop TB Partnership, and Coalition for Epidemic Preparedness Innovations (CEPI).

16.2.2 Historical Context

The present situation of relatively low ODA investment in health is partially related to the history of ODA in Japan and the emergence of Japan as a significant donor in the period after 1970 (Figure 16.1).

The evolution of Japanese health ODA has been reviewed by Kitaoka.[13] Japan joined the Colombo plan, an organization to promote economic development in the Asia-Pacific region, in 1954, when Japan was still recovering from the aftermath of World War II. After regaining sovereignty and ending the allied post-war occupation in 1951 by signing the San Francisco Peace Treaty, Japan needed to rebuild trust among Asian countries. The ODA was part of the package of war reparations. Therefore, the focus was Asia geographically, centering on reconstruction of infrastructure destroyed during the war and on industrial sectors as the engine for future growth. Often, aid was tied to Japanese trading and construction companies. As a result, there was little space for health, except hospital construction projects with some provision of technical advisors as follow-up of initial investment and receiving trainees.

Other characteristics of Japan's ODA until the 1990s[14] were (1) non-interventional but request-based assistance; (2) a greater focus on loans rather than grants (reflecting the 'self-help' spirit); (3) more projectized than

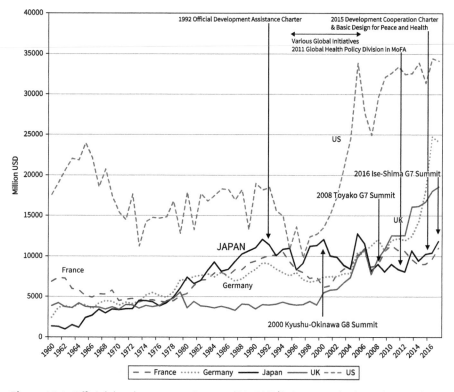

Figure 16.1 Official development assistance (2015 US$), Japan and selected countries, 1960–2016

Source: OECD (2016). Net ODA (1960-2016). https://data.oecd.org/oda/net-oda.htm. Accessed 5 September 2019.

programmatic aid; and (4) exclusive relationships with recipient governments and few collaborative initiatives with other donors and NGOs. As the volume of Japanese ODA grew, particularly after 1990 when Japan became the largest donor in volume, this inward-looking stance received heavy criticism from international development communities, depicting Japanese aid as an 'outlier'. Furthermore, Japan's inability to offer non-monetary support to international collaboration in the Gulf crisis triggered by Iraq's invasion of Kuwait in 1990 was perceived by Japanese leaders as a diplomatic defeat. It signified that allies saw Japan as a mercantilist and self-centred country.

These sentiments turned out to be a critical opportunity for Japan to review the philosophy of ODA. This led to development of Japan's ODA Charter in 1992, emphasizing its commitment to universal values such as democracy, the rule of law as a symbol of good governance, and the market economy. Such commitments were reiterated in the revised Charters of 2003 and 2015. Under the 2015 Charter, area- and region-specific action plans were developed.

In the case of health, Basic Design for Peace and Health (Global Health Cooperation)[15] was developed by the foreign ministry and approved by the Cabinet Office 'with a view to further contributing to global efforts to address health issues by fully mobilizing Japan's experience and expertise'. During the early stage of the development process, a supporting concept for the ODA Charter was sought. The proposed concept of 'human security'[16] was perceived as useful and was adopted as the backbone of the new ODA paradigm. Indeed, human security is defined in the UN General Assembly resolution 66/290, as 'an approach to assist the Member States in identifying and addressing widespread and cross-cutting challenges to the survival, livelihood, and dignity of their people'. And, it calls for 'people-centered, comprehensive, context-specific, and prevention-oriented responses that strengthen the protection and empowerment of all people'. This resolution was the prelude of the SDGs adopted by all UN member states in 2015. Japan sees that SDGs provide a shared blueprint for peace and prosperity for the people and the planet now and into the future, and a call for action by all countries—developed and developing—in a global partnership. They recognize that ending poverty and other deprivations must go hand-in-hand with strategies that improve health and education, reduce inequality, and spur economic growth. All these ideas resonate very well with the advocacy of the human security concept.

16.3 The Evolution of Global Health and Health Diplomacy in Japan

Despite the low level of interest in matters related to international health among the general public and mainstream healthcare professionals, as well as relatively modest resource allocation of ODA, Japan managed to present itself fairly well internationally in terms of global health activity. This section aims to discuss how several events have cumulated to advance Japanese commitment to global health.

In recent years, Japan has adopted its own ODA Charters that broadly define the scope and priority of ODA and allocate space for specific sectors to elaborate Japan's engagement strategy. After the first ODA Charter was adopted in 1992, the first commitment was the Global Issues Initiative on Population and AIDS in 1994, which pledged US$3 billion in seven years. This was succeeded by the Okinawa Infectious Diseases Initiative in 2000–2004 investing US$3 billion on three major infections (HIV/AIDS, TB, and malaria), parasitic diseases, and polio. This was followed by the Health and Development Initiative in 2005, pledging US$5 billion for 2005–2010, which emphasized

Japan's contribution to achieving health-related MDGs. These serial commitments were continued with the Global Health Policy 2011–2015 that invested US$5 billion to accelerate achievement of health MDGs.

During this period, Japanese initiatives evolved from vertical initiatives targeting specific health issues such as maternal and child health and infectious diseases, to more horizontal approaches such as health systems and health security, taking into account the concept of human security. The game changer appeared in 2013 when the Economic Cooperation Committee chaired by the Chief of Cabinet adopted a policy to includeglobal health as one of the pillars of Japanese foreign policy and to mainstream UHC on that agenda. Since then, UHC has become a flagship subject of Japanese health diplomacy. Prime Minister Abe and Finance Minister Aso contributed an article to the *Lancet* on this subject.[17,18]

These efforts supported and were in turn reinforced by the Japan-initiated health agendas in global meetings hosted by Japan, such as G7/8 summits and UN high-level meetings. For example, at the Kyushu-Okinawa G8 Summit held in 2000, leaders agreed to strengthen the response to HIV/AIDS, tuberculosis, and malaria, and to add numerical targets. In 2008, health system strengthening was included in the communique of the G8 Hokkaido Toyako Summit. Finally, at the G7 Iseshima Summit in 2016, the leaders agreed to strengthen support for global health, health emergencies, UHC, and antimicrobial resistance, and an immediate follow-up meeting was organized by Japan, the World Bank, the WHO, and others in 2017.

All these efforts have been coordinated by the Ministry of Foreign Affairs in collaboration with the Ministry of Health, Labour and Welfare, and the involvement and influence of new players have become visible. Since the 2008 Toyako Summit, a forum of NGOs has gained momentum and an information platform organized by the Japan Centre for Information Exchange[19] has been active.

Since 2013, when Abe was elected Prime Minister for the second time, economic revitalization has become a priority for his cabinet. The Headquarters of Health Care Policy[20] was established in the Cabinet Office with the aim to coordinate policies among relevant ministries. The characteristic of the headquarters is a combination of both domestic and international foci and is regarded as the first attempt to converge national and international health. Some critics argue that economic revitalization primarily motivates these efforts. The Japanese see the SDGs as another opportunity to engage with the world as well as to transform Japanese society in forthcoming years when greater international competition is expected. In 2016, the Cabinet established the 'SDGs Promotion Headquarters' to effectively achieve the SDGs. The Headquarters is headed by Prime Minister Abe to ensure a whole-government approach to implementing relevant policies domestically and internationally. Also, the Japan Business Federation (Keidanren) launched 'Toward the Realization of Society 5.0 for SDGs'[21] in November 2018.

16.3.1 From Millenium Development Goals to Sustainable Development Goals

Both millennium development goals (MDGs) and SDGs have been useful tools for Japanese health diplomacy. The MDGs were adopted in the declaration at the UN Millennium Summit in 2000. They consisted of eight goals with measurable targets and a 2015 deadline: (1) eradicate extreme poverty and hunger; (2) achieve universal primary education; (3) promote gender equality and empower women; (4) reduce child mortality; (5) improve maternal health; (6) combat HIV/AIDS, malaria, and other diseases; (7) ensure environmental sustainability; and (8) develop global partnerships.

The SDGs consist of 17 global goals set by the UN General Assembly in 2015, as a part of Resolution 70/1 'Transforming our world: the 2030 Agenda for Sustainable Development'. Briefly, the goals are (1) end poverty; (2) end hunger; (3) ensure healthy lives and wellbeing; (4) ensure education; (5) achieve gender equality; (6) ensure clean water and sanitation; (7) ensure affordable energy; (8) promote sustained economic growth and decent work; (9) build industry, innovation, and infrastructure; (10) reduce inequality; (11) make cities and communities sustainable; (12) ensure sustainable consumption and production; (13) combat climate change; (14) conserve marine resources; (15) protect life on land; (16) promote peace, justice, and strong institutions; (17) strengthen global partnerships for sustainable development. The terminology of MDGs and SDGs appears similar, but the fundamental concepts are quite different. A comparison of MDGs and SDGs is shown in Figure 16.2.

Under the MDGs, focused investment in health was carried out through new funding mechanisms such as the Global Fund, and this brought significant improvements in three focused areas of prevention and control: malaria, HIV/AIDS, and tuberculosis, which has contributed to improvement of child and maternal health. All these were included in the ten great global public health achievements for 2001–2010.[22] These achievements contributed to poverty reduction through a productive and healthier population and brought a healthier and wealthier world. Japan was gratified by the progress made by the MDGs, particularly in view of its own post-war experience and

	MDG	SDG
	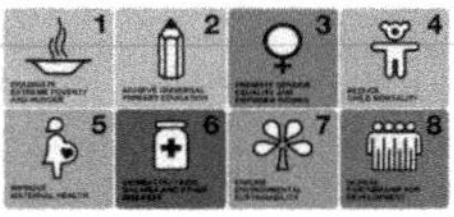	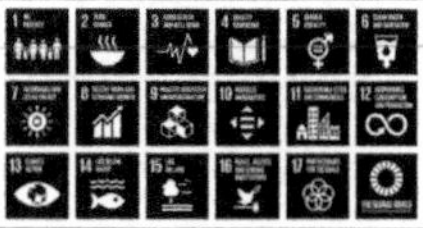
Years covered	**2000–2015**	**2016–2030**
Major Objective	Poverty Reduction	Sustainable Development
Goals & Targets	**8 Goals 18 Targets**	**17 Goals 169 Targets**
Priority Area in Health	MCH+Major Infections	Health in Life Course
Target Countries	Low Income Countries	All countries
Approach	Diseases Specific (Vertical) Realistic and Numerical Target Setting	Multisectoral Approach (Horizontal) Back-casting (Ambitious Target Setting)

Figure 16.2 Key facts comparison of Millennium Development Goals (MDGs) and Sustainable Development Goals (SDGs)

Source: Millennium Development Goals. Office of the Special Adviser on Africa. United Nations. https://www.un.org/en/africa/osaa/peace/mdgs.shtml

efforts to break the vicious cycle of poverty and ill health through heavy investment in communicable disease control, particularly in tuberculosis. Also, Japan felt proud that hosting the Kyushu-Okinawa Summit paved the way for massive and global investments in communicable diseases control worldwide.

Encouraged by such progress, Japan actively engaged in the formulation of SDGs, the next generation of global commitments, reflecting the geopolitical and situational changes after the success of its predecessor MDGs. However, the concepts of SDGs are quite different. The health challenges are wider than before. SDG3, which states 'ensure healthy lives and promote wellbeing for all at all ages', has 13 ambitious targets (nine specific and four cross-cutting). For example:

Target 3.8: 'achieve universal health coverage, including financial risk protection, access to quality essential healthcare services, and access to safe, effective, high quality, and affordable essential medicines and vaccines for all'; and

Target 3.b: 'support the research and development of vaccines and medicines for the communicable and non-communicable diseases that primarily affect developing countries, provide access to affordable essential medicines and vaccines, in accordance with the Doha Declaration on the TRIPS Agreement and Public Health, which affirms the right of developing countries to use to the full the provisions in the Agreement on Trade-Related Aspects of Intellectual Property Rights regarding flexibilities to protect public health, and, in particular, provide access to medicines for all'.

These targets call for research, and overall the SDGs urge a multisectoral approach. Reflecting these two points, many global strategies in the SDGs era make an optimistic assumption of R&D outcomes. For example, the WHO End TB Strategy[23] projects a 10% per year decline in global TB incidence rate by 2025 through optimal use of existing technologies, but an acceleration of the annual decline to 17% by 2035 through introduction of a vaccine, new drugs, treatment regimens, and point of care test for active and latent cases.

With regard to sectors that require a multisectoral approach, two typical examples in health would be non-communicable disease control, which is closely related to the social determinants of health, and lung cancer prevention, for which hefty tobacco tax is more powerful than cancer screening and treatment. All these concepts are compatible with the current Japanese political and business environment, which emphasizes R&D and society-wide approaches.

Commitment to SDGs encourages Japan to review its domestic challenges critically. For example, health inequalities were poorly recognized. The post-war, bipartisan political agenda was to generate and maintain a thick layer of the middle-class, and the idea of social gaps and their linkage with health conditions tended to be rejected. However, the long slump after the economic bubble crisis, together with globalization, diminished traditional life-long full-time employment, and blue-collar jobs were increasingly taken up by Asian neighbours. Also, there were significant changes in family structure and its value which had negative impacts on health.

Japan has a national health promotion strategy endorsed by the Cabinet since 1978, revised in 1988, and periodically updated. The third strategy 'Health Japan 21' was launched in 2000. The progress report released in 2011 showed that out of 59 targets, only 16.9% were accomplished, 42.4% showed some progress, 23.7% were unchanged, and 15.3% deteriorated. The Second Term of Health Japan 21[24] issued in 2012 has overarching objectives to improve healthy life expectancy and, for the first time, to narrow health gaps among prefectures (a difference in life expectancy of two years for men and 2.7 years for women). Other policies include prevention of onset and progression of non-communicable diseases, and maintaining physical/cognitive functions, taking into account the social determinants of health. SDGs are welcomed by Japanese public health communities as a useful platform to address the public health challenges in an ageing and rapidly changing society, domestically and internationally.

16.4 The Way Forward: New Mechanisms for Enhancing Research and Development and Human Resources

16.4.1 New Mechanisms

The discussion so far has reviewed the history and present situation of Japanese international commitments as well as challenges due to changing global issues and the landscape of international collaboration. All countries have been trying to respond to challenges and make a sustainable contribution to the health of their population as well as the rest of the world. Japan is no exception. In this section, several new mechanisms are discussed which reflect the underlying concept of convergence of domestic and international challenges, and characteristics including central coordination, promoting innovative R&D, and strengthening global health policy personnel. The ultimate goal is to realize a triple-win relationship for the world, country economy, and national interest.

The first mechanism is the Headquarters of Health Care Policy[25] as a part of the Act on Promotion of Healthcare Policy (2013) to advance R&D, promote the creation of new industries, and facilitate overseas expansion in healthcare, promote education, secure personnel working in cutting-edge healthcare, and enhance digitization and ICT use in health. This mechanism is chaired by Prime Minister Abe and has a strong coordination function across relevant ministries that used to work in silos. Role sharing by various ministries includes overall health policy under the Ministry of Health, Labour and Welfare (MHLW); R&D under the Ministry of Education, Culture, Sports, Science, and Technology (MEXT); health industries under the Ministry of Economy, Trade, and Industry (METI); health personnel under MHLW and MEXT; and digitalization under the Ministry of Internal Affairs and Communications. A major objective of the Headquarters is exploring and expanding overseas markets for Japanese healthcare and nursing care business, especially targeting the growing markets of middle-income countries in Asia.

16.4.2 Ageing, Health, and Wellbeing

In August 2019, Abe became the second longest serving prime minister in post-war Japan. His priority domestic policies are economic revitalization and active measures to address ageing and low birth rate. Moreover, he views these also from an international perspective, particularly focusing on Asia, where rapid ageing is progressing. Japan has relative advantages in this field, being the forerunner of population ageing in the world and possessing medical and healthcare technologies, products for promoting health and longevity, and a universal long-term care insurance system (Chapters 8 and 9). In this context, a typical example of the Headquarter work is the Asia Health and Wellbeing Initiative,[26] launched in 2016. The aim is to enhance international cooperation to meet the common challenges of ageing by (1) sharing Japanese experience (both positive and negative); (2) expanding services with the concept of UHC; (3) training care workers in Japan who will return home to serve their own ageing populations; and (4) R&D taking advantage of Japanese health services and products. The Cabinet Office coordinates this initiative across ministries. One development was to amend the Immigration Act in 2018 to increase the number of migrant care workers.

The second mechanism is the Global Health Innovative Technology (GHIT) Fund.[27] The Fund, the first Japan-initiated international partnership, was launched in 2013 to develop new medicines, vaccines, and diagnostics for neglected tropical diseases. As of 2018, GHIT has allocated US$170 million for 80 projects. R&D is focused on areas in which market mechanisms are inadequate. Those affected may be neglected populations in developing countries unable to afford drugs. Without GHIT support, industry lacks economic incentives. Another feature is financial partnership. Fifty percent of resources come from the Japanese foreign ministry and MHLW, and the remaining 50% from philanthropic organizations and industry. More specifically, 25% of the total is from the Bill and Melinda Gates Foundation and the Wellcome Trust, and the remaining 25% from pharmaceutical companies. This government to non-government contribution ratio is extremely high if one compares it with the ratio of the Global Fund. According to the pledges and contribution report of the Global Fund,[28] the government contribution from 2001 to 2019 is US$51 billion and the contribution from the private and non-governmental sectors is US$2.8 billion. The Board and team of the GHIT Fund are international, with the CEO and Vice-chair of the Board being non-Japanese nationals. This funding model had great impact on subsequent R&D mechanisms such as CEPI and the Light Fund of the Republic of Korea.

Third, the Human Resource Centre for Global Health (HRC-GH)[29] was commissioned by the MHLW to increase the number of Japanese nationals working in international organizations. HRC-GH was established at the recommendation of the MHLW Working Group on Human Resource Development in Global Health Policy, which reported in May 2016. The report pointed out the under-representation of Japanese nationals in international organizations; currently the Japanese occupy about 2% of senior positions in UN systems while Chinese and Korean representation is growing.

As a means to encourage Japanese nationals to take up international positions, the HRC-GH offers an information platform of vacant positions, organizes training workshops, advises on career development, and advocates appointments to international agencies.

16.5 Conclusion

Table 16.1 represents a summary of global health engagement in Japan.

Countries are divided into high-, middle-, and low-income groups, and types of engagement into services (including development aid), R&D, and policy development and coordination. The grey cells are traditional foci of international health for Japan. R&D is a new space rapidly being developed following the Act on Promotion of Healthcare Policy 2013. The three new mechanisms underlined in Table 16.1 occupy different cells and play unique roles. Furthermore, the Cabinet Office through the Headquarters of Health Care Policy has been active in coordination for a previously unaddressed area of the growing market in middle-income countries.

Table 16.1 Concept Model of Global Health Engagement in Japan.

	Services	R&D	Policy development and coordination
High-income countries	Private and academic sector engagements	Private and academic sectors, bilateral agreements with foreign countries	Headquarters of Health Care Policy/ Cabinet Office, MHLW, MoFA (OECD, G7/8 Summits)
Middle-income countries	In-bound/out-bound medicine provided by both public and private sectors coordinted by Medical Excellence Japan, Asia Health and Wellbeing Initiative	- Research grants from AMED - Participation of private companies in Access Accelerated Initiatives to improve access to medicine	Headquarters of Health Care Policy/ Cabinet Office, METI, MHLW, MoFA, MOF, (G20 Summit, ASEAN Summit), HRC-GH
Low-income countries	JICA, some NGOs, (implementation-oriented UN agencies such as UNICEF)	GHIT Fund	Headquarters of Health Care Policy/Cabinet Office, MHLW/WHO, MoFA, MOF/World Bank, HRC-GH

Grey cells = traditional activities. White cells = recent policy developments.

MHLW: Ministry of Health, Labour, and Welfare; MoFA: Ministry of Foreign Affairs; AMED: Japan Agency for Medical Research and Development; METI: Ministry of Economy, Trade, and Industry; MOF: Ministry of Finance; HRC-GH: Human Resource Centre for Global Health; JICA; Japan International Cooperation Agency; GHIT Fund: Global Health Innovative Technology Fund.

The Japanese commitment to global health is evolving and expanding. The current engagements depart from the traditional concept of international health addressing the under-served populations in low income countries. SDGs offer good opportunities for action. As described above, synergetic works coordinated by the Cabinet Office to achieve convergence of domestic and international health have begun. Such movement is echoed by a wide range of stakeholders including the government, NGOs/NPOs, experts, private sectors, international organizations, and domestic organizations. Synergetic efforts made by both public and private sectors have started to address both domestic and international health challenges. Sustainable Development Goals catalyse collective efforts toward sustainable development and surely will occupy a central position in future health agendas in Japan and beyond.

References

1. Cabinet Office, Government Of Japan. *Yoron Chosa* (in Japanese) (Opinion Poll Portal). Available at: https://survey.gov-online.go.jp/h30/h30-gaiko/2-2.html [last accessed 8 March 2020].
2. Ministry of Foreign Affairs. Financial year telephone survey report, March 2019 (in Japanese). Available at: https://www.mofa.go.jp/mofaj/files/000469693.pdf [last accessed 8 March 2020].
3. Ando N. Prospect of development assistance: Japan's opinion poll and burden sharing, March 2012 (in Japanese with English abstract). Available at: http://www.grips.ac.jp/r-center/wp-content/uploads/11-30.pdf [last accessed 8 March 2020].
4. Yoshimizu K, Kodama T, Oguri S, Fujimoto Y, Kanzaki N, Umezaki S, He BJ, Shinchi K. Images of international health and nursing in college students of Fiji, Japan and Taiwan. *Journal of International Health* 2011;26(1): 21–8.
5. Japan Association for International Health. *Kokusai Hoken Iryou Gaku* (*Textbook of Global Health*) Tokyo: Kyorin-shoin 2013.
6. Brown TM, Cueto M, Fee E. The World Health Organization and the transition from 'international' to 'global' public health. *Am J Public Health* 2006; 96:62–72.
7. HM Government. Health is global: a UK Government strategy 2008–2013. COI for the Department of Health 2008.
8. Institute of Medicine. The U.S. commitment to global health: recommendations for the public and private sectors. The National Academies Press 2009.
9. Koplan JP, Bond TC, Merson MH, et al. Towards a common definition of Global Health. *Lancet* 2009;373:1993–5.

10. The European Commission. Communication from the Commission to the council, the European parliament, the European economic and social committee and the committee of the regions: the EU role in global health, March 2010. Available at: http://aei.pitt.edu/id/eprint/37945 [last accessed 24 March 2020].

11. Donor Tracker. Supporting evidence -based advocacy for global development. Available at: https://donortracker.org/ [last accessed 8 March 2020].

12. Financing Global Health | Viz Hub. Institute for Health Metrics and Evaluation, University of Washington. Available at: https://vizhub.healthdata.org/fgh/ [last accessed 8 March 2020].

13. Kitaoka S. Sustainable development goals and Japan's official development assistance policy: human security, national interest, and a more proactive contribution to peace. *Asia-Pacific Review* 2016;23:32–41.

14. Menocal AR, Denney L. Informing the future of Japan's ODA part one: locating Japan's ODA within a crowded and shifting marketplace. Overseas Development Institute, JICA, July 2011. Available at: https://www.files.ethz.ch/isn/141036/7363.pdf [last accessed 8 March 2020].

15. The Cabinet Office, Government of Japan. Basic design for peace and health (Global Health Cooperation), 11 September 2015. Available at: https://www.mofa.go.jp/mofaj/files/000110234.pdf [last accessed 8 March 2020].

16. Commission on Human Security. Human security now: protecting and empowering people, New York 2003. Available at: https://reliefweb.int/sites/reliefweb.int/files/resources/91BAEEDBA50C6907C1256D19006A9353-chs-security-may03.pdf [last accessed 8 March 2020].

17. Abe S. Japan's vision for a peaceful and healthier world. *Lancet* 2015;386:2367–8.

18. Aso T. Crucial role of finance ministry in achieving universal health coverage. *Lancet* 2017;390:2415–17.

19. Japan Center for Information Exchange. Available at: http://www.jcie.or.jp/ [last accessed 8 March 2020].

20. Headquarters of Healthcare Policy, Cabinet Office. The healthcare policy and the new system of medical R&D. Available at: https://www.kantei.go.jp/jp/singi/kenkouiryou/en/pdf/doc1.pdf [last accessed 8 March 2020].

21. Japan Business Federation (Keidanren). Toward the realization of Society 5.0 for SDGs. Available at: https://www.keidanren.or.jp/en/speech/2019/0101.html [last accessed 24 March 2020].

22. Centers for Disease Control and Prevention: Ten great public health achievements — worldwide, 2001–2010. MMWR 2011;60(24):814–18. Available at: https://www.cdc.gov/mmwr/preview/mmwrhtml/mm6024a4.htm?s_cid=mm6024a4_w [last accessed 8 March 2020].

23. WHO. The End TB Strategy 2015. Available at: https://www.who.int/tb/strategy/End_TB_Strategy.pdf?ua=1 [last accessed 8 March 2020].

24. National Institute of Health and Nutrition. Health Japan 21 (the second term). Available at: http://www.nibiohn.go.jp/eiken/kenkounippon21/en/kenkounippon21/index.html [last accessed 8 March 2020].

25. Prime Minister of Japan and His Cabinet. Headquarters of Health Care Policy. Availale at: https://www.kantei.go.jp/jp/singi/kenkouiryou/en/ [last accessed 8 March 2020].

26. Headquarters for Healthcare Policy. Basic Principles of the Asia Health and Wellbeing Initiative. Available at: https://www.kantei.go.jp/jp/singi/kenkouiryou/en/pdf/2018_basic-principles.pdf [last accessed 8 March 2020].

27. Global Health Innovative Technology Fund. GHIT Fund: annual report 2018. Available at: https://www.ghitfund.org/assets/othermedia/GHIT_Fund_Annual_Report_2018_eng.pdf [last accessed 8 March 2020].

28. The Global Fund. Financials, 3 June 2019. Available at: https://www.theglobalfund.org/en/financials/ [last accessed 8 March 2020].

29. Human Resource Strategy Center for Global Health. Newsletter No. 0, October 2017. Available at: https://hrc-gh.ncgm.go.jp/files/uploads/newsletter_vol.0.pdf [last accessed 8 March 2020].

17

Geographic Disparities in Health

Tomoki Nakaya and Tomoya Hanibuchi

17.1 Introduction

Geographic disparities in health that are evident with worse population health in socially disadvantaged areas, have been widely observed at different geographic coverages and scales in different societies.[1] As well as resident's personal lack of resources, such as low income and assets, area-related environmental factors, such as poor access to community resources and increased stress related to unsafety or discrimination may explain the poor health of socioeconomically disadvantaged regions. Today there is a renewed interest in the environmental factors that hinder healthy living in residential spaces creating geographic health disparities.[2] For example, urban development creates public health challenges like unwalkable built environments or food deserts— areas in which purchasing fresh, healthy, and affordable food is made difficult due to the lack of supermarkets in the neighbourhood— as unintentional consequences. In short, where people live affects their health in multiple ways, and geographical disparities in health reflect the role of socially structured geographical environments in shaping population health.[1] Reducing such geographic disparities is part of public health promotions such as the Health Japan 21 (Secondary Term), which began in 2013.

It is important to note that disparities in health appear differently depending on the geographic scales/resolutions. With a population of 127.1 M in 2015, Japan is divided into 47 prefectures, i.e. large-scale administrative units with populations ranging from 13.4 M in Tokyo to 0.573 M in Tottori Prefecture. Each prefecture consists of smaller geographic units like municipalities (cities, towns, and villages) and neighbourhoods called *chocho-aza*. In the post-war period, Japan experienced rapid economic growth and improvements in sanitary environments through urbanization, particularly during the period of high economic growth from the mid-1950s to the early 1970s, which resulted in improved population health. While the water-supply system coverage rate was about 25% in 1950, it reached 90% in the late 1970s. The population

Tomoki Nakaya and Tomoya Hanibuchi, *Geographic Disparities in Health* In: *Health in Japan*. Edited by: Eric Brunner, Noriko Cable, and Hiroyasu Iso, Oxford University Press (2021). © Oxford University Press. DOI: 10.1093/oso/9780198848134.003.0017.

living in urbanized areas, which are called Densely Inhabited Districts in the Japanese census, increased from 43.7% in 1960 to 57.0% in 1975 and 68.3% in 2015. During the high growth period, geographical differences in living standards changed a great deal to become more equal, accompanied by massive rural to urban migration at the prefecture level. At the same time, as the metropolitan areas greatly expanded in terms of population size, socially segmented areas emerged with varying population health at the neighbourhood level inside the metropolitan areas.

This chapter highlights the geographical aspects of health disparities in Japan at different levels, beginning with (1) disparities in life expectancy in the post-World-War-II period in the 47 national prefectures, (2) health disparities among socioeconomically segregated neighbourhoods within metropolitan areas, (3) discussion on the factors that may have given rise to such relationships between Japanese neighbourhoods and health impacts, and (4) the challenges in tackling health disparities across all social levels in the era of a super-ageing society with the threat of re-widening social inequalities.

17.2 Reduced Prefectural Disparities in Life Expectancy

Persisting geographic health disparities have been observed in many countries. For example, in England and Wales (E&W), despite the drastic reduction in mortality throughout the twentieth century, the north-south divide—with northern areas more socioeconomically deprived and having higher mortality rates compared to southern areas, which were more affluent and had low mortality rates—has been firmly grounded for over a century, at least into the 2000s.[3] Unlike the history of E&W, Japan, another island developed country, has experienced more drastic changes in the geographic patterns of health disparities. This section summarizes the transformation of geographic health disparities after World War II at the level of 47 prefectures.

Figure 17.1 shows the trends in the prefectural-based gaps in per capita income and net in-migration to three major metropolitan areas—Tokyo, Nagoya, and Osaka—from 1955 to 2015 in the top box (a), and demonstrates the gaps in life expectancy (LE) per prefecture and the rankings of Tokyo and Osaka's LEs. Coefficients of variation (CV), defined as the standard deviation divided by the average, are used as a measure of prefectural income gaps. A larger CV means a larger variation of LE among prefectures. Distribution during the high economic growth period (mid-1950s–early 1970s) shows a sharp decline in the mortality rate in the country, demonstrating a clear

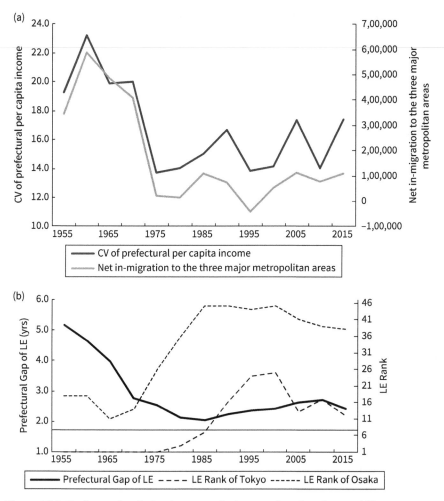

Figure 17.1 Prefectural variation in per-capita income, in-migration, and life expectancy at birth, Japan, 1955–2015

(a) Coefficient of variation (CV) of prefectural per capita income and net migration to the three major metropolitan areas (persons).

(b) Maximum difference of prefectural life expectancies at birth (LE), and LE ranks of Tokyo and Osaka prefectures.

Source: Annual Reports of Prefectural Accounts (Cabinet Office), for prefectural per capita income; Report on Internal Migration in Japan (Ministry of Internal Affairs and Communications), for the migration data based on basic resident registration information; Shigematsu, T. et al. (1996), Shinban Mizushima todofukenbetsu seimeihyo, Public Health Department at Fukuoka University, for the data on life expectancies of 1954-56 and 1959-1961, Prefectural Life Tables (Ministry of Health, Labour, and Welfare), for the data on life expectancies from 1965-2015.

core-peripheral pattern of LE that corresponds to regional economic/income levels. The populations of the metropolitan areas with the highest income per capita also enjoy the longest lives. The LE of Tokyo in 1965 is the longest among the prefectures for both sexes. Overall, the industrialized areas called the *Taiheiyo-belt* (Pacific belt), stretching from Tokyo through Aichi, Osaka, and Hiroshima to the Fukuoka Prefecture by connecting rapid transportation networks, also attained better health, reflecting regional economic growth.

During the early phase of the high-growth period, the gap in income levels between metropolitan and non-metropolitan areas widened significantly, after which large-scale population movements occurred from non-metropolitan areas to metropolitan areas, reducing the economic gap.[4] The direction of the migration toward metropolitan areas was also to 'move to a healthy place' at the time. A study estimated regional disparities in health caused by differences in the average income level of prefectures and examined its temporal trend from 1955 to 2000.[5] It found that the socioeconomic disparity in LE among the prefectures decreased substantially during the period from the 1960s to the early 1970s.

As the income gap between metropolitan and non-metropolitan areas has shrunk and the population movement towards large metropolitan areas has also subsided, it is no longer possible to find a clear health gap between metropolitan and non-metropolitan areas at the prefectural level after the 1990s.

The absolute difference of LE is substantially diminished at the prefectural level. While the gap between the longest and shortest prefectural LE was 5.37 years for men and 5.13 years for women around 1955, they are recorded at 3.11 years for men and 1.74 years for women in 2015. While the sex-averaged LE of Tokyo in 2015 was 84.2 years (81.1 years for men and 87.3 years for women), which is ranked twelfth, Osaka is ranked thirty-eighth among the 46 prefectures excluding Okinawa. It should be noted that statistics from Okinawa are not available for the years 1955 to 1970. While Okinawa has been economically one of the least developed prefectures, the region used to be well known as 'longevity place'. When Okinawa was included for the prefectural comparison of LEs, the ranking of LE in Okinawa was first among the 47 prefectures for both sexes in 1985 but dropped to thirty-sixth for men and seventh for women in 2015. The Okinawan mystery—least developed but longevity place— is no longer observed for men (Chapter 19).

The Japanese egalitarian system of social welfare which was introduced before World War II, including compulsory primary education, a social insurance system, and the universal health insurance established in 1961, may have promoted regional equalization of health.[6] Further, to reduce income disparities across prefectures, the national government adopted a financial adjustment policy to assist local governmental revenue. This has helped to reduce regional disparities in living standards and public health resources, thereby contributing to the reduction of geographical disparities in health levels.[7] In addition, the Comprehensive National Development Plans and related acts tried to reduce regional economic inequalities by lessening overcrowding in metropolitan areas and promoting the development of industries outside existing metropolitan areas. An international comparison of regional socio-economic disparities in mortality between Japan and E&W showed that the degree of disparity was much smaller in Japan than in E&W around 1990.[8]

However, this regional equalization trend in Japan has been obscured since the latter half of the 1990s. Some argue that in recent decades, the health disparity between regions has been gradually widening, in line with the widening trends of socioeconomic disparities in society.[5,9]

In sum, the decrease in geographical inequalities in LE was accompanied by a significant extension of LE from the high-growth period that began in the mid-1950s until the mid-1990s. This was a great achievement for improvements in the health of the Japanese population in the post-war period, indicating that national strategies to equalize the regional financial imbalance of local governments as well as their economic activities were beneficial in reducing regional health disparities and creating better conditions for the health of the general population of the entire country. However, we need to exercise some caution owing to the recent trend of regional polarization in Japan.

17.3 Socioeconomic Segregation and Health Disparities in Metropolitan Areas

17.3.1 Looking through a Cartogram Lense

In response to the reduction in economic disparities between major metropolitan and non-major metropolitan areas, health disparities on the spatial scale of prefectures have been largely diminished in the long-term. However, as a result of large-scale migration towards metropolitan areas from rural areas throughout the high-growth period, the population of the three major metropolitan areas reached 51.8% in 2015 in terms of the population nationally, and continues to increase, particularly in the Tokyo metropolitan area. There are then large populations with different demographic and socioeconomic characteristics, depending on their locations within the metropolitan areas.

To see more detailed geographic disparities in health, the municipality distribution of male LE as of 2015 was displayed by using conventional (Figure 17.2a), and alternative projections (population cartogram) which scaled the areas up or down according to their population size (Figure 17.2b). The conventional-style map showed that regional differences of LE are large between non-metropolitan prefectures. For example, areas with shorter LE

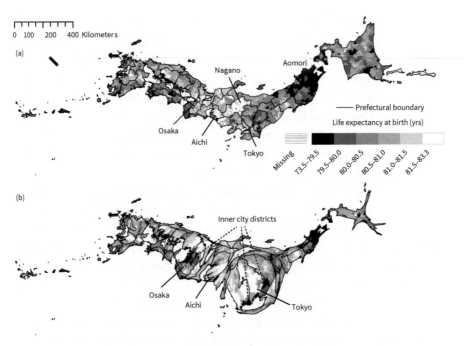

Figure 17.2 Municipal distribution of life expectancy at birth in 2010
(a) Distribution based on traditional map projection.
(b) Distribution based on population cartogram.
Source: 2010 Municipal Life Tables, Ministry of Health, Labour, and Welfare

are distributed in the northern part of the main island, such as the Aomori Prefecture, and areas with longer LE are distributed mainly in the central part of the main island, such as the Nagano Prefecture. However, although municipalities with low population densities may have a large area size affecting the visual impression on the distribution map, their existence is overemphasized because they include mountains and rural areas with significantly smaller populations. On the other hand, in the LE distribution map by cartogram, the Tokyo, Aichi, and Osaka Prefectures, which are densely populated metropolitan core regions, are greatly expanded, and the large disparities in health hidden in them becomes apparent.[10]

The most obvious feature of this cartogram-based map is the magnitude of health disparities within the metropolitan area. The eastern and coastal areas of Tokyo and the central part of Osaka are highlighted as areas with a shorter LE (dark colour) while the surrounding suburbs are coloured in white indicating the longest LE. Note that on the cartogram, the size of an areal unit on the map corresponds to the size of the population. Thus, enlarged areas of dark and white coloured regions within the metropolitan areas suggest that there are both large sized healthy and unhealthy residential populations within the areas. Their population size can be larger than a rural prefecture, such as the Nagano Prefecture.

17.3.2 Association of Health Disparities with Socioeconomic Segregation

These geographical disparities in health within metropolitan areas correspond well with socioeconomic differences in residential areas, which feature contrasts between affluent uptown and the relatively deprived inner-city districts. Such differentiation of residents based on their socioeconomic attributes is called socioeconomic segregation within a metropolitan area and has been observed in major Japanese metropolitan areas,[11–12] particularly at small area levels, such as neighbourhoods.

How then have health disparities associated with socioeconomic segregation formed within metropolitan areas? Domestic migrants into metropolitan areas during the high-growth period began to flow into the centre of metropolitan areas, where employment and school opportunities were concentrated, and then migrated to the suburbs in search of better living environments after getting married and having children. In addition, the remoteness of land developed for housing in large metropolitan areas advanced rapidly in response to the surge in housing prices, which was itself a response to the increase in office demand in central Tokyo and Osaka, which occurred during the bubble economy of the 1980s. As a result, households with relatively high incomes moved to outer wards, and the suburban areas with good health levels (longer LE) expanded extensively within the metropolitan area. On the other hand, areas with low health levels tend to be localized in the outermost edges of metropolitan areas, and in the inner-city regions near metropolitan centres where relatively deprived people live.[13]

To associate such socioeconomic characteristics of residential areas with health outcomes, area deprivation indices (ADI) are often used in many countries to measure area-level poverty by using census indicators.[1,14] Figures 17.3a and b show the distribution of all-cause mortality measured by standard mortality ratio (SMR) and ADI at the level of small areas, or neighbourhoods (*chocho-aza*), in the Osaka Prefecture. High ADI areas—socioeconomically disadvantaged/deprived neighbourhoods—are distributed in the central part of the Osaka Prefecture in a ring-shape surrounding the city centre, and in such deprived areas there is a tendency for the mortality ratios to be high.[10]

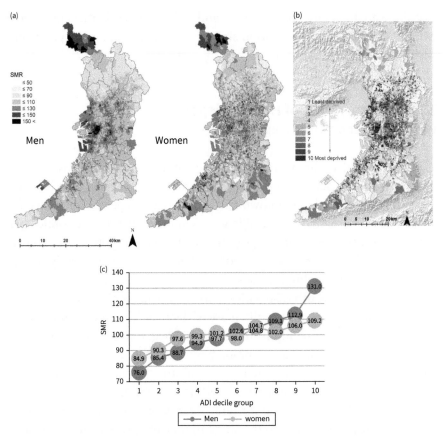

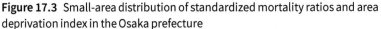

Figure 17.3 Small-area distribution of standardized mortality ratios and area deprivation index in the Osaka prefecture

(a) Distribution of standardized mortality ratios.

(b) Distribution of area deprivation index (ADI).

(c) Standardized mortality ratios by ten decide groups of ADI.

Source: Nakaya, T. and Ito, Y. The Atlas of Health Inequalities in Japan, Springer. 2019.

Figure 17.3c indicates that there is a clear gradient in mortality along the area deprivation, particularly for men as compared to women. The SMRs in the most deprived decile group in the least deprived segments are about 1.72 times higher for men and 1.29 times higher for women as compared to those in the most deprived areas, respectively. Another study showed that the survival rates of cancer patients tended to be lower in higher ADI groups of small areas[15] (see Chapter 12).

Another study linking a social area typology of residential composition, called 'geodemographics', to the nationwide social survey data reported distinctive differences in self-rated health and health behaviours among different neighbourhood types.[16] Such social area classification was originally conducted in the fields of urban sociology and geography by grouping small areas that have similar demographic and socioeconomic attributes of residents from small area indices, such as occupation, housing, and family composition, by utilizing cluster analyses.[17] The study shows that while the most affluent residential neighbourhood type, 'Corporate Success', distributed mainly in metropolitan suburbs, not only has the highest income levels, but also the lowest rate of poor self-rated health (14%), a higher percentage of social participation (37%), a high rate of regular exercise habits (46%), and the lowest smoking rate (27%).[16] By contrast, the low-income 'Social Housing' neighbourhood type showed the highest percentage of the poor self-rated health (23%) as well as a low rate of social participation (25%) indicating social isolation, a low rate of regular exercise habits (19%), and the highest smoking rate (40%).

In summary, these studies indicated that the socioeconomic segregation of residential areas is closely associated with the health and health-related behaviours of their residents. This is observable even in Japanese society with its egalitarian nature and more socioeconomically mixed residential structure in comparison with Western societies.[11]

17.4 Environmental Factors that Create Neighbourhood-scale Health Disparities

Several studies have pointed out the area-level factors affecting health in the context of Japanese neighbourhoods. These include place-based discrimination, built environments of urban design and food deserts, some of which are strongly related to socioeconomic segregation and the development histories of the metropolitan areas described above.

A study highlighted an aspect of the social environment of deprived inner-city neighbourhoods in Osaka City where residents faced discrimination based on their place of residence that affected their health.[18] The study revealed that the experience of such discrimination was strongly associated with poor self-rated health. In addition, the higher the proportion of residents who experienced place-based discrimination, the poorer the self-rated health of residents, even after adjusting for individuals' experience of such discrimination. Such place-based discrimination occurs partly because of people's perceptions of the supposed unsanitary or unsafe conditions of deprived areas, particularly for areas with high concentrations of day-labourers and homeless people, such as in Nishinari Ward, Osaka City. At the same time, such discrimination is related to *Buraku* discrimination, which is a long-persisting discrimination against perceived out-caste people, historically originating in pre-modern society. There remain many *Buraku* districts in Osaka. Irrespective of the different reasons for discrimination, neighbourhoods with a high percentage of place-based discrimination correspond to highly deprived areas. It was thus considered that in areas with deprived neighbourhoods, even if the residents were not conscious of it, they were susceptible to disadvantage and psychological stress from socially embedded discrimination. Although the study highlighted a specific case of place-based discrimination rooted in the history of Japan, other forms of the relationship between social environments and residential health may be widely observed. For example, there are reports that cooperative neighbourhood social environments are likely to promote better residential health because of the effects of social capital on health.[19]

Built environments of residential areas can also affect resident's health. Access to parks is argued to be unequally distributed among neighbourhoods depending on their socioeconomic level. A longitudinal survey on environmental equity in park access in Yokohama City[20] indicated that in areas where more people of higher socioeconomic status live, there are both more and larger parks available, with more new parks being constructed in those neighbourhoods. This study suggests the possibility that people living in affluent neighbourhoods are more likely to have the ability to change the living conditions of their neighbourhoods which have more desirable environmental characteristics. Importantly, access to parks and green spaces has been found to be associated with a variety of health benefits, such as increased opportunities for physical activity and social interaction.[21]

As well as parks, living in neighbourhoods with good access to facilities for daily activities, such as shopping or commuting, are considered to contribute to health by increasing physical activity, i.e. walking. Walkable environments are characterized by high density, mixed land-use, and well connected pedestrian-friendly road networks. The relationship between the individual elements of walkable environments and walking or physical activity are commonly observed in many aspects in both Japan and Western societies,[22] but the major difference lies in the exposed environment. In the US, suburban areas are considered as unwalkable environments with low density, single-purpose land-use, and car-oriented road networks, contributing to the obesity epidemic in the country.[23] On the other hand, the suburbs of large metropolitan areas in Japan are more densely inhabited compared to the 'motorized'

US major cities, with well developed public transportation and more mixed land-use under weak land-use regulations.[24] Suburban development by railroad companies may have contributed to the expansion of metropolitan areas while maintaining high residential density and the availability of public transportation. Low crime rates in Japan may also contribute to more people walking outside (see Chapter 13).

Access to daily food supplies may be another built-environment characteristic related to geographic disparities in health, particularly in the countries like the US where food deserts are often associated with urban poverty concentrations and are another cause of the obesity epidemic.[23] On the contrary, better access to supermarkets is associated with the probability of being overweight for Japanese elderly.[25] Considering this, in Japan, being underweight, rather than overweight, is associated with a higher risk of mortality.[26] Namely, a poor diet relating to being underweight, associated with poor food access, could be more important in considering the food environmental effects in Japan.[27] Although, in general, food deserts are serious for mobility-impaired elderly persons (people without cars) living in Japanese rural or metropolitan fringe areas where many local stores were closed due to depopulation and the ageing of local populations, it has become a concern even in metropolitan areas, particularly for elderly residents who are socially isolated.[28] According to a recent nationwide survey conducted by the Ministry of Economy, Trade, and Industry in 2010, 17.1% of the elderly aged 60 or older felt some difficulty in shopping for their daily needs, and approximately 7 M elderly throughout Japan may suffer from the problem of limited access to shopping facilities. Due to the country's rapid ageing population, the number is estimated to keep rising.

17.5 Challenges

As discussed in this chapter, geographical health disparities exist at multiple levels, from nationwide disparities between metropolitan/urban and non-metropolitan/rural areas to local disparities between urban centres and suburbs within metropolitan areas. In the era of the threat of re-widening social inequalities and a super-ageing society, it is important to consider the issues of health disparities and challenges in building health-supportive environments in each geographical setting.

In the centres of major metropolitan areas such as Tokyo and Osaka, population re-centralization has occurred since the late 1990s with the rise in income levels of the new residents in central Tokyo, a process known as gentrification. Urban geographers have also become concerned about widening socio-spatial income gaps, or polarization under globalization, which has occurred in central urban areas.[29] As introduced by the relative income hypothesis, a large social disparity between rich and poor could deteriorate residents' health by causing a great deal of chronic stress and a weakening of social cohesion.[30] In addition to the widening disparities between metropolitan and non-metropolitan areas, those within metropolitan areas may have widening health concerns in different neighbourhoods in major Japanese cities.

Suburbs of large metropolitan areas, which once achieved good health levels, are now facing serious environmental challenges. When Japanese metropolitan areas rapidly expanded through an influx of young migrants, and because of the scarcity of undeveloped open lands, housing developments on hilly lands have been carried out since the 1960s to solve the housing shortage problem. Such hill development used slopes, steps, and stairs, which make the neighbourhoods unwalkable for older residents. The large number of residents who moved to the suburbs are mostly of the baby-boomer generation, now retired, while many of their children have moved out to urban centres. This rapid declining and ageing population, together with decreasing income levels, has caused a shrinkage of stores including supermarkets and has turned some places into food deserts. The problem underscores the importance of considering the long-term effects of land development and city planning on sustaining healthy lives in residential areas.

In non-metropolitan regions, including rural areas, population decline and ageing are continuing and will gradually worsen both the built and social environments in relation to health. For example, many rural settlements face a lack of social infrastructure, including hospitals and supermarkets, making medical care and healthy food inaccessible to local residents. The deterioration of the urban centre in small- and middle-sized cities has been prevalent in non-metropolitan areas. In particular, the decay of the shopping centre district, which was triggered by the easing of regulations for large-scale retail stores in the 1990s, has caused a geographical dispersion of commercial functions, which resulted in a more car-oriented society in non-metropolitan areas. Currently, unwalkable spaces are expanding further in non-metropolitan regions because of the decline in both residential density and accessibility to destinations, which may contribute to regional disparities in health between metropolitan and non-metropolitan areas. It is vital for policymakers to support residents' access to health-supportive resources, including healthy food (delivery or mobile catering) and environments enabling physical activity, as well as healthcare services, to promote successful ageing.

17.6 Conclusions

As Japan has attained the longest longevity rates in the world, the country has successfully reduced geographical gaps in longevity at the larger geographic level through area socioeconomic equalization via national policies and migration. However, at the smaller geographic level, Japanese metropolitan areas now have more salient health disparities associated with the socioeconomic segregation of residential places. A number of environmental characteristics of Japanese neighbourhoods, including social discrimination, access to community resources, walkable built environments, and food deserts are associated with neighbourhood-scale disparities in health in different geographical settings. In the era of a super-ageing society that contains the threat of re-widening social inequalities, Japan faces challenges to build health-supportive environments for tackling multiscale disparities.

Importantly, the ways to tackle disparities at different levels are not independent of each other. For instance, national strategies to equalize the regional financial balances of local governments may be necessary for building health-supportive environments at the local level in less developed areas to reduce health disparities. At the same time, urban planning concepts such as smart shrinking or compact city policies, restricting further city expansion and maintaining public services, have become increasingly important for public health policies, since a population decline is inevitable in most areas. Prioritizing such planning actions may contribute to reducing broader regional health disparities between large cities and small towns. Thus, it is insufficient to focus on the associations between neighbourhood and health in specific areas when considering possible options for improving or sustaining population health. Rather, we need to consider the problems and policies at multiple levels and in different geographical settings simultaneously.

Acknowledgements

TN and TH have been supported by the JSPS KAKENHI (#JP15H02964, #JP20H00040) and the JSPS KAKENHI (#JP17H00947) respectively.

References

1. Kawachi I, Berkman LF. *Neighborhoods and Health*. Oxford: Oxford University Press 2003.
2. Roux AVD, Mair C. Neighborhoods and health. *Ann N Y Acad Sci* 2010;1186(1):125–45.
3. Gregory IN. Comparisons between geographies of mortality and deprivation from the 1900s and 2001: spatial analysis of census and mortality statistics. *BMJ* 2009;339:b3454.
4. Tabuchi T. Interregional income differentials and migration: their interrelationships. *Reg Stud* 1988;22(1):1–10.
5. Fukuda Y, Nakao H, Yahata Y, Imai H. Are health inequalities increasing in Japan? The trends of 1955 to 2000. *Biosci Trends* 2007;1(1):38–42.
6. Ikeda N, Saito E, Kondo N, Inoue M, Ikeda S, Satoh T, et al. What has made the population of Japan healthy? *Lancet* 2011;378(9796):1094–105.
7. Takano T, Nakamura K. The national financial adjustment policy and the equalisation of health levels among prefectures. *J Epidemiol Community Health* 2001;55(10):748–54.
8. Nakaya T, Dorling D. Geographical inequalities of mortality by income in two developed island countries: a cross-national comparison of Britain and Japan. *Soc Sci Med* 2005;60(12):2865–75.
9. Nomura S, Sakamoto H, Glenn S, Tsugawa Y, Abe SK, Rahman MM, et al. Population health and regional variations of disease burden in Japan, 1990–2015: a systematic subnational analysis for the Global Burden of Disease Study 2015. *Lancet* 2017;390(10101):1521–38.
10. Nakaya T, Ito, Y (eds.). *The Atlas of Health Inequalities in Japan*. Dordrecht: Springer 2019.
11. Fielding T. Social class segregation in Japanese cities: the case of Kyoto 2003. *Transactions of the Institute of British Geographers, New Series* 2004;29(1):64–84.
12. Kurasawa S, Asakawa T (eds.). *New Social Atlas of Metropolitan Tokyo: 1975–90*. Tokyo: University of Tokyo Press 2004.
13. Nakaya T. An information statistical approach to the modifiable areal unit problem in incidence rate maps. *Environ Plan A* 2000;32(1):91–109.
14. Nakaya T, Honjo K, Hanibuchi T, Ikeda A, Iso H, Inoue M, et al. Associations of all-cause mortality with census-based neighbourhood deprivation and population density in Japan: a multilevel survival analysis. *PloS One* 2014;9(6):e97802.

15. Ito Y, Nakaya T, Nakayama T, Miyashiro I, Ioka A, Tsukuma H, et al. Socioeconomic inequalities in cancer survival: a population-based study of adult patients diagnosed in Osaka, Japan, during the period 1993–2004. *Acta Oncol* 2014;53(10):1423–33.

16. Nakaya T, Hanibuchi T. Neighbourhood inequalities in health and income in Japan. *Annals of the Japan Association of Economic Geographers* 2013;59(1):57–72.

17. Harris R, Sleight P, Webber R. *Geodemographics, GIS and Neighbourhood Targeting*. West Sussex: John Wiley & Sons 2005.

18. Tabuchi T, Nakaya T, Fukushima W, Matsunaga I, Ohfuji S, Kondo K, et al. Individualized and institutionalized residential place-based discrimination and self-rated health: a cross-sectional study of the working-age general population in Osaka city, Japan. *BMC Public Health* 2014;14(1):449.

19. Ichida Y, Kondo K, Hirai H, Hanibuchi T, Yoshikawa G, Murata C. Social capital, income inequality and self-rated health in Chita peninsula, Japan: a multilevel analysis of older people in 25 communities. *Soc Sci Med* 2009;69(4):489–99.

20. Yasumoto S, Jones A, Shimizu C. Longitudinal trends in equity of park accessibility in Yokohama, Japan: an investigation into the role of causal mechanisms. *Environ Plan A* 2014;46(3):682–99.

21. Takano T, Nakamura K, Watanabe M. Urban residential environments and senior citizens' longevity in megacity areas: the importance of walkable green spaces. *J Epidemiol Community Health* 2002;56(12):913–18.

22. Inoue S, Ohya Y, Odagiri Y, Takamiya T, Kamada M, Okada S, et al. Perceived neighborhood environment and walking for specific purposes among elderly Japanese. *J Epidemiol* 2011;21(6):481–90.

23. Pearce J, Witten K (eds.). *Geographies of Obesity: Environmental Understandings of the Obesity Epidemic*. London: Routledge 2016.

24. Sorensen A. *The Making of Urban Japan: Cities and Planning from Edo to the Twenty-first Century*. London: Routledge 2005.

25. Hanibuchi T, Kondo K, Nakaya T, Nakade M, Ojima T, Hirai H, et al. Neighborhood food environment and body mass index among Japanese older adults: results from the Aichi Gerontological Evaluation Study (AGES). *Int J Health Geogr* 2011;10(1):43.

26. Inoue M, Sobue T, Tsugane S. Impact of body mass index on the risk of total cancer incidence and mortality among middle-aged Japanese: data from a large-scale population-based cohort study–the JPHC study. *Cancer Causes Control* 2004;15(7):671–80.

27. Nakamura H, Nakamura M, Okada E, Ojima T, Kondo K. Association of food access and neighbor relationships with diet and underweight among community-dwelling older Japanese. *J Epidemiol* 2017;27(11):546–51.

28. Iwama N. Daitoshi-kogai niokeru fudodezato-mondai no genjyo to kadai (Current situations and challenges of the food desert problem in metropolitan suburbs). *Operations Research* 2012;57(3):112–18.

29. Toyoda T. Spatial structure of income inequality in metropolitan cities: a comparative analysis of Tokyo and Osaka. *Nihon Toshigakkai Nenpou (Annals of the Japanese Association of Urban Studies)* 2011;44:219–26.

30. Wilkinson R, Pickett K. *The Spirit Level*. London: Allen Lane 2009.

18

Disaster and Health

What Makes a Country Resilient?

Naoki Kondo and Jun Aida

18.1 Introduction

Like many countries in East Asia, Japan is a showcase of natural disasters, where every year ten typhoons or more hit every corner of the land, causing serious flooding and landslides. Thousands of earthquakes happen every year. In 2018, Japan experienced 2,179 quakes, including 11 strong quakes, with intensity level five or more on the Japanese earthquake scale.[1] The Japanese islands have 111 active volcanos,[2] and a total of 488 people have died or disappeared due to volcanic eruptions since 1900. The 2011 Great East Japan Earthquake, the biggest in Japan's history, resulted in 18,446 dead or missing, mainly from the tsunami after the quake, and a further 3,701 deaths from other earthquake-related causes.[3] The Great Hanshin-Awaji Earthquake of 1995 killed 6,437 people,[4] most of them due to the collapse of their homes.[5]

Disasters are not necessarily caused by nature; they can also be caused by humans. Violent conflicts are typical and terrible human-made disasters. The Japanese Constitution bans war, and most people have been treasuring long-standing peace since the end of World War II. However, the impact on human health of another type of man-made crisis also needs to be seriously considered: economic crisis. Since the end of World War II, Japan has repeatedly experienced economic crises: in 1973 ('the oil shock'), 1997 (Asian Financial Crisis), and 2008 (Global Financial Crisis). Japan has also experienced a lingering economic downturn since the late 1980s, termed 'the lost decades' and triggered by the bursting of the 'bubble economy' (see Chapter 1.5 and Chapter 6.1).

Resilience is a key concept in considering the impacts of these disasters on people's lives. Resilience reflects the capability of individuals and social groups of all kinds to resist, cope with, continue functioning in, and recover

Naoki Kondo and Jun Aida, *Disaster and Health* In: *Health in Japan*. Edited by: Eric Brunner, Noriko Cable, and Hiroyasu Iso, Oxford University Press (2021). © Oxford University Press. DOI: 10.1093/oso/9780198848134.003.0018.

from a disaster.[6] The concept of resilience is applicable to all parts of society—individual, family, organizations, and community.[7] Understanding the factors that determine the resilience of communities should be an important topic for public health, because of its implications for building a resilient social environment in which people can survive and maintain their health throughout disasters. Moreover, because resource scarcity after a disaster in the community has a greater impact on those with existing socioeconomic difficulties, community resilience is associated with health inequality across communities and individuals under various socioeconomic statuses in disaster settings.

Many resources can determine community resilience that include strong infrastructure or well-built physical environments, a vigorous economy, and effective governmental policies.[8] To make countries resilient, governments invest to strengthen infrastructure, such as building strong levees. However, these government-supplied resources are not sufficient. For example, when a natural disaster happens, in the immediate aftermath, we need to help each other before the arrival of governmental support to survive. Even after formal disaster-relieving support becomes available for the recovery process, those formal supports may not be enough. As described later in this chapter, many epidemiological studies point to the importance of social capital and the structural and cultural aspects of society that foster social capital.

In this chapter, we present findings from recent epidemiological studies relevant to disaster resilience in Japan, and we discuss the roles of social and cultural factors, such as social capital, in disaster resilience.[6,9-11] We also take a deeper look at trends in health inequality during periods of disaster. When a disaster happens, some societies can recover with relatively low levels of health inequality, but others, less so. A good understanding of the impacts of those societal characteristics on population health and inequality should contribute to building a resilient society. In this chapter, we focus on recent natural and human-made disasters in the last 30 years in Japan, including two mega-earthquakes: the 2011 Great East Japan earthquake and the 2015 Kumamoto Earthquake; and two economic crises: the 1997 Asian Financial Crisis and the 2008 Global Financial Crisis.

As stated in Chapter 1, the general health status of the Japanese has continuously improved despite the occurrence of these macroeconomic hardships and natural disasters. So, we can say that Japanese society is resilient in general. Nonetheless, when looking into health inequality, or the health gaps across subpopulations, we can describe more detailed and interesting pictures. Hence, we introduce relevant evidence on how population health and its inequality changed during and after these disasters. Then we discuss what lessons can be drawn from those experiences to make our society more resilient.

18.2 Population Health in Natural Mega-disasters: Evidence from the 2011 Great East Japan Earthquake and Tsunami

Natural disasters occur suddenly and change physical and social environments. Disasters such as earthquakes, tsunamis, floods, volcanic eruptions, heat/cold waves, and mountain fires directly kill and injure people. In addition to these direct effects, natural disasters can affect health through the change of social determinants. For example, relocation because of destruction of homes changes neighbourhood environments. Loneliness because of the death of family members or separation from friends due to relocation may affect mental health and increase the risk of mortality. Various studies have reported the importance of social relationships for health.[12,13] Social capital, of individuals and of groups/communities, is considered an important factor for disaster preparedness, aiming to reduce the damage caused by and to promote recovery from disasters.[9,10] For disaster responses, infrastructural technical solutions have been emphasized,[14] but research has indicated the importance of social solutions.[6,9-11] Therefore, this section focuses on social solutions relating to disaster risk reduction and social determinants of health.

The 2011 Great East Japan Earthquake and Tsunami destroyed many houses and killed people living in coastal areas. Because of its huge scale, there have been many studies reporting on the health effects of the disaster. The majority of such studies have focused on the effects of the disaster on mental health, e.g. outcomes such as post-traumatic stress disorder (PTSD), and they have evaluated the effects immediately after disasters.[15] However, there is also evidence of the medium- and long-term effects of disasters, not only on mental health but also various other health issues, including dementia, disability, tooth loss, and obesity.

18.2.1 Determinants of Mental Health among the Disaster Survivors

As has also been shown in previous studies elsewhere in similar situations, PTSD and depression increased among the survivors following the Japanese earthquake and tsunami.[16–20] The loss of social relationships, most typically as a result of experiencing the deaths of family or friends and the destruction of housing by the tsunami, increased the risk of PTSD.[19] However, studies of the 2011 Great Earthquake have suggested the importance of social relationships *before* the disaster as a determinant of PTSD. In addition, pre-disaster community characteristics, i.e. whether or not living in a community where many residents had social relationships, also reduce the risk of PTSD, regardless of individuals' levels of social connectedness after the disaster.[19] Social support in communities can promote recovery after disaster and protect the mental health of residents.

Though most studies focus on the survivors' mental health in the immediate aftermath, the effects of disaster on mental health are long lasting. Some studies have examined the mental health of survivors three years after the disaster in Japan. Survivors whose homes were destroyed had to relocate to prefabricated temporary housing. The physical environment of this housing was poor, e.g. thin walls. Such individuals were at increased risk of depression compared to relocated survivors whose housing conditions were better.[16] After three years, property loss as a result of the disaster was still associated with depression,[18] despite the loss of loved ones which was not statistically associated with it. Poor living environments and economic difficulties due to loss of housing can cause continuous mental stress. Therefore, they seem to affect mental health for a longer time than bereavement caused by a disaster.

Factors that bolster mental health are also reported. Participation in group exercises or regular walking may reduce the risk of depression among survivors.[17] In public prefabricated temporary housing, the opportunities for public health interventions to improve social participation were greater due to the collective living situation than they were for survivors living in private housing. This more frequent social participation may reduce psychological distress among survivors living in prefabricated temporary housing.[21] These studies suggest the importance of social relationships **both** before and after disasters to mitigate the disaster's impact on mental health among survivors.

18.2.2 Impact of the Disaster on Health Outcomes other than Mental Health

Studies after the 2011 disaster reported various health impacts arising as a result.[22–25] Housing damage due to the tsunami increased dementia about three years after the disaster among some older survivors.[22] Depression and a decrease in social relationships due to the disaster were part of the mechanism linking housing damage and dementia.

Instrumental activities of daily living (IADL) are activities relating to independent living. Because a decline of physical and cognitive status among older people causes disability and dependent living, IADL are often measured in health studies. Housing damage and disruption of access to medical services after the disaster decreased IADL among older disaster survivors.[23] Decreasing social interaction due to relocation and exacerbation of medical conditions, in part due to difficulties accessing medical care after the disaster, are considered possible mechanisms in IADL decline.

Disaster damage was also reported to be associated with oral health problems, with economic deterioration and housing damage leading to increased tooth loss after the disaster.[24] Social inequalities in oral health have been widely reported worldwide, and psychological distress, lower accessibility to dental care, and poorer health behaviours are major contributors to these inequalities. These mechanisms of social inequality may be exacerbated after disasters and later economic difficulties, which may in turn lead to a widening of social inequalities in health. Relocation due to the disaster also changed food access. Coastal residents in Iwanuma City were relocated after the disaster and their access to supermarkets and bars rapidly improved. As a result, obesity increased among study participants who were 65 years or older.[25]

These studies on various post-disaster health outcomes suggest such events have a wide-ranging impact. For several decades, studies have emphasized that social relationships, economic difficulties, and living environments are important social determinants of health. Disasters change these important social determinants and affect various aspects of people's health status in both the medium- and the long-term after disasters. Public health interventions are required to protect the wellbeing of disaster survivors, including mental health and a broad spectrum of health issues.

18.2.3 Determinants of Social Relationships after the Disaster

As mentioned, social relationships are important determinants of health among disaster survivors.[26] To maintain social relationships amidst natural disasters, studies suggest several successful solutions.[17,21,27,28]

When survivors must relocate due to the destruction of their housing, 'group relocation' is a good option to maintain relationships.[27,28] After the

2011 disaster, some Iwanuma City survivors moved into a prefabricated temporary housing village, and local government and the survivors tried to maintain social relationships. To achieve this, survivors from the same local communities before the disaster moved into the same sections of the temporary facility. As a result, the impact on and damage to social networks was greatly reduced. Other municipalities, mostly in large cities, decided where to relocate people by lottery. In such cases, most of the relocated neighbours were strangers to each other.

Social participation is also an important determinant of health.[13,29] After the disaster, local governments and volunteer groups created opportunities for social participation in the public housing communities. A study examining mental health among 10,880 survivors in 306 housing communities reported social participation statistically, which significantly explained differences in mental health between the communities.[30] In the temporary housing communities, the prevalence of social participation was higher than among the survivors living in private rented housing, and the contribution of social participation to health was larger among those living in the prefabricated housing.[21] In the prefabricated communities, because such interventions for improving social participation were widely implemented, they probably contributed to improving the health of the survivors in those communities.[21] Examples of such interventions in the communities included exercise programmes[17] and farming programmes.[31]

In a non-disaster setting, community 'salon' programmes (pronounced *saron* in Japanese) have been reported as effective for preventing functional disability[29] and cognitive decline,[32] and many municipality governments have implemented programmes creating such salons in the community. A salon is voluntarily run by local residents, with the support of local government and other public and private organizations. Such social gathering interventions may also be effective in public prefabricated temporary housing communities.

18.2.4 The Dark Side of Social Relationships and Social Capital in Disaster Settings

While there are many benefits of social capital, as mentioned, there is also a dark side.[33] After the 2011 disaster, several episodes involving negative aspects of social relationships were reported.[34] For example, the survival of the social norms of gender inequality in rural coastal communities meant that men's higher social position in the temporary shelters led to the female survivors having to cook all the meals. The fact that men were largely in control of the distribution of supplies to temporary shelters meant that supplies specifically needed by women (e.g. menstrual sanitary products) were either inadequately supplied or overlooked altogether. In these cases, women could not escape from the social norms formed from men's behaviour because of their strong social capital. Another factor is that in a community with solid social relationships, it may be difficult for outsiders to join in or find acceptance. These aspects of the dark side of social capital need to be carefully considered in post-disaster communities.

18.3 Population Health and Health Inequality in Two Recent Economic Crises during 'the Lost Two Decades'

Japan experienced a major economic boom in the late 1980s and early 1990s, when stock market and real estate prices rose to unprecedented heights. The end of this economic boom, called the burst of the 'bubble economy', triggered a long-lasting recession. As it continued for nearly twenty years, the period is also called 'the lost two decades' (see also Chapter 6). Although there was a temporary period of recovery between 2002–2008, actual annual growth was less than 3%, and it was not enough to create a major recovery. The period saw two serious economic crises, the Asian Financial Crisis in 1997 and the Global Financial Crisis in 2008. This ongoing economic hardship led to the emergence of vulnerable populations. Recent studies evaluating population health trends during this period have suggested some atypical patterns of health inequality.[35-38]

18.3.1 Increased Job Strain among Managers and the Suicide Epidemic

In general, a macroeconomic hardship makes many people unemployed, causes financial difficulties, and leads to mental stress. It is likely to disproportionately affect socially vulnerable people and widen health inequality. However, Hiyoshi and colleagues[35] found that overall, the prevalence of poor health (self-rated health) fell during the late 1980s and the middle of the 2000s, but that the pace was slower among higher-income groups. Consequently, income-based inequality in the prevalence of poor self-rated health shrank (Figure 18.1) A recent analysis updating these longitudinal observations found that there were possible increasing inequalities in men and women in the decade before 2013 (Chapter 10.3.1; Figure 10.3).

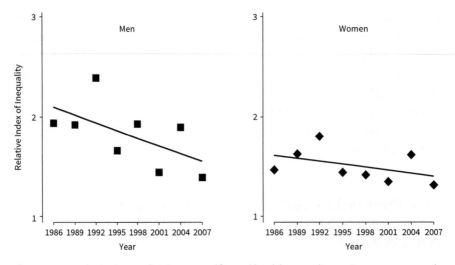

Figure 18.1 Relative inequality in poor self-rated health according to income, men and women, Japan, 1986–2007

Relative Index of Inquality is the ratio of the proportion reporting poor health at the bottom of the income distribution, versus the top.

Source: Comprehensive Survey of Living Conditions. Hiyoshi A et al. J Epidemiol Community Health 2013;67:960-965.

The slower improvement in health among wealthier workers may be linked to high rates of work-related strain among corporate managers and professional workers. The lingering economic recession since the 1990s led many male corporate managers to commit suicide, and the Asian Financial Crisis in 1997 triggered a suicide epidemic among men of working age (see Chapter 6, Chapter 15, and Figure 15.2). Although the mortality rate for men was lowest among managers and professionals, their mortality, especially in the form of suicide, started to increase in the late 1990s.

Female managers are not an exception; they may also have suffered from job-related stress, depending on the workplace environment. Data from 2010 shows that in workplaces where the company provided unfair working environments (e.g. insufficient support for employees), more workers, both men and women, suffered from psychological distress, while among women, the prevalence of smoking was higher among female managers and professionals than it was among other working women.[39]

18.3.2 Child Poverty and Health after the Global Financial Crisis

In Japan, the issue of child poverty has been actively debated in recent years. In particular, the poverty rate for single-parent working families was 50.8%, the highest for any of the member states of the Organization for Economic Co-operation and Development.[40] The reasons for this high poverty rate include low wages for uncertain work, the major job status of parents who rear children alone, and shortage of childcare services in Japan.[41] These stressful conditions for single-parent families may result in their children's health being poor: our study identified increased obesity risks among children in low-income and single-parent households as a potential impact of the 2008 Global Financial Crisis[42,43] (Figure 18.2).

18.4 Building Resilience: Lessons Learned in Japan

In earlier sections, it has been shown that natural disasters damage a wide range of social determinants of health and affect both mental and physical health. Good individual social relationships and community social capital can protect population health. The evidence regarding population health trends during the long-lasting economic recessions in Japan reveals an atypical patterning of health inequality after the recent economic crises in Japan: a narrowing of income-based health inequality. The emergence of new vulnerable populations, including corporate managers and children in single-parent households, is another thing to consider. Here are the messages and lessons we can learn from Japan's experiences.

18.4.1 Community Preparedness Counts

Disasters and crises can happen anywhere and anytime, regardless of a country's developmental and financial status. The first lesson from Japan is the importance of community preparedness: that is, building good social and physical community environments. As discussed earlier, in a disaster situation, good pre-disaster social relationships reduce the detrimental effects on population health. Community efforts to enrich positive community social capital are important. Activities such as community salons and strategies such as group relocation may facilitate an enrichment of this capital.[29,32]

Concrete actions for community organizing or building partnerships across divisions and organizations in cities should produce effective social capital that yields fruit when disasters happen.[44] When such an event occurs, everything should progress as fast as possible. It is very difficult to provide sufficient resources for each division or organization to build such partnerships after a disaster has taken place. After the 2011 Earthquake, the health division of a city

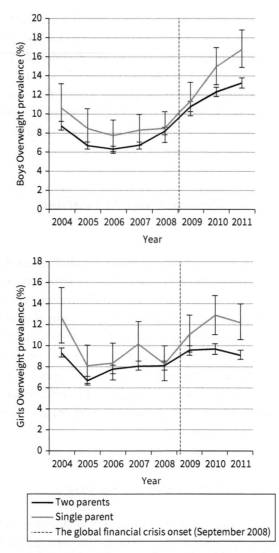

Figure 18.2 Overweight prevalence by type of parenthood, boys and girls, Japan, 2004–2011

Overweight prevalence adjusted for baseline (before 2008) household income. Error bars show 95% confidence intervals.

Source: Longitudinal Survey of Newborns. Shiba K and Kondo N. Int J Environ Res Public Health. 2019;16:1001

affected by the disaster tried to negotiate with the facilities division in charge of building disaster relocation housing, asking them to consider the design of the housing so that it would foster interpersonal exchanges among the residents. However, the negotiation failed because it was too late. According to a member of the health division, one reason for this failure was limited regular communications between divisions in the city. Making effective response, recovery, and business continuity plans for disaster and routine drilling and simulations are another community action for disaster preparedness.

18.4.2 Monitoring Health across Subpopulations and Assessing the Effects of Actions

From the studies of economic crises in Japan discussed in this chapter, we learn the importance of monitoring population health and health inequality. Continuous monitoring over time means we can understand who suffers from disasters and crises the most. As the experience of Japan shows, in some cases it is not only the lower social classes but also privileged populations (e.g. managers) who can be at great risk. Japan has long been considered a country having good welfare systems but given the widening inequality in obesity risks among children, Japan's current health and welfare systems may not be able to cope. To address the health issues of children in poverty and single-parent households, policy reforms across multiple dimensions are needed, including stronger social security for child-rearing families, more child-care resources, and better job regulations that facilitate more job opportunities for people with various living conditions. Monitoring schemes for health and health inequalities can be used to assess the effectiveness of policy reforms in response to a disaster or crisis.

Monitoring the effects of intervention is especially important to evaluate any possible 'side effects'. For example, we should prevent the effects of the dark side of social capital, e.g. overly strong social norms and potential social exclusion of 'outsiders', which could be harmful to health outcomes. Interventions to promote social interactions in the community could have such negative impacts. However, as it is difficult to predict if such side effects will occur when initiating community interventions. Again, careful and continuous monitoring of the positive and negative effects of these interventions is essential.

18.4.3 Align Central and Regional Policies to Improve Recovery from a Disaster

Central government measures have an enormous impact on local communities. It is therefore important that the central government align its measures with local actions, ensuring they support and promote effective community actions rather than inhibit them with unnecessary regulations. For example, legally grounded measures by the central government in promoting social participation among disaster survivors could improve survivor health. After disasters, if there has been large-scale housing damage and survivors have to relocate to temporary housing, group relocation to maintain pre-disaster social relationships is a good option.

In Japan, local governments determined the relocation strategy in recent disasters, and the variations in policies among municipalities might induce health inequalities among victims. Hence, legally grounded standard actions and guidelines by the central government regarding relocation policy could be effective in preventing such inequality. Central government aid to create better living environments could also contribute to maintaining survivors' health. For example, a policy of reducing disaster survivors' out-of-pocket health insurance expenses would result in improved access to healthcare.[45] Such a policy could reduce the harmful effects of disruption to access of medical services due to a disaster, because such harmful effects have been reported.[18,23]

References

1. Meteorological Agency of Japan. Earthquakes in Japan in 2018. Available at: https://www.jma.go.jp/jma/press/1901/11a/1812jishin2018.pdf [last accessed 9 March 2020].

2. Meteorological Agency of Japan. About volcano 2019. Available at: https://www.data.jma.go.jp/svd/vois/data/tokyo/STOCK/kaisetsu/katsukazan_toha/katsukazan_toha.html [last accessed 9 March 2020].

3. Reconstruction Agency of Japan. About deaths related to the Great East Japan Earthquake 2019. Available at: http://www.reconstruction.go.jp/topics/main-cat2/sub-cat2-6/20140526131634.html [last accessed 9 March 2020].

4. Cabinet Office, Government of Japan. White paper on disaster management 2017. Available at: http://www.bousai.go.jp/kaigirep/hakusho/index.html [last accessed 9 March 2020].

5. Tanida N. What happened to elderly people in the great Hanshin earthquake? *BMJ* 1996;313(7065):1133–5.

6. Castleden M, McKee M, Murray V, Leonardi G. Resilience thinking in health protection. *J Public Health* 2011;33(3):369–77.

7. Weems CF. The importance of the post-disaster context in fostering human resilience. *Lancet Planet Health* 2019;3(2):e53–e54.

8. Committee on Measuring Community Resilience, National Academies of Sciences. *Building and Measuring Community Resilience: Actions for Communities and the Gulf Research Program*. Washington, DC: National Academies Press 2019.

9. Nakagawa Y, Shaw R. Social capital: a missing link to disaster recovery. *Int J Mass Emerg Disasters* 2004;22(1):5–34.

10. Aida J, Kawachi I, Subramanian SV, Katsunori K. Disaster, social capital, and health. In: Kawachi I, Takao S, Subramanian SV (eds.). *Global Perspectives on Social Capital and Health*. New York: Springer 2013:167–87.

11. Aldrich DP, Meyer MA. Social capital and community resilience. *Am Behav Sci* 2015;59(2):254–69.

12. Holt-Lunstad J, Smith TB, Baker M, Harris T, Stephenson D. Loneliness and social isolation as risk factors for mortality: a meta-analytic review. *Perspect Psychol Sci* 2015;10(2):227–37.

13. Holt-Lunstad J, Smith TB, Layton JB. Social relationships and mortality risk: a meta-analytic review. *PLoS Med* 2010;7(7):e1000316.

14. Xiao Z, Wang G, Zhu J. Model and algorithm for rescue resource assignment problems in disaster responses based on demand-ability-equipment matching. Paper presented at the International Conference on Queueing Theory and Network Applications 2017.

15. Uscher-Pines L. Health effects of relocation following disaster: a systematic review of the literature. *Disasters* 2009;33(1):1–22.

16. Sasaki Y, Aida J, Tsuji T, et al. Does type of residential housing matter for depressive symptoms in the aftermath of a disaster? Insights from the Great East Japan Earthquake and Tsunami. *Am J Epidemiol* 2018;187(3):455–64.

17. Tsuji T, Sasaki Y, Matsuyama Y, et al. Reducing depressive symptoms after the Great East Japan Earthquake in older survivors through group exercise participation and regular walking: a prospective observational study. *BMJ Open* 2017;7(3):e013706.

18. Tsuboya T, Aida J, Hikichi H, et al. Predictors of depressive symptoms following the Great East Japan earthquake: a prospective study. *Soc Sci Med* 2016;161:47–54.

19. Hikichi H, Aida J, Tsuboya T, Kondo K, Kawachi I. Can community social cohesion prevent posttraumatic stress disorder in the aftermath of a disaster? A natural experiment from the 2011 Tohoku Earthquake and Tsunami. *Am J Epidemiol* 2016;183(10):902–10.

20. Inoue Y, Stickley A, Yazawa A, et al. Adverse childhood experiences, exposure to a natural disaster and posttraumatic stress disorder among survivors of the 2011 Great East Japan earthquake and tsunami. *Epidemiol Psychiatr Sci* 2019;28(1):45–53.

21. Kusama T, Aida J, Sugiyama K, et al. Does the type of temporary housing make a difference in social participation and health for evacuees of the Great East Japan

Earthquake and Tsunami?: a cross-sectional study. *J Epidemiol* 2019;29(10):391–8. doi: 10.2188/jea.JE20180080.

22. Hikichi H, Aida J, Kondo K, et al. Increased risk of dementia in the aftermath of the 2011 Great East Japan Earthquake and Tsunami. *Proc Natl Acad Sci U S A* 2016;113(45): E6911–E6918. doi: 10.1073/pnas.1607793113

23. Tsuboya T, Aida J, Hikichi H, et al. Predictors of decline in IADL functioning among older survivors following the Great East Japan earthquake: a prospective study. *Soc Sci Med* 2017;176:34–41.

24. Matsuyama Y, Aida J, Tsuboya T, et al. Are lowered socioeconomic circumstances causally related to tooth loss? A natural experiment involving the 2011 Great East Japan Earthquake. *Am J Epidemiol* 2017;186(1):54–62.

25. Hikichi H, Aida J, Kondo K, Tsuboya T, Kawachi I. Residential relocation and obesity after a natural disaster: a natural experiment from the 2011 Japan Earthquake and Tsunami. *Sci Rep* 2019;9(1):374.

26. Aida J, Hikichi H, Matsuyama Y, et al. Risk of mortality during and after the 2011 Great East Japan Earthquake and Tsunami among older coastal residents. *Sci Rep* 2017;7(1):16591.

27. Hikichi H, Sawada Y, Tsuboya T, et al. Residential relocation and change in social capital: a natural experiment from the 2011 Great East Japan Earthquake and Tsunami. *Sci Adv* 2017;3(7):e1700426.

28. Koyama S, Aida J, Kawachi I, et al. Social support improves mental health among the victims relocated to temporary housing following the Great East Japan Earthquake and Tsunami. *Tohoku J Exp Med* 2014;234(3):241–7.

29. Hikichi H, Kondo N, Kondo K, Aida J, Takeda T, Kawachi I. Effect of a community intervention programme promoting social interactions on functional disability prevention for older adults: propensity score matching and instrumental variable analyses, JAGES Taketoyo study. *J Epidemiol Community Health* 2015;69(9):905–10.

30. Matsuyama Y, Aida J, Hase A, et al. Do community- and individual-level social relationships contribute to the mental health of disaster survivors?: a multi-level prospective study after the Great East Japan Earthquake. *Soc Sci Med* 2016;151:187–95.

31. Takahashi S, Ishiki M, Kondo N, et al. Health effects of a farming program to foster community social capital of a temporary housing complex of the 2011 great East Japan earthquake. *Disaster Med Public Health Prep* 2015;9(2):103–10.

32. Hikichi H, Kondo K, Takeda T, Kawachi I. Social interaction and cognitive decline: results of a 7-year community intervention. *Alzheimers Dement (NY)* 2017;3(1):23–32.

33. Villalonga-Olives E, Kawachi I. The dark side of social capital: a systematic review of the negative health effects of social capital. *Soc Sci Med* 2017;194:105–27.

34. Hikichi H, Kondo K, Aida J, Kondo N. Social capital in disaster medicine: group interviews with public health nurses working in areas stricken by the Tohoku earthquake (in Japanese). *Jap J Disast Med* 2015;20:51–6.

35. Hiyoshi A, Fukuda Y, Shipley MJ, Brunner EJ. Inequalities in self-rated health in Japan 1986–2007 according to household income and a novel occupational classification: national sampling survey series. *J Epidemiol Community Health* 2013;67(11):960–5.

36. Wada K, Kondo N, Gilmour S, et al. Trends in cause specific mortality across occupations in Japanese men of working age during period of economic stagnation, 1980–2005: retrospective cohort study. *BMJ* 2012;344:e1191.

37. Kachi Y, Inoue M, Nishikitani M, Tsurogano S, Yano E. Determinants of changes in income-related health inequalities among working-age adults in Japan, 1986–2007: time-trend study. *Soc Sci Med* 2013;81:94–101.

38. Kondo N, Subramanian S, Kawachi I, Takeda Y, Yamagata Z. Economic recession and health inequalities in Japan: analysis with a national sample, 1986–2001. *J Epidemiol Community Health* 2008;62:869–75.

39. Kobayashi Y, Kondo N. Organizational justice, psychological distress, and stress-related behaviors by occupational class in female Japanese employees. *PLoS One* 2019;14(4):e0214393.

40. OECD. Child poverty: OECD Family Database. Available at: http://www.oecd.org/els/soc/CO_2_2_Child_Poverty.pdf [last accessed 9 March 2020].

41. Nohara Y. In one of the world's richest countries, most single mothers live in poverty. *Bloomberg*, 25 June 2018.

42. Ueda P, Kondo N, Fujiwara T. The global economic crisis, household income and pre-adolescent overweight and underweight: a nationwide birth cohort study in Japan. *Int J Obes* 2015;39(9):1414.

43. Shiba K, Kondo N. The global financial crisis and overweight among children of single parents: a nationwide 10-year birth cohort study in Japan. *Int J Environ Res Public Health* 2019;16(6):1001.

44. Minkler M. *Community Organizing and Community Building for Health and Welfare 3rd edn.* London: Rutgers University Press 2012.

45. Matsuyama Y, Tsuboya T, Bessho SI, Aida J, Osaka K. Copayment exemption policy and healthcare utilization after the Great East Japan Earthquake. *The Tohoku Journal of Experimental Medicine* 2018;244(2):163–73.

19

Social Determinants of Health on the Island of Okinawa

Kokoro Shirai

19.1 Introduction

Okinawa was declared a 'World Longevity Area' in 1995. Life expectancy and the number of centenarians per 100,000 were the highest of any prefecture when it reverted to Japanese political control in 1972. However, life tables showed Okinawa's life-expectancy ranking of men had dropped from first to twenty-sixth of 47 prefectures by 2005. Men's life expectancy was 78.6 years and women's was 86.9 years.[1] This was the last year when women in Okinawa prefecture had the longest life expectancy in Japan; since then relative ranking of longevity has gradually declined.

In 2017, prevalence of overweight and obesity (BMI ≥ 25) in Okinawa was the highest in Japan (38.4% among men and 25.9% among women), although still lower than in Western countries. According to the Ministry of Health, Labour and Welfare, prevalence of metabolic syndrome at prefecture level is also highest in Okinawa (33.8% in Okinawa and 26.4% nationally). Mortality from alcohol-related liver disease is the highest in Okinawa, while hepatitis B- and C- related liver disease are more common in mainland Japan. The need for renal dialysis, due to diabetic nephropathy, is 1.85 times higher in Okinawa than in Japan as a whole. Okinawans are now at higher risk of premature death among those 40–65 years of age than their mainland Japan counterparts.[2]

How did Okinawa become the island with the highest longevity in the world? And why did it then become an island with a high premature death rate and high risks of life-style related diseases among those people of middle and young old age? Reasons for longevity include genetic factors and life-style related factors such as diet, drinking habit, smoking, physical exercise, stress and sleep pattern. Environmental factors, the healthcare system, socioeconomic status, social and economic inequalities, social relations, and other

Kokoro Shirai, *Social Determinants of Health on the Island of Okinawa* In: *Health in Japan*. Edited by: Eric Brunner, Noriko Cable, and Hiroyasu Iso, Oxford University Press (2021). © Oxford University Press. DOI: 10.1093/oso/9780198848134.003.0019.

Table 19.1 Life Expectancy in Okinawa, Japan, and Aomori, Men and Women, 1965–2015

	Year	1965	1975	1985	1995	2000	2005	2010	2015
Men	Okinawa	—	72.2	76.3	77.2	77.6	78.6	79.4	80.3
	Japan	67.7	71.8	75.0	76.7	77.7	78.8	79.6	80.8
	Aomori	65.3	69.7	73.1	74.7	75.7	76.3	77.3	78.7
Women	Okinawa	—	79.0	83.7	85.1	86.0	86.9	87.0	87.4
	Japan	72.9	77.0	80.8	83.2	84.6	85.8	86.4	87.0
	Aomori	71.8	76.5	79.9	82.5	83.7	84.8	85.3	85.9

Source: Ministry of Health, Labour and Welfare, 2017

*1965 data for Okinawa is not available (under US occupation). Aomori is the prefecture with the shortest life expectancy, located in the north of Japan.

psychosocial factors are related. This chapter explores the social determinants of good and bad health in Okinawa based on its historical, social, and cultural characteristics.

19.2 Health and Demographic Status in Okinawa

Life expectancy in Japan is the longest in the world, 81.3 for men and 87.3 for women in 2018. In 1947, it was 50.1 for men and 53.9 for women, and extended to 71.8 and 77.0 in 1975. It reached 80.8 and 87.0 respectively in 2015. In 60 years, life expectancy increased by 30 years in Japan. In Okinawa, it was 72.2 and 78.0 years for men and women in 1975, reaching 80.3 and 87.4 years in 2015. In 1978, when Japan first became a nation of the longest life expectancy in the world, Okinawa had the longest one among all prefectures in Japan, which was one year longer for men and women respectively, than the Japanese average. Since then, up to 2010, Okinawan women had the highest life expectancy in Japan (Table 19.1).[1] Compared with other areas, Okinawa showed a small increase on past longevity and the extension rate of life-span is now the lowest in the country. In the past, the age-adjusted mortality rate in Okinawa for all age groups was lower than other areas in Japan. However, it increased to the same level as the mainland in 2003 among men and in 2014 among women. Since 2007, the age-adjusted mortality rate among men in Okinawa has been higher than the mainland: 498.5 per 100,000 population in Okinawa and 486.0 per 100,000 in Japan according to recent national statistics. Among women it is 251.7 and 255.0 per 100,000 for Okinawa and Japan, respectively. Furthermore, the age-adjusted mortality rate in the 30–64 age group is now higher in Okinawa than Japan at 265.4 for men and 129.7 for women and 214.3 for men and 106.8 for women respectively.[1]

The year 2010 was significant for Okinawa, marking its transition from an island of longevity to one with high risk for premature deaths. In the same year, women's relative ranking of longevity dropped from the first place to the third among 47 prefectures for the first time and men in Okinawa moved from the middle group to the bottom group in terms of life expectancy in Japan. In 1995, life expectancy at birth for women was 79.0 in Okinawa and 77.0 in Japan, and for men, 72.2 and 71.8. However, by 2010, it was 79.4 for men and 87.0 for women in Okinawa, while the national averages were 79.6 and 86.4 respectively.

The generational disparity in Okinawa between the middle-aged and the older population, as well as the gender gap in life expectancy and health, is large. Mortality rates in the middle-aged population have increased. Furthermore, the difference in life-expectancy between men and women of 7.6 years is greater than the 5.3 years gained in 30 years between 1980–2010.

Okinawa was unusual in having the lowest proportion of older people, despite long life expectancy and many centenarians. The combination of low birth rate and increasing aged population is a characteristic of Japan and other ageing societies. In Okinawa, long life expectancy combined with a high birth rate. This might be considered an ideal population composition in the sense that old people live long lives as individual level but the ageing rate is low as the society level.

Okinawa is the youngest prefecture in terms of age structure of its residents, average age of the prefecture is the youngest as 40.75 years, and the proportion of the population under 16 years is 17.4%, the highest in Japan in 2017. Levels of 'ageing society' is defined by the percentage of its population aged 65 and over: 7% is deemed an 'ageing' society, 14% 'aged', and 21% as 'super-aged'. Japan is a super-aged society with 27.4% of the population aged 65 and over, while Okinawa is 20.5% and still 'aged society' unlike the rest of Japan. The total fertility rate in Okinawa in 2017 is the highest in Japan at 1.96 births per woman (1.43 nationally). However, the divorce rate, proportion of single parents, relative poverty rate among children, and average number of dental caries among children under 12 years old in Okinawa are also the highest in Japan. On a small island, with a population of less than 1.5 million, Okinawa has many of the best and the worst demographic characteristics in Japan.

19.3 Social Determinants of Health in Okinawa

Why Okinawan residents born 80 years ago have relatively long and healthy lives, while those born 50 years ago have shorter life-spans and higher risks of diseases? This pattern of change suggests that their life-span is not determined by genetic factors alone but also by changes in their socio-environment and life-style related factors which influence their health status. From a historical perspective, the region has experienced a significant level of enforced change in its social and cultural environment, related to changes of government and overseas influence. The singer Yutaka Sadoyama comes from *Koza* in Okinawa city, an area which has been highly influenced by the presence of the US military base. In his song *Dochumuini* (Talking to myself), Sadoyama describes Okinawa as being thrown from one superpower to another: 'From Tang Dynasty (China) to Yamato reign (Japan), Yamato reign to America reign, from America reign to Yamato reign again Okinawa changed too many times'.

This song describes the resilience of the people of Okinawa, saying that despite the rapid shifts in rulers, Okinawan didn't really change. However, from the health status point of view, these historical transitions of power delivered considerable effects as part of the social determinants of health in Okinawa.

Before 1879, Okinawa existed as the independent Ryuku Kingdom, the three polities of the Ryukus, Nanzan, Chuzan and Hokuzan were unified under King Sho-Hashi in 1429.[34] At this time Ryuku Kingdom joined the powerful Chinese tributary system and became a successful trading nation. In 1609 however, the Ryuku Kingdom was invaded by the Shimazu clan from the Satsuma domain in Japan who subsequently dominated. When Commodore Perry's US fleet of 'black ships' arrived in 1853, he negotiated the US-Ryukyu Treaty of Amity and Commerce before reaching an agreement with Japan. Ryukyu Kingdom was also requested to sign the Ryukyu-France and Ryukyu-Dutch Treaty of Amity in 1855 and 1859 as an independent nation closely related with Japan as part of diplomatic negotiation between Japan and Western countries. However, in 1879, Ryuku was annexed by Japan and it lost its status as an independent nation. After World War II, it was occupied by the US. Infrastructure development, including currency, education, health, and transport, was promoted for 30 post-war years. Residents of Okinawa were required to use passports to visit mainland Japan and used different currency and social systems. After US Naval Government (1 April 1945 to 30 June 1946) and US Army Government (1 July 1946 to 14 December 1950) rule, US Civil Administration of the Ryukyu Islands (USCAR) was established. Okinawa was returned to Japan on 15 May 1972, but, as in the words of Sadoyama's song, for the people of Okinawa the dramatic changes they experienced in social systems, everyday life, values, and social norms had not occurred through their own choices but through the waves of change caused by superpowers.

The sweeping changes of social environment caused by external pressures appear to have influenced the health of the Okinawan people both negatively and positively. A positive influence was seen in relation to prevention and treatment of communicable diseases during US Army control. In addition to effective countermeasures against tuberculosis, Japanese encephalitis, and filariasis, positive effects were reported on malaria control, and reduction in the infant mortality rate due to rapid improvements in post-war nutrition and sanitary conditions. On the other hand, in terms of non-communicable diseases (NCD), the health of Okinawans now in mid-life and early old-age became the subject to negative influences. Okinawans who spent their childhood under US rule are currently aged about 50s and 60s and may now see negative effects on their health.

The rapid influx of American life-style was not experienced elsewhere in Japan. Some Micronesian islands such as Palau experienced similar situation. Its influence is linked to higher risks of lifestyle-related NCDs, including increased rates of mortality, morbidity and obesity, incidence of diabetes, alcohol-related liver disease, renal disease, colon cancer, and colorectal cancer. This, in turn, may explain the reduction of life expectancy extension rate as a mid- to long-term result. Ironically, the nutritional transition which occurred earlier in Okinawa than mainland Japan may have helped extend the life span of the population heading into older age in the post-war decades because of increased protein and total energy intake. It seems the health effect of the dramatic societal change during the US occupation was dependent on their life stage, meaning that there was a negative impact on the health of younger generations, but a positive effect on the older population in relation to life extension. Further research examining age, cohort and period effects of society changes of Okinawa and its effects on their health based on the life course perspectives is required.

19.4 Diet and Societal Change on Okinawa

According to the National Health and Nutrition Survey, for many years salt intake in Okinawa was the lowest in Japan. In 2010, it was 9.5 g/day for men and 8.1 g/d for women, compared with 10.6 g/d for all Japan. However, salt intake has been increasing in Okinawa, making the gap between Okinawa and mainland Japan smaller. This is especially true among the younger generation whose intake is now similar to mainland Japan. Among the older generation, salt intake remains low.

One possible reason for this low intake among older people is the use of flavouring other than salt. Fish (bonito) and kelp broth are key elements of the traditional Okinawan diet which enhance *umami* and reduce salt intake. But nowadays consumption of chemical seasoning is increasing and kelp and bonito are consumed less often. Okinawa used to be a high consumer of kelp, as reported in the annual household survey in 1980, which shows mean consumption at 1405 g/year in Naha city (capital of Okinawa) compared to 596 g/year for all of Japanese. Although kelp consumption in Naha was once the highest in Japan, it decreased by two-thirds in just two decades between 1980 and 1999.[3] High kelp consumption in Okinawa was considered as a reflection of the history of an active sea-trade in the Ryukyu Dynasty, since kelp cannot be collected in the Okinawan Sea. Increasing salt intake in Okinawa was associated with changing life-styles including modernized cooking, Japanized and Westernized food culture.

In the 1950s, Okinawans were exposed to Western-style food, such as canned processed pork ('spam') just after experiencing low-nutritional circumstances during the war period. In 1960s, steak houses and Western-style restaurants were opened under the US occupation. Hamburger shops and many fast food chains started trading on the mainland in the 1970s, however the first hamburger shop ('A&W') opened in 1963 on Okinawa. Fast food culture quickly became popular among Okinawans, and mixed food culture of traditional Okinawan with Asian and Western countries were blended together. Later, in the 1980s, commercialized Japanese food became popular after Okinawa reverted to Japan. Savoury food such as sushi and ramen noodles were introduced, broiled meat restaurants appeared, and gradually levels of salt and energy intake increased. The first wave of change, leading to higher fat and energy intakes, was introduced with US culture after the World WarII, and the second wave leading to increased salt intake was introduced with Japanese food culture after Okinawa was returned to Japan.

Changes in diet and life-style are ultimately the choice of individuals, but differences of availability and accessibility of food and economic pricing greatly influence individual choices and behaviours.[4] A meta-analysis showed that a 10% increase in the price of soft drinks resulted in an 8–10% reduction in consumption.[5] Similarly, a price increase of one dollar for a soft drink and pizza led to a 124 kcal total energy reduction, 1.05 kg weight loss, and reduction of insulin resistance.[4,6,7] In Okinawa, dietary changes towards high fat, salt, and total energy intake followed the postwar change in governance.

Currently, Okinawa has the highest number of hamburger shops per capita in Japan. The total number of shops in Japan is 5,972, which equates to 4.7 per 100,000 people, but in Okinawa there are 9.4 shops per 100,000 while Tokyo, with the second highest density, has 6.7 shops. The 2000 domestic consumption report, shows that consumption volume per population of processed meat such as canned pork and corned beef is also highest in Okinawa. As noted above, individual preferences are influenced by environmental factors and socioeconomic incentives. Furthermore, Okinawa is small in size, with dense community and family networks, and these factors appear to have led to effects of changes of social environment into life-style and health status of individuals in a short period of time.

The traditional Okinawan diet was rich in vegetables, potatoes, pork and fish but had less salt and fat; it was similar to the Mediterranean and DASH diet.[8] The traditional Okinawan diet was low-calorie, nutrient-dense, fiber-rich and antioxidant-rich.[9] It can therefore be said that changes away from this diet may be involved in the changes in health and longevity statistics.[10] The patterns of food supply, food behaviors and other cultural transitions, as well as shifting chronic disease rates over the past 70 years in Okinawa, all provide a powerful example of the relationship between changes in social environment and health.

19.5 Social Gradient and Socioeconomic Status in Okinawa

The economic differences across the islands of Okinawa as well as gap between mainland Japan and Okinawa are both substantial. According to a wage survey in 2017 by the Ministry of Health, Labour and Welfare, the average annual income of company employees (excluding self-employed or government employees) in Japan is 4,726,500 yen (£35,328, $44,126) per year. It is 3,389,400 yen (£25,330, $31,641) per year in Okinawa (the lowest in Japan) and 5,823,600 yen (£43,521, $54,382) per year in Tokyo (the highest in Japan). Similarly, according to the Cabinet Office annual report on prefectural accounts, in 2017, average prefectural income per capita is lowest in Okinawa at 210,1700 yen (£19,625, $19,626) and highest in Tokyo at 443,4500 yen (£33,149, $41,410) while the average throughout Japan is 306,700 yen (£22,879, $28,584). Based on the regional minimum wage report in 2018, Okinawa had the lowest minimum wage between 2009 and 2017, and the highest unemployment rate in the same period (Ministry of Internal Affairs and Communications Statistics Bureau Labour Survey, fiscal 2018).

Okinawa is also one of the highest three prefectures for income inequality based on the GINI coefficient. As surveys of family income and expenditure have shown, the GINI coefficient can vary significantly from one year to another, so this index should be used carefully. However, in 2004, the national average was 0.308 while on Okinawa it was 0.340, and later surveys (2009, 2014) again showed Okinawa to have one of the three highest levels of inequality. Thus it can be said that Okinawa is a region with significant economic disparity both within and between prefectures. Increased risk of mortality due to disparities within the community based on the GINI index, after adjusting for individual incomes, has been observed in the US.[11] It may be that even high-income individuals have higher risk of mortality when they live in a community with large economic disparities.[12-14] In the case of Okinawa, however, the mortality rate was low and life expectancy was high despite the absolutely and relatively deprived socioeconomic situation indicated by the low income, high unemployment and high GINI coefficient. It could be explained by suggesting that social resources in Okinawan society could have weakened the negative cycle of social disadvantages and poor health, thus buffeing and reducing health inequalities in Okinawa. If these social resources are now decreasing, or negative in their effects, it may be that they contribute to the recent decline in the health of Okinawans.

19.6 Social Capital and Health in Okinawan Culture

Diet pattern, socioeconomic disparities, physical inactivity due to limited access to public transportation, low and late health screening participation, smoking habit, high alcohol consumption, and suicide among men could be one of the factors related to elevated risk of health status in Okinawa. In this section, unexamined factor, social capital and social connectedness are considered as another aspect of the social determinants of health in Okinawa. The impact on health of social capital, social support, social networks, and the way in which people interact, will be discussed in this section.

Based on close ties and networks in the community, associations and volunteer groups for health promotion and self-support groups are very active in some areas of Okinawa. These factors, such as participation in volunteer groups, social activities and maintaining variety of networks in the community are well discussed as factors related to better physical and mental conditions of older population.[15-17] At the same time, these close ties and networks can encourage sharing of unhealthy life-styles such as smoking and high alcohol consumption.[18] Both positive and negative aspects of close networks, social supports and social capital can be observed in Okinawa.

Could it be that the social resources that remain common in Okinawa influence the achievement and impairment of health and longevity? Okinawa presents a dual aspect, maintaining the traditional resources of Japanese society and keeping its own distinctive heritage originated in Ryukyus.

The traditional word *yui-maru* remains a part of daily life in Okinawa, and even the younger generations have opportunities to use it in everyday conversation. *Yui-maru* is a phrase that symbolizes the local society's spirit of mutual aid and sense of trust and reciprocity. The combination of *yui* (connection, mutual help, exchange of labour) and *mawaru* (goes round), expresses a cycle of mutual aid and reciprocal labour exchanges. For example, in labour sharing, as a *yui-maru* activity, small farmers used to share one combine harvester and work together one by one, with a famer in each field. *Yui-maru* is well-known concept throughout the worldwide Okinawan diaspora—so that in locations such as Brazil and Hawaii the spirit of *yui-maru*, together with Okinawa's characteristic local events and customs, remains strong among offsprings of immigrants from Okinawa.[35] A relatively new network-building event (the Worldwide Uchinanchu Festival) for people with Okinawan roots is held every five years. Approximately 420,000 people including second and third generation of immigrants from overseas have gathered under the word of *yui-maru* as a slogan on each occasion since the first such event was held in 1990.[36]

19.6.1. *Moai* as One Example of Local Social Capital

Another local form of social capital is *moai*, a unique social resource in the community. *Moai* is a type of micro-financing known as ROSCA (Rotating Savings and Credit Association). As an alternative to banks and forma financial resources, ROSCA allows access to funds without significant collateral by collecting small sums of money from family, friends, and acquaintances.[19] It can be thought of a financial arrangement based on relationships, with social trust as collateral, and capitalized by these relationships. The spirit of trust and mutual aid among the members is a form of 'social collateral' that prevents defaults on loans.[20] In this context, *moai* is a system offering mutual aid based on community ties and widespread friendships, and has persisted to the present day in Okinawa, despite changing major objectives and forms, such as social gathering and friendship ties so-called *shinboku-moai*.

Similar mutual help groups with a credit function including ASCA (Accumulating Savings and Credit Association) have been observed in other parts of the world.[20] Analogous groups also exist in mainland Japan. For example, *Mujinko*, in Yamagata prefecture[21] and *Tanomoshiko* in Okayama prefecture. Epidemiological surveys have examined their links with health, and have reported the positive influence of these organizations.[22,23]

The participation rate in *moai* exceeded 60% based on the local governmental survey conducted by Okinawa Development Bureau in 1974, and was still around 40% in 2006. People of all generations, from 20 to 90 years, participate in *moai*, and among women aged 60 and older, 61% reported participation.[24]

Regular participation in *moai* was associated with lower risk of declining IADL level,[25] and higher cognitive function (after considering baseline health conditions and other psychosocial background).[26] Furthermore, types of moai, bridging and bonding showed different effects on health based on gender in Okinawa. For women aged over 65, participating in *moai*, ROSCA like a financial co-support group, especially defined as bridging type of moai that connects people with diverse social demographic characteristics such as age, gender, or occupation promoted the health and well-being of those women. For men, a bonding social capital, where persons of similar sociodemographic background come together, was associated with reduced risk of ill health conditions.[26]

19.6.2 Possible Pathways between *Moai* and the Health of Okinawans

Moai as social capital resources in Okinawa have worked through multiple pathways both in positive and negative links. Some examples, such as 1) providing opportunity of social participation and maintaining social network, 2) weaken visible social disparity, 3) psychological distress and emotional & appraisal support, 4) information exchanges via networks will be discussed in the following section.

Participation in *moai* gives opportunities to interact regularly. It is frequently argued that social participation is beneficial for physical and cognitive health among older people. It allows individuals to maintain friendship and acquaintance networks and to give and receive social support; each of these activities has a positive influence on health.[16,27–29] Regular monthly *moai* meetings constitute a system that incorporates interactions with others. Unlike the usual drinking parties and social gatherings, by engaging in transfers of money, participation in *moai* fosters a shared understanding of responsibilities and roles. It gives members a reason to leave the house which is easily accepted by family and community. For those who often do not go out, these groups offer regular meetings and help maintain their relationships with others. Through this interaction, the sense of mutual support is reconfirmed and this positively influences the health and psychological stability of the older population.[17]

Moai, as a form of social capital, can protect individuals as well as the community. It functions to disperse the risk of economic disadvantage within the community, preventing concentration in any one sector, and thus protecting the community and its health.[30] Speculatively, *moai* may have decoupled economic disparities and health disparities, and contributed to the health and longevity of the island inhabitants. In addition to *yui-maru* and *moai*, other traditional practices such as *kyodo-baiten*—a system of cooperative sales stalls—and *monchū clan*—extended family groups and ancestor worship—contribute to the social capital which has been skillfully deployed in a community of limited resources.

Nowadays, while the practice and financial significance of *moai* has decreased, the importance of its social networking function has increased, providing a safety net of emotional and functional support. In *moai*, the order in which participants receive funding can be adjusted depending on members' request or needs. Mutual support groups composed of friends can respond to life events such as children starting school, parents requiring nursing care, or family members being hospitalized, and distributing funds on a monthly basis. Even if the role of financial assistance is small, the process of sharing emotional support and being judged deserving of assistance is beneficial. As social capital reduce psycho-social stress;[30] *moai* in Okinawa may work as a buffer to the stresses caused by social disparities.

There is also the possibility that *moai* can be detrimental to health by reinforcing unhealthy behaviours.[18] *Moai* can be a context for the regular exchange of information including health-related messages. Within networks, information received from trusted partners is often treated as important and trustworthy information or norms, which can be adopted and passed on to others not merely depending on the quality of information. In communities with low levels of social capital, and lower level of trust in others, there is a tendency for individuals not to heed warnings and advice given by others.[31] In a widely cited analysis, based on the Framingham Heart Study, Christakis and Fowler (2007, 2008), examined social networks to demonstrate the high probability that obesity, propensity to smoke, and life satisfaction tend to be correlated between members of networks.[32,33]

Regular meeting events, such as *moai*, with trusted fellow members can work as a hub for intensive information exchange. Social capital is a transferable neutral resource based on social relationships. Therefore, both good and bad influence on health and well-being can be brought, depending on context. If information beneficial to health is transmitted through social networks and comes from trustworthy partners, it is effectively internalized with benefits for health. On the other hand, detrimental information and behaviours inimical to health, such as substance abuse, drinking and smoking habits, can be reinforced along the same lines, and promoted to be internalized. In the case of Okinawa, close social networks and social capital may have been beneficial in reducing social and economic disparities and buffering negative effects on health through mutual help and support. However, at the same time, harmful information and behavioural norms for health may also have been distributed through these tight networks.

While *moai* appears to have a positive influence on health and longevity in older generations, it is also possible that it is linked to unhealthy status and behaviours among younger generations. Given the relationship between alcohol consumption and liver disease, kidney disease, and accidental mortality, there is cause for concern in regard to the improvement of health among the middle-aged and young-old population. In addition, many *moai* meetings are held in venues such as pub-restaurants that serve alcohol, and it is not uncommon to see parents with young children, under school age, at evening meetings; this latter issue has caused concern about parental influence on the life-style and health of children. The report Healthy Okinawa 21 identified obesity, high alcohol consumption, and low participation in regular health checkups as three points to be targeted. People sometime discuss the reason of worsening health status in Okinawa can be related to the decrease of social capital in the community. However, it might be related to changes in the role and effect of social capital rather than its decline as an influence in the community. Negative aspect of social capital in rich social connectedness might be one of the reasons of worsening health status in Okinawa as one of the resources among several other factors. There is a need for further investigation to determine causal links between such social resources and health on Okinawa.

19.7 Conclusion

Okinawan people have for many decades had the longest life expectancy in Japan, and indeed worldwide. However, extension of longevity has slowed, and there are large gaps between male and female average lifespans, as well as intergenerational health gaps. Okinawa is a small island with a population under 1.5 M. There is a major gap between the longevity and health of people born 80 years ago, who are relatively healthy and long lived, and those born 50 years ago, who are less healthy and live shorter lives. Okinawa has experienced major changes in its social environment. In this chapter, possible social determining factors for health, such as changes in life-style habits, the socioeconomic environment, and the strength of local attachments in the area have been examined.

Okinawa exhibits both a positive aspect in the maintenance of the health and longevity of the older generation and a negative aspect of worsening indices for lifestyle-related disease among the middle-aged and young-old generation. The latter has now become the focus of an urgent need for intervention and policymaking to improve health status. As a focus of attention for preventable health problems in Japan, it can be said that Okinawa is a front runner, facing both good and bad conditions earlier than mainland Japan.

Although Okinawa is significant as a location for academic verification of determinants of population health, large-scale cohort studies are lacking, and there is a dearth of coherence among the multiple small-scale research projects in existence. In future, locally based studies with well-structured research designs, together with collaboration between external research groups, is required to fill the gaps in evidence and to support policy intervention.

Acknowledgement

The original manuscript of this chapter was written during a period when author worked as an associate professor in University of the Ryukyus in Okinawa. Author is grateful to her colleagues in Okinawa for their inspiring discussions and fruitful suggestions.

References

1. Ministry of Health, Labour and Welfare. Life tables of prefectural levels in Japan 2015. Available at: https://www.mhlw.go.jp/toukei/saikin/hw/life/tdfk15/index.html.
2. Okinawa Prefecture. Kenko-Okinawa21. Available at: http://www.kenko-okinawa21.jp/090-docs/2018020100011/files/nenreichouseisibouritsu-suii.pdf

3. Todoriki H, Shirai K. Well-being transition and social capital in post-war Okinawa. *Intern Rev Ryukyu Oki Studies* 2012;1(1):9–28.

4. Meyer KA, Guilkey DK, Ng SW, et al. Sociodemographic differences in fast food price sensitivity. *JAMA Intern Med* 2014;174(3):434–42.

5. Andreyeva T, Long MW, Brownell KD. The impact of food prices on consumption: a systematic review of research on the price elasticity of demand for food. *Am J Public Health* 2010;100(2):216–22.

6. Duffey KJ, Gordon-Larsen P, Shikany JM, et al. Food price and diet and health outcomes: 20 years of the CARDIA Study. *Arch Intern Med* 2010;170(5):420–6.

7. Brownell KD, Farley T, Willett WC, et al. The public health and economic benefits of taxing sugar-sweetened beverages. *N Engl J Med* 2009;361(16):1599–605.

8. Willcox DC, Scapagnini G, Willcox BJ. Healthy aging diets other than the Mediterranean: a focus on the Okinawan diet. *Mech Ageing Dev* 2014;136–7:148–62.

9. Willcox BJ, Willcox DC, Todoriki H, et al. Caloric restriction, the traditional Okinawan diet, and healthy aging: the diet of the world's longest-lived people and its potential impact on morbidity and life span. *Ann N Y Acad Sci* 2007;1114: 434–55.

10. Moriguchi EH, Moriguchi Y, Yamori Y. Impact of diet on the cardiovascular risk profile of Japanese immigrants living in Brazil: contributions of World Health Organization CARDIAC and MONALISA studies. *Clin Exp Pharmacol Physiol* 2004;31(2):S5–7.

11. Lochner K, Pamuk E, Makuc D, et al. State-level income inequality and individual mortality risk: a prospective, multilevel study. *Am J Public Health* 2001;91(3):385–91.

12. Kawachi I, Kennedy BP. *The Health of Nations: Why Inequality is Harmful to Your Health*. New York: The New Press 2002.

13. Evans RG, Barer ML, Marmor TR. *Why Are Some People Healthy and Others Not? The Determinants of Health of Populations*. New York: Aldine de Gruyter 1994.

14. Wilkinson RG, Pickett KE. Income inequality and population health: a review and explanation of the evidence. *Soc Sci Med* 2006;62(7):1768–84.

15. Kawachi I. Social capital and community effects on population and individual health. *Ann NY Acad Sci* 1999;896:120–30.

16. Hughes TF, Chang CC, Vander Bilt J, et al. Engagement in reading and hobbies and risk of incident dementia: the MoVIES project. *Am J Alzheimers Dis Other Demen* 2010;25(5):432–8.

17. Nyqvist F, Forsman AK, Giuntoli G, et al. Social capital as a resource for mental well-being in older people: a systematic review. *Aging Ment Health* 2013;17(4):394–410.

18. Lindström M. Social capital and health-related behaviors. In: Kawachi I, Subramanian SV, Kim D (eds.), *Social Capital and Health*. New York: Springer 2008:215–38.

19. Besley T, Coate S. Group lending, repayment incentives and social collateral. *J Dev Econ* 1995;46:1–18.

20. Besley T, Loury, G. Rotating Savings and Credit Associations, Credit Market and Efficiency. *Rev Econ Studies* 1994;61:701–19.

21. Kondo N, Minai J, Imai H, et al. Engagement in a cohesive group and higher-level functional capacity in older adults in Japan: a case of the Mujin. *Soc Sci Med* 2007;64(11):2311–23.

22. Iwase T, Suzuki E, Fujiwara T, et al. Do bonding and bridging social capital have differential effects on self-rated health? A community based study in Japan. *J Epidemiol Community Health* 2012;66(6):557–62.

23. Kondo N, Shirai K. Microfinance and social capital. In: Kawachi I, Takao S, Subramanian SV (eds.), *Social Capital and Health from Global Perspectives*. New York: Springer 2013.

24. Shirai K. Older population and social capital in the Okinawan community. In: Todoriki H, Kawachi I (eds.), *Social Capital and the Community in Okinawa*. Tokyo: Nihon-hyoron 2013.

25. Avlund K, Lund R, Holstein BE, et al. The impact of structural and functional characteristics of social relations as determinants of functional decline. *J Gerontol B* 2004;59(1):S44–51.

26. Shirai K. Social capital and health in Okinawa. In: Fujita YT, Karimata S (eds.), *New Perspectives for the Health and Well-being of the Island Region*. Kyusyu: Kyusyu University Press 2014:1–382.

27. Emmons KM. Health behaviors in a social context. In: Berkman L, Kawachi I (eds.), *Social Epidemiology*. New York: Oxford University Press 2000:242–66.

28. Fratiglioni L, Paillard-Borg S, Winblad B. An active and socially integrated lifestyle in late life might protect against dementia. *Lancet Neurol* 2004;3(6):343–53.

29. De Silva MJ, McKenzie K, Harpham T, et al. Social capital and mental illness: a systematic review. *J Epidemiol Community Health* 2005;59(8):619–27.

30. Cramm JM, Nieboer AP. Relationships between frailty, neighborhood security, social cohesion and sense of belonging among community-dwelling older people. *Geriatr Gerontol Int* 2013;13(3):759–63.

31. Vaske J, Kobrin K. Place attachment and environmentally responsible behavior. *J Environ Educ* 2001;32(4):16–21.

32. Christakis NA, Fowler JH. The collective dynamics of smoking in a large social network. *N Engl J Med* 2008;358(21):2249–58.

33. Christakis NA, Fowler JH. The spread of obesity in a large social network over 32 years. *N Engl J Med* 2007;357(4):370–9.

34. Takara K. *Ryukyu Okoku*. Tokyo: Iwanami Shoten 1993:1-178.

35. Hamasaki M. A mass of Shijyukunichi of an Okinawaken in Sao Paulo. *Immigration Studies* 2010;6:71–82.

36. Kato J, Maemura N, Kinjo H, et al. Okinawan Identity and Okinawan network based on the survey result of the 6th Worldwide Uchinanchu Festival. *Immigration Studies* 2018;14:1–20.

20

Japan in Long View

Eric Brunner, Noriko Cable, and Hiroyasu Iso

20.1 The First Super-ageing Epidemiological Transition

During the 56 years and two generations between 1964 and 2020, headline health indicators for the Japanese population improved dramatically. There was exponential economic growth until 1990 (Section 1.5). Health screening and universal health care were introduced in 1961 (Chapters 11 and 12). Health inequalities were narrower in Japan than in many other countries, particularly in the first half of this time period (Chapter 10). Since 2000, health inequalities have increased slightly, as demographic and economic pressures have increased. Rapid ageing of the population, and a slowdown in the economy, partly as a result of growing external competition, has meant that Japan is entering a new epidemiological era, of wealth, low growth, high technology, long life expectancy, and super-ageing. In this new era, living with disease or disability among older people and the need for social care have become important policy issues, even in healthy populations such as Japan's.[1,2]

The super-ageing epidemiological transition has come to Japan ahead of other countries. In 2020, one in three Japanese people are aged over 60, compared to one in four or five in Europe and the US. Infectious disease is unusual and heart attacks are rare. Since the first Tokyo Games, the stroke mortality rate, taking population ageing into account, has declined from 200 to 30 per 100,000/year. In the past 25 years, the cancer mortality rate has decreased by one third. These favourable changes in disease and death rates are indicators of strong positive health trends, with great benefits for individuals who live a much longer disease-free life, on average, than their parents and grandparents.

If we want to understand the epidemiology of the Japanese population in a holistic way, we need to think about health and disease at social as well as individual levels. This consideration is important for two reasons. First, the size of the older population of Japan has grown fast in recent decades, and second, rates of chronic disease and physical and mental impairment increase with

Eric Brunner, Noriko Cable, and Hiroyasu Iso, *Japan in Long View* In: *Health in Japan*. Edited by: Eric Brunner, Noriko Cable, and Hiroyasu Iso, Oxford University Press (2021). © Oxford University Press. DOI: 10.1093/oso/9780198848134.003.0020.

age. These two influences, population ageing and prevalence of age-related conditions, combine to produce an important characteristic of Japan in the twenty-first century. There is a large proportion, and a large number, of older people living with frailty and dementia in communities across Japan. The related volume of need for social care is an important concern for Japanese policymakers even though a universal system of long-term care insurance (LTCI) was introduced in 2000.

20.2 Policy-making in Super-ageing Japan

The demographic trend in Japan has added to the challenges of its ageing society. The number of live births in Japan has fallen since 1973, from just above 2 M to less than 1 M in 2017. There are social, economic, and other reasons for this decline, the clearest being the decline in fertility rate, the number of children born to a woman during reproductive years (ages 15–49), which has not been at or above replacement level since 1973 (Figure 2.1). One result of this almost five-decade long trend is a shrinking population, from its peak of 128.1 M in 2010 to 126.5 M in 2018. The impact on society is profound. Older people outnumber those of working age, and it is unclear how Japan will look after the dependent part of its older population as it increases. Indeed, the headline of a 2018 *Japan Times* article suggested the country needed to recognize the crisis of population decline, and politicians need to take action.[3]

In one important way, the article exaggerated the problem. Universal LTCI provides a comprehensive system of care according to individual need. Japan is far ahead of the UK and China in its consideration of the need to make fair arrangements for its super-ageing population (Chapters 8 and 9). The system is under pressure, with about 6 M people eligible for care in 2017.[4] Increases in insurance premiums, user copayments, and sales tax have sustained the LTCI system up to now. Further revisions of the system may follow, due to its high cost and the shrinking Japanese workforce.[5]

In 2019, the political response to the growing shortage of workers was to increase the number of visas. This new policy means that by 2024 at least 350,000 additional unskilled and skilled workers will have come to live and work in Japan for up to five years. Those in shortage occupations will be able to apply to bring their families, and after ten years will be able to apply to remain on a permanent basis. Significantly, the largest visa quota, among 14 occupational groups, is allocated to caring and nursing (N = 60,000). The planned increase in work visas is not trivial, however one forecast of the shortage of workers in Japan by 2030 is 6.4 M.[6]

Another official response to the ageing challenge is to promote increased community involvement and engagement with older people. The aim is to support independent living at home for as long as possible. A survey in 2011 in a town near Kyoto found that among respondents around age 74, 9.3% were certified to receive LTCI benefits. Prevalence of frailty (based on Fried phenotype) in this group was four times higher than in those without LTCI certification (40% versus 10%).[7] Community involvement, including organized community activities, as an effective approach to help prevent or delay loss of independence, and to solve other social challenges of ageing, is being tested in the JAGES study and elsewhere (Chapter 9).

20.3 Health and Wellbeing in Japan

The reader may have the thought that population health in Japan is a puzzle, with important inconsistencies. Life expectancy is high, mortality rates due to common causes except suicide are low, yet several authors have emphasized problems and challenges to the health of Japanese people, which remain to be fixed. Mental health is important in this respect. Social stigma continues to be attached to mental illness, and the transition from hospital-based to community-based care is slow (Chapters 5 and 15). Child poverty is relatively common, and corporal punishment, bullying, social withdrawal (*hikikomori*), overwork and *karōshi*, and insecure work are among other concerns authors describe that are related to health (Chapters 4, 5, 6, 7, and 15).

A general response to the puzzlement is that every society, however developed and sophisticated, has imperfections. One of the tasks of the contributors to this book, working in epidemiology and public health, is to identify such imperfections through their research, in order that the process of social development can continue.

A more particular response is that Japan was and continues to be a collective society. This situation has its strengths and weaknesses. Wellbeing is more strongly defined in terms of relationships in Japan than in Europe and the US. There is an expectation, learned at home and at school, that adjusting to people around you brings harmony. This expectation is a powerful source of wellbeing and collective, enlightened self-interest, or social capital (Chapter 9) which is weaker in Western culture. On the other hand, a less positive aspect of social harmony, historically, has been a preference for conformity over diversity, for example legal discrimination against gay marriage and same-sex adoption.

Not everyone can conform, and groups who did not fit the mainstream, perhaps due to mental illness or physical disability, were likely to experience social exclusion. Social inclusion is an important contributor to positive well-being, and vice versa, social exclusion is likely to have adverse effects on well-being. The mainstream itself in Japan is in a state of change. Since 1980, when it was the mainstream, the three-generation household (6.9% of households in 2015), has all but disappeared.

20.4 Change and Continuity

Japanese youth culture, ageing of the population, and increasing exposure to cultures and values outside Japan means that some long-held social norms are in the process of changing. An opinion poll in 2015 suggested a majority support same-sex marriage.[8]

Disability rights are now recognized by Japan, as thinking has shifted away from a medical understanding and towards a social understanding. The United Nations *Convention on the Rights of Persons with Disabilities* (CRPD) became law in 2014. CPRD values are embodied in the policy set out in the accessibility guidelines for the Tokyo Olympics/Paralympics. The guidelines confirm the intention to deliver inclusive Games accessible to everyone regardless of physical or intellectual impairment.[9] A visible product of inclusive thinking is the new accessible Tokyo taxi (Figure 20.1).

Japanese population health is in a new epidemiological era for rich countries of wealth, low economic growth, high technology, long life expectancy, and super-ageing. The challenges of this new era are recognized by the World Health Organization, which set up a department of social determinants of health in 2019 to develop sustainable policies promoting global health equity.[10] The evidence from Japan presented in this book shows improvement of healthy life expectancy is able to continue in the future low-growth world.

20.5 Messages and Research Questions

The messages and research questions that follow provide a sample of the contents of each chapter in this book. They summarize only a small part of the evidence assembled and synthesized in the 19 chapters.

EXCELLENT POPULATION HEALTH in high income countries does not depend on continuing economic growth (Chapter 1).

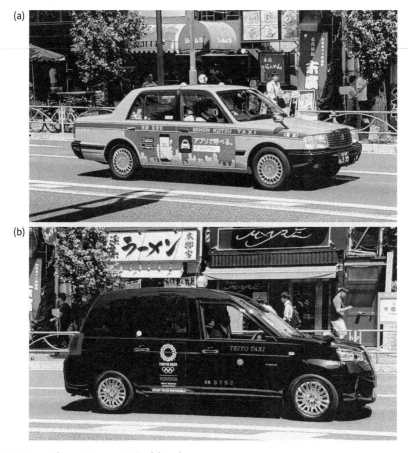

Figure 20.1 The Japanese taxi, old and new

(a) Classic Japanese yellow taxi.

(b) New accessible taxi with sliding door, high roof, and interior space for a wheelchair.

The Chinese ONE CHILD POLICY was probably not necessary. The Japanese fertility rate decline took place as soon as social and economic development was established (Chapter 2).

World-leading life expectancy of Japanese women is thought-provoking, in the context of the POSITION OF WOMEN in Japanese society. GENDER INEQUALITY has narrowed, but it continues (Chapter 3).

The Japanese infant mortality rate is the lowest in the world. Some Japanese children continue to face challenges to their health, including CHILD POVERTY, VACCINATION HESITANCY, and PHYSICAL and PSYCHOLOGICAL ABUSE (Chapter 4).

Individuals with mental health problems or disability have been subject to SOCIAL EXCLUSION. Recent INCLUSIVE policies suggest a CULTURAL SHIFT is in motion (Chapter 5).

Japanese work culture in the economic miracle years was characterized by solidarity and reciprocal commitment between companies and SALARYMEN. Income inequality was low and men's health improved progressively, despite widespread PRESENTEEISM, which continues today (Chapter 6).

Between 1990 and 2020, less secure, NON-STANDARD EMPLOYMENT e.g. part-time and agency work, increased to 22% in men and 56% in women. Such workers have reduced rights to health insurance and screening. Evidence about the health of non-standard workers is sparse (Chapter 7).

Universal HEALTH CARE was introduced in 1961. Japan is a super-ageing society with 35 M people aged 65 or older in 2020. In response to population ageing, universal SOCIAL CARE was introduced in 2000, based on insurance, taxation, and user copayment (Chapters 8 and 9).

HEALTH INEQUALITY WAS LOW in the post-war period but started to grow as the economy slowed down after 1990. Occupational inequality in male mortality in Japan is unique, in that managers and professionals experienced relatively high mortality rates (Chapter 10).

REDUCTION OF STROKE and coronary disease mortality over the past six decades made important contributions to longevity. Economic development, cardiovascular screening, and treatment contributed to the reduction. The enduring RICE-BASED DIET is evidence of Japanese cultural resilience (Chapter 11).

DECREASING INCIDENCE of STOMACH AND LIVER CANCER, CANCER SCREENING, and TREATMENT have contributed to major reduction in Japanese cancer mortality in the past 20 years. The impact of cancer screening on health inequality remains unclear (Chapter 12).

The Tokyo OLYMPIC and PARALYMPIC GAMES have potential to widen social participation in sport, exercise, and physical activity (Chapter 13).

Japanese TOBACCO CONTROL has been weak by international standards, with interference from the tobacco industry. Socioeconomic inequalities in smoking increased as smoking prevalence has decreased (Chapter 14).

Wellbeing in Japan is based on social relationships, and it is collective in scope. Japanese SUICIDE rates remain HIGH compared to other countries. The long economic recession around 2000 was associated with a rise in suicide among men but not women (Chapter 15).

Japan is the FOURTH LARGEST PROVIDER of Official Development Assistance internationally. It has been said that Japan is an invisible champion of global health (Chapter 16).

Geographic (prefectural) HEALTH INEQUALITIES have been REDUCED over the past 60 years, despite major migration into the mega-cities of Tokyo, Nagoya, and Osaka (Chapter 17).

The value of collective action and SOCIAL RESILIENCE is readily observable in Japan, where natural disasters and economic stagnation have only modest effects on population health (Chapter 18).

OKINAWA was the healthiest Japanese prefecture until 1995. Younger generations are experiencing the negative health effects of MODERNIZATION (Chapter 19).

References

1. Chatterji S, Byles J, Cutler D, et al. Health, functioning, and disability in older adults: present status and future implications. *Lancet* 2015;385(9967):563–75. doi: 10.1016/s0140-6736(14)61462-8 [published Online First: 4 December 2014].

2. Chen BK, Jalal H, Hashimoto H, et al. Forecasting trends in disability in a super-aging society: adapting the future elderly model to Japan. *Journal of the Economics of Ageing* 2016;8:42–51. doi: 10.1016/j.jeoa.2016.06.001 [published Online First: 6 June 2017].

3. *Japan Times*. We need a sense of crisis over depopulation. Available at: https://www.japantimes.co.jp/opinion/2018/09/05/commentary/japan-commentary/need-sense-crisis-depopulation/#.Xcmdpfn7SUk [last accessed 10 March 2020].

4. Curry N, Castle-Clarke S, Hemmings N. What can England learn from the long-term care system in Japan? Research report, Nuffield Trust 2018. Available at: https://www.nuffieldtrust.org.uk/research/what-can-england-learn-from-the-long-term-care-system-in-japan [last accessed 10 March 2020].

5. Takasaki Y, Kawachi I, Brunner EJ. Japan's answer to the economic demands of an ageing population. *BMJ* 2012;345:e6632. doi: 10.1136/bmj.e6632 [published Online First: 19 October 2012].

6. World Economic Forum. How Japan can take the lead with an ageing workforce. Available at: https://www.weforum.org/agenda/2019/05/japan-reskilling-aging-workforce [last accessed 10 March 2020].

7. Yamada Y, Nanri H, Watanabe Y, et al. Prevalence of frailty assessed by Fried and Kihon Checklist Indexes in a prospective cohort study: design

and demographics of the Kyoto-Kameoka longitudinal study. *Journal of the American Medical Directors Association* 2017;18(8):733.e7–33.e15. doi: 10.1016/j.jamda.2017.02.022 [published Online First: 16 May 2017].

8. Bloomberg News. Majority of Japanese support same-sex marriage, poll shows. Available at: https://www.bloomberg.com/news/articles/2015-11-29/majority-of-japanese-support-same-sex-marriage-poll-shows [last accessed 10 March 2020].

9. Tokyo 2020 Organizing Committee. The Tokyo 2020 Accessibility Guidelines. Available at: https://tokyo2020.org/en/organising-committee/accessibility/ [last accessed 10 March 2020].

10. WHO. Social determinants of health. Available at: https://www.who.int/social_determinants/en/ [last accessed 10 March 2020].

Index

For the benefit of digital users, indexed terms that span two pages (e.g., 52–53) may, on occasion, appear on only one of those pages.

Tables, figures and boxes are indicated by *t*, *f* and *b* following the page number